1001
TIPS
for Living Well
with Diabetes

▲®American Diabetes Association®
Cure • Care • Commitment®

Director, Book Publishing, John Fedor; *Associate Director, Consumer Books,* Sherrye Landrum; *Composition,* American Diabetes Association; *Associate Director, Book Production,* Peggy M. Rote; *Cover Design,* Koncept, Inc.; *Printer,* Transcontinental Printing.

Printed in Canada
1 3 5 7 9 10 8 6 4 2

The suggestions and information contained in this publication are generally consistent with the *Clinical Practice Recommendations* and other policies of the American Diabetes Association, but they do not represent the policy or position of the Association or any of its boards or committees. Reasonable steps have been taken to ensure the accuracy of the information presented. However, the American Diabetes Association cannot ensure the safety or efficacy of any product or service described in this publication. Individuals are advised to consult a physician or other appropriate health care professional before undertaking any diet or exercise program or taking any medication referred to in this publication. Professionals must use and apply their own professional judgment, experience, and training and should not rely solely on the information contained in this publication before prescribing any diet, exercise, or medication. The American Diabetes Association—its officers, directors, employees, volunteers, and members—assumes no responsibility or liability for personal or other injury, loss, or damage that may result from the suggestions or information in this publication.

The paper in this publication meets the requirements of the ANSI Standard Z39.48-1992 (permanence of paper).

ADA titles may be purchased for business or promotional use or for special sales. To purchase this book in large quantities, or for custom editions of this book with your logo, contact Lee Romano Sequeira, Special Sales & Promotions, at the address below, or at LRomano@diabetes.org or 703-299-2046.

American Diabetes Association
1701 North Beauregard Street
Alexandria, Virginia 22311

Library of Congress Cataloging-in-Publication Data

1,001 tips for living well with diabetes.
    p. cm.
  Includes index.
  ISBN 1-58040-218-6 (pbk. : alk. paper)
    1. Diabetes--Popular works. I. Title: One thousand one tips for living well with diabetes.
  II. American Diabetes Association

  RC660.4.A175 2004
  616.4'62--dc22

                                                            2004052980

1,001 TIPS FOR LIVING WELL WITH DIABETES

▼

TABLE OF CONTENTS

101 TIPS FOR IMPROVING YOUR BLOOD SUGAR

▲

A project of the
American Diabetes Association

▼

Written by

The University of New Mexico Diabetes Care Team

David S. Schade, MD, *Editor in Chief*
Patrick J. Boyle, MD
Mark R. Burge, MD
Carolyn Johannes, RN, CDE
Virginia Valentine, RN, MS, CDE

101 TIPS FOR IMPROVING YOUR BLOOD SUGAR

▼

TABLE OF CONTENTS

Chapter 1
GENERAL TIPS

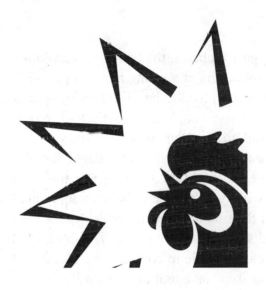

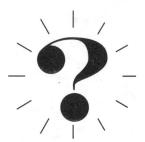

How do I know whether I have type 1 or type 2 diabetes?

▼

TIP:

With type 1 diabetes, the body stops making insulin. This usually occurs at a young age. People with type 1 diabetes will require insulin for life because insulin is essential for using and storing food. These people are usually lean and, if they did not have insulin, would go into diabetic coma within a day or two. In the past, this disease was called insulin-dependent diabetes mellitus (IDDM). The proper name is now type 1 diabetes.

People with type 2 diabetes have enough insulin early in the disease, but their bodies are unable to use the insulin correctly to lower blood sugar. They are *insulin resistant*. Many people with type 2 diabetes are able to control their blood sugar with diet and exercise, and some take oral diabetes pills. In the past, this type of diabetes was called non-insulin-dependent diabetes mellitus (NIDDM). The correct term is now type 2 diabetes. After several years with type 2 diabetes, many people will need insulin, but they still have type 2 diabetes, it's just insulin-requiring. Most people with type 2 diabetes are overweight and more than 30 years old.

*I*f I didn't have diabetes, what would my
normal blood sugar be?

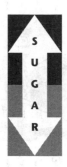

TIP:

The answer to this question depends on whether you have eaten
food in the last 6 hours. Before breakfast, when you have not
had food for 8 or more hours, normal blood sugar would be
between 70 and 100 mg/dl. However, after a meal, normal blood
sugar rarely goes above 200 mg/dl. People who do not have diabetes don't have problems associated with high blood sugar (diabetic complications). That is why your blood sugar goal is to stay close
to the upper limit of normal blood sugar ranges.

NORMAL BLOOD GLUCOSE LEVELS

Fasting blood glucose	<100 mg/dl
After-meal blood glucose (2-h)	140 mg/dl
Bedtime glucose	<120 mg/dl
A1C	<6%

< means less than

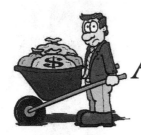

As a resident of the United States, how much does diabetes cost me?

▼

TIP:

In the United States, total medical costs to care for diabetes in 1997 were approximately $98 billion. These costs are usually divided into two parts: direct medical costs and indirect costs. Direct medical costs are those that are paid directly for either hospitalization, nursing, or treatment at home. Indirect costs are costs from a diabetes-caused disability such that a person cannot go back to work or from premature death and loss of a productive citizen. On a per-person basis, health care for a person with diabetes costs approximately $10,000 per patient per year compared with $2,600 for people who do not have diabetes. In other words, health care for a person with diabetes costs four times as much as health care for a person without diabetes. This is one reason why great emphasis is placed on preventing diabetes and improving the treatment of patients to prevent diabetic complications.

What are my blood sugar goals if I have diabetes?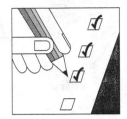

TIP:

We encourage you to try for nearly normal blood sugar levels with few episodes of low blood sugar. The American Diabetes Association (ADA) goals are listed below. If you are persistently outside of these goals or have low blood sugar too often, you need to discuss changing your diabetes therapy with your health care team. These goals are determined from studies that examined the effects of near-normal blood sugar levels on the rates of diabetic complications.

BLOOD SUGAR GOALS FOR PEOPLE WITH DIABETES (mg/dl)

	Nondiabetic	Good	Action Needed
Before-meal blood sugar	<100	90–130	<70 or >200
After-meal blood sugar	<140	160	<100 or >180
A1C	<6%	7%	8%

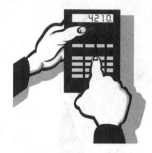

*H*ow can I tell if my diabetes program is
successful?

▼

TIP:

Keep track of your diabetes the same way you do your checking
account—by keeping tabs on the balance. With diabetes, the
balance is the sum of
■ Your blood sugar
■ Your daily weight
■ Your blood pressure
■ Your exercise
■ How you feel
If all of these items meet your goals, then you are doing fine.

Keep a daily record of your blood glucose and weight. You can
check your blood pressure at home or have it done at shopping
centers, pharmacies, etc. Make daily exercise one of your goals.
When you monitor your health daily, you help yourself succeed.

EXAMPLE RECORD

Date	Wt	Blood Pressure	Average Glucose	Feelings	Exercise
6/1	150	122/80	102	Good	Yes
6/2	151	120/75	111	Good	No
6/3	149	115/80	98	So/So	Yes

What determines when type 1 diabetes develops?

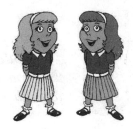

▼

TIP:

We don't understand all of the factors that lead to type 1 diabetes. Until very recently, it was believed that type 1 diabetes did not occur in susceptible individuals until they were exposed to some specific environmental trigger that initiated an immune response against the insulin-producing cells of the pancreas. Years later, when almost all of the insulin-producing cells were destroyed, diabetes would develop. Possible trigger events include viral infections or drinking cow's milk as an infant. A recent study, however, suggests that genetics may have more to do with when type 1 diabetes develops than was previously thought. Scientists compared the age at onset of type 1 diabetes among a group of identical twins to groups of nonidentical twins and non-twin siblings who also had diabetes. The study showed that the development of type 1 diabetes in one identical twin predicted the development of type 1 diabetes in the other twin much more accurately than when one nonidentical twin or non-twin sibling developed type 1 diabetes. Because identical twins are genetically identical, this study suggests that genetics play a stronger role than previously thought in the development of type 1 diabetes.

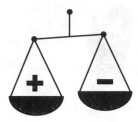

If I follow all the advice in this book and my blood sugar control improves, are there drawbacks that I should be aware of?

▼
TIP:

Yes, there are. However, these are usually not bad enough to discourage you from keeping your blood sugar near normal. The two main concerns are frequent episodes of low blood sugar and a tendency to gain weight. You can head off low blood sugar by monitoring carefully. You can keep your weight in line by watching the number of calories you eat and by increasing the amount of exercise you do. Overall, the disadvantages are minor compared to the benefits you gain from lowering your blood sugar.

Why should I work so hard to improve my blood sugar level?

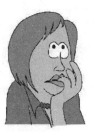

▼
TIP:

Because you'll feel more energy and a greater sense of well-being when your blood sugar enters the normal range. In addition, you'll delay or prevent problems with your eyes, kidneys, and nerves as your blood sugar improves. Many doctors also believe that problems with heart disease, strokes, and hardening of the arteries may be delayed by good blood sugar control. If you do not get any complications of diabetes, you'll live a longer, healthier life.

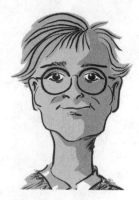

Will controlling my blood sugar prevent my recently diagnosed diabetic eye disease from getting worse?

▼ TIP:

Yes. Although improving your blood sugar control may temporarily make your eye disease worse, over the long term, it will help. The Diabetes Control and Complications Trial (DCCT) monitored patients with mild diabetic eye disease for years. This study showed that the diabetic eye disease of patients with good blood sugar control progressed much more slowly than the eye disease of similar patients with poor blood sugar control. This is a major reason to strive for excellent blood sugar control, particularly if you have mild to moderate complications of diabetes. Another long-term study called the United Kingdom Prospective Diabetes Study (UKPDS) focused on people with type 2 diabetes and found the same beneficial effects of good blood sugar control.

*D*o I have to use alcohol on my *finger before checking my blood sugar like the nurses at the hospital do?*

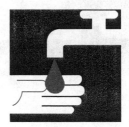

TIP:

No. Using alcohol is not necessary before checking your sugar level. Washing and drying your hands is enough. Just be sure that there is no soap left on your hands and they are dry. Test strips for determining the glucose (blood sugar) in your blood have a substance in them that causes sugar to turn into a colored chemical. Alcohol can destroy this substance and cause a false low blood sugar reading. Alcohol is drying and can lead to broken skin near nails. Also, if all the alcohol doesn't evaporate before you stick your finger, you may feel stinging as well as the discomfort of the poke.

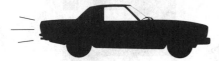

*H*ow should I prepare for a long car trip alone so I don't get high or low blood sugars?

TIP:

The best way to approach a long driving trip alone is to establish a routine. Start your day early so that you can arrive at your destination early. Because you are less active while driving, exercise before you leave or stop along the way at a park or rest area and take a walk. You might also consider either slightly increasing your daily insulin or decreasing the amount of food that you eat. Because hypoglycemia (low blood sugar) is particularly dangerous when you are driving, plan on checking your blood sugar levels frequently (every 2–4 hours) and always have some form of sugar in the car with you. Choose something that won't melt and be messy, such as glucose tablets, a bottle of regular soda, or vanilla wafers.

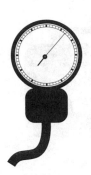

*W*hy did my doctor recently start me on a blood pressure medication even though my blood pressure is only slightly elevated?

▼

TIP:

High blood sugar combined with high blood pressure increases your risk of getting diabetic kidney disease. Kidney disease can lead to kidney failure and the need for either dialysis or a kidney transplant. Doctors can identify diabetic kidney disease at a very early stage, when small amounts of protein appear in the urine (microalbuminuria). Certain drugs that lower blood pressure, such as ACE inhibitors, also lower microalbuminuria and can slow down the development of kidney disease. A lower-protein diet may also be beneficial in preventing kidney problems.

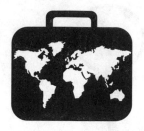

What if my blood glucose meter quits working while I am on an out-of-town trip?

▼

TIP:

Continue monitoring your blood sugar with visual test strips (BetaChek, Uni-Check, Glucostix). These are available without a prescription at most pharmacies. In the meantime, call the toll-free number, which can usually be found on the back of the meter. Most companies will try to replace the meter within a day or two.

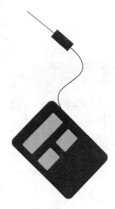

Will an insulin pump improve my blood sugar control?

▼ TIP:

Maybe, maybe not. It depends on the individual. These devices require you to pay close attention to your blood sugar levels and to adjust your insulin, food, and exercise to achieve good readings. With an insulin pump, you can vary your mealtime schedule more readily than with insulin injections, and you can skip a meal when you must. There is more flexibility for people with unpredictable mealtimes. Discuss the pros and cons of using an insulin pump and whether you are a good candidate for having one with your health care team before purchasing one. Also, because they are expensive, check whether your insurance company will help cover the cost.

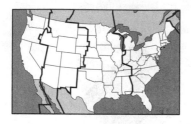

How do I make adjustments in my insulin when I travel across several time zones?

▼
TIP:

The easiest approach is to omit your intermediate- or long-acting insulin on the morning of the trip and rely on regular insulin to keep your blood sugar normal. You will have to test your blood sugar frequently (every 4 hours) and take regular insulin frequently (every 4 hours, adjusting the insulin dose to your blood sugar level). When you arrive at your destination and change your watch to the new time zone, go back on your usual insulin and meal schedule.

*I*s there a level of average blood
sugar below which I do not have to
worry about complications from
diabetes?

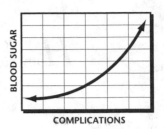

TIP:

No. There is no safe threshold. The DCCT looked at the relationship between average blood sugar levels (as measured by A1C) and the beginning of complications. There is no level below which the risk disappears. However, the lower your A1C (also known as hemoglobin A_{1c}), the lower your risk of eye, kidney, and nerve disease. Therefore, you should try for the best average blood sugar that you can (but still avoid seriously low blood sugars) to reduce your risk of having diabetic complications.

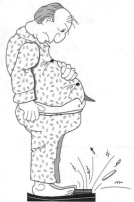

*H*ow does the fact that I am overweight affect my ability to obtain normal blood sugars?

TIP:

Being overweight causes resistance to insulin. This means that any insulin that your body may make (or that you inject) will have a hard time lowering your blood sugar. This makes it difficult for you to control your blood sugar. In addition, being overweight may raise your blood pressure, which makes you prone to kidney disease and stroke. Being overweight may also be associated with high blood fat levels, which makes you susceptible to hardening of the arteries. If you reduce your weight, your blood sugar levels and your health will improve.

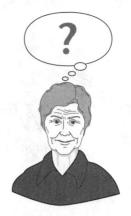

*A*t age 72, why should I worry about blood sugar control?

▼
TIP:

*A*ge alone is not a reason to ignore your diabetes control. You may live to be 90 or 100 years old. This is enough time for complications of diabetes to develop. The better your blood sugar control, the lower your risk of developing complications.

People are lowering their risk of diabetic complications through intensive diabetes management. They do have more frequent low blood sugars, but that is riskier for some people than for others. People with heart disease and people who do not feel warning signs when they develop low blood sugar (for example, shakiness, sweating, or increased heart rate) need to be careful. People who live alone also need to be careful. Tight blood sugar control is not for everyone (and may even be dangerous for some). You and your health care team should determine what blood sugar levels are right for you.

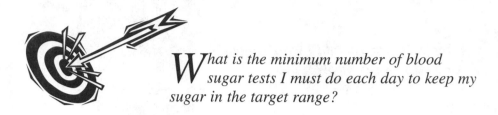

What is the minimum number of blood sugar tests I must do each day to keep my sugar in the target range?

TIP:

The answer depends on the type of diabetes you have. Most people with type 1 diabetes and people with type 2 who require insulin need to test their blood sugar four times a day (before each meal and at bedtime) to allow them to adjust their premeal insulin dose. People with type 2 diabetes may need to test only before breakfast each day. Occasionally, people with type 1 or type 2 diabetes should test their blood sugar 2–3 hours after a meal (postprandial) to find out whether it is going too high or in the middle of the night to see whether it is going too low. If so, the amount of food, exercise, or medication may need to be adjusted. All people with diabetes should test their blood sugar any time they think it may be too high or too low. The symptoms of being high or low may be similar (see page 29), or these symptoms may not be due to blood sugar at all!

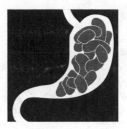

Will my blood glucose be affected if my stomach empties slowly?

▼
TIP:

Yes. If it takes many hours for your stomach to empty and food to be absorbed after a meal, you risk low blood sugar when you take your insulin 45 minutes before you eat. The insulin will peak before the food is absorbed, and you may have high blood sugar many hours later when your stomach finally empties. The common cause of slowed digestion in people who have had diabetes for many years is damage to the nerves affecting stomach muscle activity. This condition is called gastroparesis. Unpredictable stomach emptying makes it difficult to achieve near-normal blood sugars. There are several medications now available that may improve the motion of your stomach, and you should discuss these with your health care team.

Chapter 2
HIGH BLOOD SUGAR TIPS

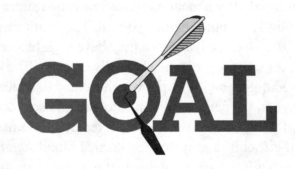

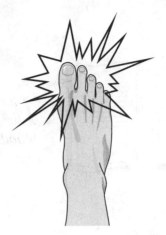

*D*oes the pain in my feet have anything to do with high blood sugar?

TIP:

Probably, especially if you have had high blood sugar for many years and the pain has lasted for several months. Nerves work better when they are surrounded by normal rather than high blood sugar. Discuss your pain with your health care team. Some people find the pain in their feet and legs will decrease when their blood sugar is brought closer to normal. Others find it painful for bed-sheets to touch their feet. If you experience this, placing a hoop over the end of the bed so that the sheet is kept off of your feet will provide relief until your blood sugars can be lowered. If the problem doesn't go away with improved blood sugar control, then putting capsaicin cream (which is made from chili peppers) on the affected skin may help. Other therapies (especially medication) are also available, so you need to discuss the various choices with your diabetes health care team.

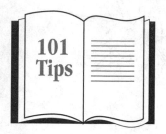

I have read this book, so why do I need help from anyone else to control my high blood sugars?

TIP:

Although books on diabetes have many good, helpful suggestions to control your blood sugar, there are many situations in which you need additional advice. Your doctor and health care team can

1. Help you choose the blood sugar goal that is appropriate for you
2. Teach you how to care for your diabetes and keep you up to date on new treatments
3. Help you develop a meal plan
4. Check your medications so they don't interfere with each other
5. Design a physical activity program specifically for you
6. Review your blood sugar records with you and make suggestions on how to improve your sugar control
7. Help you manage your diabetes when you become ill and thereby prevent more serious health problems

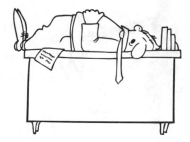

*W*hat are the symptoms of high blood sugar?

▼

TIP:

Symptoms of high blood sugar may vary from person to person or even in one person from day to day. But, in general, a person will

1. Feel more hungry or thirsty than usual
2. Have to urinate more frequently than normal
3. Have to get up at night several times to go to the bathroom
4. Feel very tired or sleepy or have no energy
5. Be unable to see clearly or see "halos" when looking at a light

If you have any of the above symptoms, locate your glucose meter and check immediately. Do not treat these symptoms with additional insulin unless you are certain that they are due to high blood sugar. There arc other conditions that cause similar symptoms.

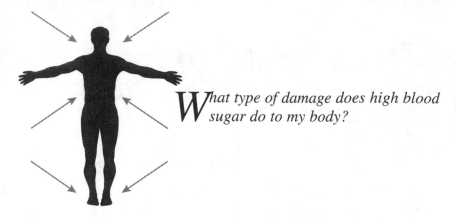

What type of damage does high blood sugar do to my body?

▼ TIP:

Over time, high blood sugar levels can damage both blood vessels and nerves in your body. This can result in poor blood flow to your hands and feet in addition to your legs, arms, and vital organs. Poor blood flow to these areas increases your risk of infections, heart problems, stroke, blindness, foot or leg amputation, and kidney disease. In addition, you can either lose the feeling in your feet or have increased pain in your feet and legs. Damage to your feet can occur from mild injuries, and you may not know it. Finally, damage to blood vessels and nerves can lead to sexual problems that are difficult to treat. For all these reasons, you should make a major effort to avoid high blood sugars in your body.

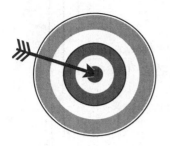

Why is my A1C high when my average blood sugar is in my target range?

▼

TIP:

Your average blood sugar is probably based on your premeal blood sugars. While this usually works well, it does not take into account the level of your blood sugar after you eat. It may be that your blood sugar is rising unexpectedly after your meal because you are either not taking enough insulin or not taking insulin far enough ahead of eating your meal. To see if this is the reason that your A1C is high, measure your blood sugar 2 hours after breakfast, lunch, and dinner for several days (in addition to your premeal blood sugars). Blood sugar that is more than 200 mg/dl 2 hours after a meal is too high. In addition, your blood sugar may be high throughout the night, when you are asleep. To find out, wake yourself up at 4:00 A.M. several times during the week to check your blood sugar. At 4:00 A.M., blood sugar that is higher than 150 mg/dl is too high. Continue to check your blood sugar 2 hours after meals and in the middle of the night once a month to be certain that you are not having unexpected high blood sugars at these times.

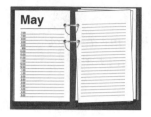

*H*ow can I evaluate my blood sugar
control when my doctor does an A1C
only every 6 months?

▼
TIP:

Y ou can use your self-monitored blood glucose results to predict
your A1C (also known as hemoglobin A_{1c} and HbA_{1c}). Here's
how. Average all your blood sugar check results each week. Find
your average on the table below. Read across to the A1C number.
This will give you an idea of your A1C range, before your doctor
measures it. Your blood sugar ranges might be slightly different if
the normal range of your laboratory's A1C is different from ours.
Our nondiabetic range of A1C is 4.5–6.5%. Find out your laboratory's normal A1C range and use it to revise this table. If you have
type 1 diabetes, have an A1C test done every 3 months.

Average Glucose (mg/dl)	Predicted A1C %
<100	<6.5
100–120	6.5–7.0
121–140	7.0–7.5
141–160	7.5–8.0
161–180	8.0–8.5
>180	>8.5

*W*hy would my blood sugar be high before supper when I use regular insulin before each meal and NPH at night?

TIP:

A verage doses of regular insulin last only 4–6 hours. Because the time between lunch and supper can often be 6 or 7 hours, it is not surprising that your lunchtime insulin is wearing off before supper.

An ideal insulin regimen is flexible to allow for whatever changes come up in your day-to-day schedule. You should be able to make adjustments to correct for unusual swings in your blood sugar that result from known or unknown causes. The regimen you describe is very popular, but many people find that not having an intermediate- or long-acting insulin during the day limits how flexible they can be. As you can see, your regimen is not dealing with the blood sugar rise before supper. Talk to your health care team about this pattern you see developing, so they can suggest ways to prevent it.

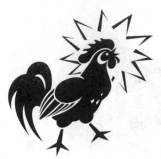

Why are my morning blood sugars usually the highest of the day?

▼
TIP:

The reason for high morning blood sugars may be related to how long your insulin covers your body's needs overnight. For many, NPH is too short-acting because it may last only 6–8 hours. This may not be long enough to maintain good blood sugar levels overnight if you take your NPH at suppertime. Try moving your evening NPH injection to bedtime. If this change doesn't work, you may need to consider switching to a longer-acting insulin, such as ultralente or glargine. Many people who use two injections of ultralente per day (in addition to rapid-acting insulin before each meal) see improvement in their morning blood sugars. Or you may need to increase your dose. To see if you have nighttime lows, check your blood sugar between 2:00 and 4:00 A.M. Starting off the day with a blood sugar close to normal is a key to good overall blood sugar control.

APPROXIMATE INSULIN ACTION

	Onset	Peak	Duration
Lispro	15–30 min	0.5–2.5 h	≤5 h
Aspart	<12 min	1–3 h	3–5 h
Regular	0.5–1 h	2–3 h	3–6 h
NPH	2–4 h	4–10 h	10–16 h
Lente	3–4 h	4–12 h	12–18 h
Glargine	2–4 h	—	20–24 h
Ultralente	6–10 h	10–16 h	18–20 h

Should I take large doses of regular insulin when my blood sugar is high?

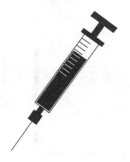

▼

TIP:

For an adult, very high blood sugars do not necessarily require very large doses of regular or lispro insulin. While it makes sense to increase your insulin when your blood sugar is high, increasing your regular dose by 1 or 2 units is unlikely to make your blood sugar come down much faster. In fact, the main effect of taking larger dosages of regular insulin is that the insulin works over a longer period of time. For example, a large morning dose of regular insulin may result in mid-afternoon hypoglycemia. If you are using lispro insulin, you may be able to bring your blood sugar down faster by taking a larger dose, but you may also have mid-afternoon hypoglycemia. Thus, if you are using regular insulin, when your blood sugars are very high,

1. Take your regular insulin dose immediately.

2. Drink large amounts of water to stay well hydrated.

3. Delay your next meal until your blood sugar is below 200 mg/dl. This may mean waiting 1 or 2 hours (or more) after injecting your insulin before eating.

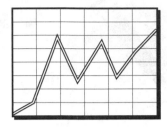

Why do my blood sugar levels vary so much since I switched to ultralente insulin?

▼
TIP:

One of the reasons may be because you do not always get the same concentration of insulin crystals into the syringe. One basic instruction that is often overlooked when patients start on ultralente insulin is how to mix the crystals correctly. After you rock the bottle between your palms, you must immediately draw the dose out of the bottle. The weight and shape of these crystals cause them to settle rapidly back to the bottom of the bottle. If you set the bottle down to draw your regular insulin and then return to the ultralente, the amount of insulin suspended may be quite different from that in the dose you drew up immediately.

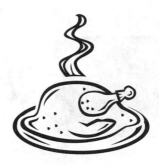

*W*hat should I do when it's getting
close to my mealtime and my
blood sugar is above 240 mg/dl?

▼

TIP:

High blood sugar before a meal tells you that your liver is making too much glucose and needs to be told to slow down! The signal it needs is insulin. Because it takes time for insulin to be absorbed from the skin and additional time to reduce the liver's glucose production, we suggest that you take your usual dose of insulin and wait 60–90 minutes (instead of the usual 30–45 minutes) to eat. This will allow your blood sugar level to fall toward the normal range before you eat, giving the insulin a "head start." The goal is not to become low before eating but to regain control over high blood sugar. An alternative is to take lispro insulin 15–30 minutes before your meal, which should lower your blood sugar more rapidly than regular insulin.

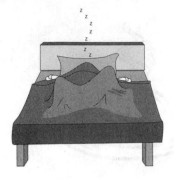

How can I sleep late on weekends without waking up with high blood sugar?

▼
TIP:

If you want to sleep late (for example, until 10:00 or 11:00 in the morning), then set your alarm for 6:00 A.M., go to the bathroom, and check your blood sugar. If your blood sugar is high, take a couple of units of rapid-acting insulin so that while you are sleeping late, your blood sugar will slowly decline. If your blood sugar is low, you should drink some juice or milk. If your blood sugar is normal, take 1 or 2 units of regular insulin and go back to sleep. This schedule has worked well for many people, and often they do not even remember waking up at 6:00 A.M. and taking their insulin.

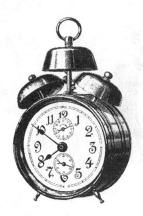

*H*ow soon after I wake up in the
morning should I check my blood
sugar?

▼
TIP:

Check your blood sugar immediately on awakening—before any morning activities, such as showering, shaving, or putting on makeup. The reason for this schedule is that if your blood sugar is low, you can drink some juice or milk. If it is high, you can take your insulin immediately and allow it to work at least 1 hour before breakfast. It is important to get into this habit, because if you start the day with a normal blood sugar level before breakfast, keeping your blood sugar under control throughout the day is much easier. Monitoring your sugar immediately on awakening does not take a major change in lifestyle, but it is very effective in improving your blood sugar control.

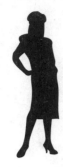

Why do my blood sugars run high before I have my menstrual period?

▼
TIP:

Many women with diabetes have swings in blood sugar control around the time of menstruation. There are many possible reasons for this, from changes in behavior (eating more food) to hormonal changes (high estrogen levels before the period begins can increase your insulin requirements). Young women seem to have the largest swings in blood sugar during their monthly cycle and need to adjust their insulin. Older women also have erratic swings in hormone levels and may have a challenge with maintaining blood sugar control. As you become familiar with your body's rhythm, you may find that the changes in your insulin needs become predictable from month to month. Monitor your blood sugar often and adjust your insulin as necessary during your menstrual period.

*W*hy do I get high blood
*sugar levels after I treat a
low blood sugar reaction?*

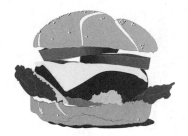

▼
TIP:

Two factors raise your blood sugar after a low blood sugar reaction. First, the hormones that your body naturally releases into
your blood to combat low blood sugar slowly raise the level of blood
sugar. Second, the food you eat raises your blood sugar. Many people with diabetes eat or drink too much after a low blood sugar reading. Low blood sugar causes intense hunger. All of these factors can
cause high blood sugars 2–4 hours or longer after eating. It's important to drink only a small amount (1/2 glass) of juice or milk, or eat
glucose tablets, and then recheck your blood sugar in 30 minutes. If
you eat a larger amount of food, then cover the food with extra regular insulin.

Chapter 3
LOW BLOOD SUGAR TIPS

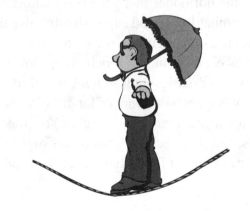

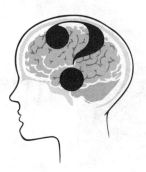

Will repeated low blood sugars damage my ability to think clearly?

▼
TIP:

We don't know. A recent large study of people with repeated moderate low blood sugars did not show a decrease in the brain's functioning. But low blood sugar levels can be dangerous, particularly if they are very low or last for a prolonged period of time. The brain uses blood sugar for energy, and if it is without fuel for longer than a few minutes, it can suffer damage. For this reason, treat low blood sugars rapidly, so that no damage occurs. Take special care to quickly treat low blood sugar in children to avoid damage to their growing brains.

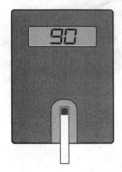

Why do I feel like my blood sugar is low when my meter says it is normal?

▼
TIP:

There are several possibilities. First, your glucose meter may be broken, dirty, or the battery may be low. Repair it, clean it, and change the battery. (Call the manufacturer if you need help.) Have your health care team check the accuracy of your meter.

Second, it takes several weeks for you to get used to normal blood sugars when you have had high blood sugars for a long period of time. Your body may be sending you false signals.

Third, you can feel like your blood sugar is low if your blood sugar rapidly drops from a high level to a normal level. This usually occurs after a large dose of regular insulin. For all these reasons, don't guess what your blood sugar is—always measure it.

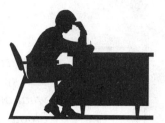

*W**hy did I have a low blood sugar this morning even though I didn't eat anything different and took my usual insulin dose?*

TIP:

E xercise can sometimes result in low blood sugar that night or the next day. This is called "delayed-onset low blood sugar." A day of skiing or 18 holes of golf can result in low blood sugar during your sleep that night or even the next day. Whenever you exercise strenuously, it's a good idea to check your blood sugar more frequently. Eat extra carbohydrates as needed during the next 24 hours or adjust your insulin dose.

Another factor is that intermediate- or long-acting insulin is absorbed at different rates from day to day. For example, injecting into your leg and then exercising can cause the insulin to be absorbed more quickly than usual. You can control this to some extent by injecting insulin into the abdominal area, because it is absorbed more evenly there.

A third factor may be that you forgot your nighttime snack. This snack is important to provide early morning sugar because the food you eat for supper is usually completely absorbed by 3:00 A.M.

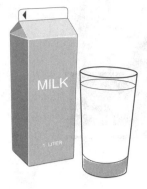

*B*esides glucose tablets (which I find too
sweet) and juice (which I'm tired of),
what other choices do I have to treat low
blood sugar reactions?

▼
TIP:

O ne of our favorite recommended treatments is a glass of milk.
Milk contains lactose that is broken down into glucose (sugar).
It also has fat and protein in it to slow down the rise in your blood
sugar and keep it steady over time. For this reason, milk is better
than juice or glucose tablets. Fat-free and reduced-fat milk have the
same amount of lactose. Other studies have found that a small
amount of ice cream will work nearly as well. You might also consider graham crackers, which are easy to keep on hand. Try to avoid
high-fat treatments, such as candy bars, because they aren't
absorbed as quickly, may lead to very high blood sugar levels in the
hours after you eat them, and can contribute to weight gain, too.

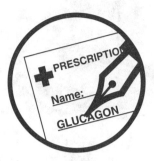

How do I protect myself against low blood sugar while I am trying for tight diabetes management?

▼
TIP:

Keep glucagon handy for emergency treatment of severe low blood sugar. If it is not an emergency, food is better and cheaper (see previous tip). Glucagon raises blood sugar. In many ways, it does the opposite of what insulin does. You get glucagon from the pharmacy with a prescription from your doctor. Someone in your household must know how to mix up the glucagon and inject it if you become severely hypoglycemic, confused, and unable to swallow food. This will need to be done quickly. Glucagon will raise your blood sugar within 10–15 minutes, but its effect doesn't last long. Eat some crackers after you become fully conscious again. Some people are nauseated after receiving glucagon. Most severe episodes of low blood sugar happen during your sleep, so to prevent your family from having to search for the glucagon, keep it in one place, such as the refrigerator door.

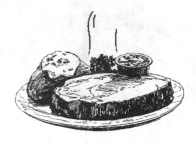

Should I take my insulin before I eat even if my blood sugar is low?

▼
TIP:

First treat the low blood sugar level with enough food to return your blood sugar to the normal range. Liquids, rather than solids, are most rapidly absorbed, and you need to drink just enough to return your blood sugar to normal. In 10–15 minutes, take your insulin and wait about 20 minutes before eating your meal. While this takes some willpower, it prevents your blood sugar from rebounding and ending up above your goal of a normal blood sugar level after a meal.

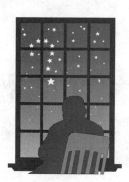

*W*hat should I do to overcome my *fear of having a low blood sugar reaction while I'm asleep?*

▼
TIP:

Many people are insecure about sleeping after having a bad time with low blood sugar during the night. It is reasonable to feel fearful. Many factors influence your blood sugar levels during the night, including how low your blood sugar level is before you go to sleep, hours worked, exercise you did during the day, changes in your insulin dose, and whether you ate or skipped a nighttime snack. If you and your physician are unable to determine why the reaction happened, try setting your alarm to wake you at 3:00 A.M. several nights in a row. If you find that your blood glucose usually falls during the night, you and your health care provider can adjust your evening insulin dose or bedtime snack. You might ask your provider about whether to try a slow-release carbohydrate snack bar, such as Gluc-O-Bar, Extend, or NiteBite.

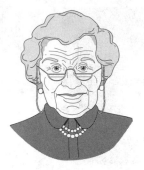

Should my 85-year-old mother try to keep her blood sugar higher than the normal target ranges?

▼
TIP:

Maybe. She and her health care team need to decide that. Each patient using intensified diabetes management has an individual blood glucose goal aimed at preventing the long-term complications of diabetes. However, asking people to come close to normal increases their risk of severe hypoglycemia (episodes of very low blood sugar). Elderly people suffer more from low blood sugars. In fact, it may increase their risk for a heart attack or cause a stroke. For some elderly people with diabetes, the risks may outweigh the benefits of trying for normal blood sugar levels. While aiming for a glucose level as close to normal as possible is ideal, maintaining a slightly higher glucose level does offer your mother some room for her blood glucose to fall into the normal range with less fear of having serious low blood sugar.

I live alone; what can I do to reduce
the risk of a severe nighttime low
blood sugar reaction?

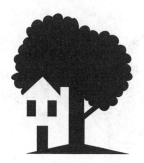

▼
TIP:

S tudies have shown that 50% of severe low blood sugars happen
between midnight and 8:00 A.M. (usually at 4:00 A.M.). Having a
normal blood sugar level before you go to sleep does not guarantee
that it won't drop too low a few hours later, especially if you use
intensified insulin treatments, such as nighttime NPH. Test your
blood sugar level before bed and have a good bedtime snack to prevent low blood sugar before 8:00 A.M. If nighttime low blood sugars
happen often, set your alarm and check your blood sugar level at
3:00 A.M. every night. Eat some food if it is below 75 mg/dl. Ask
your health care provider whether a slow-release carbohydrate snack
bar, such as Extend or NiteBite, would be a good nighttime snack
for you.

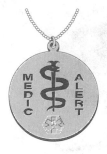

What should I do about very severe low blood sugar episodes that cause me to pass out?

▼
TIP:

Teach your family members and friends the signs and symptoms of low blood sugar, so they can help you in case you are not alert enough to tell them that your blood sugar is low. Some common symptoms are feeling shaky or lightheaded, having a rapid heartbeat, sweating, being nauseated, being confused, and having slurred speech or delayed reflexes. For those times when you may be someplace where no one knows you, carry a card in your wallet or wear a bracelet or necklace stating that you have diabetes. The card should also state whether you are on insulin and that you may become confused when you have low blood sugar. In this way, you may get help more quickly.

Work with your health care team to try to determine why you are having these episodes of low blood sugar. Keep glucagon at home or with you, and be sure a family member or friend knows how to inject it for you.

Always check your blood sugar level before you drive.

*W*hy is my blood sugar still high
this evening when my low blood
sugar occurred early this morning?

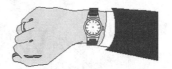

▼
TIP:

Your body reacts to low blood sugars by secreting several hormones, including growth hormone and cortisol. These hormones may not act immediately, but after several hours, they will
raise your blood sugar. Their activity may last up to 24 hours, so you
may then have to take additional insulin to keep your blood sugar
from going too high. This rebound effect is one reason why you
want to avoid very low blood sugars. Another reason for the high
blood sugar may be that you ate too much when you tried to treat the
low blood sugar reaction.

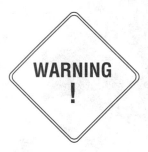

Why do I no longer feel the warning signs of low blood sugar?

▼
TIP:

Many people who have had diabetes for more than 5 years lose some of the symptoms of low blood sugar. The usual feelings of hunger, sweatiness, anxiety, and increased heart rate may fade and escape your attention. Sometimes you may just feel sleepy as your blood sugar drops. The reasons for this are complex but are related to a loss of adrenaline release in your body when your blood sugar is low. If you are unaware of low blood sugars, try not to let your blood sugar level drop below 100 mg/dl. You may need to monitor your blood glucose levels more often.

If this is a problem for you, always check your blood sugar level before you drive.

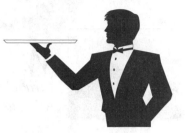

*W*hy do I develop low blood
sugar after a fancy restaurant
meal?

▼
TIP:

Perhaps you prepare for a restaurant meal by injecting extra
insulin. Restaurant meals are usually rich in fat and protein, but
these nutrients do not raise your blood sugar levels as quickly as carbohydrates do, and they don't require any extra insulin. In fact, a
problem with nicer restaurant meals is getting enough carbohydrates. To increase the carbohydrate content, eat well during the
bread course at the start of the meal (you might need to avoid the
butter), and consider ordering a glass of skim milk with your meal or
having a nonfat dessert, such as fresh fruit, or a frozen dish, such as
sherbet or sorbet.

　　If you have an alcoholic drink when you eat out, the alcohol
may be causing the low blood sugar, particularly if you eat a very
small meal.

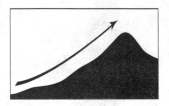

*Why do my blood sugars read
lower on my glucose meter when
I travel from Miami (sea level) to
Albuquerque (5,000 foot elevation)?*

▼
TIP:

Most blood glucose meters use a chemical reaction that requires oxygen from the air to measure your blood sugar. At high altitudes, there is less oxygen in the air, which causes the results to be lower. Thus, the results you get may be affected by altitude. You should read the instructions that came with your meter and also read the package insert in the strips. You may also call the toll-free 800 number given in your package insert or write to the company that makes your meter to find out whether its readings are affected by altitude.

Chapter 4
INSULIN TIPS

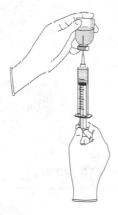

If you have type 2 diabetes, but you are taking insulin, these tips will work for you as well.

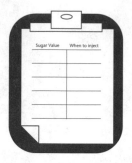

*I*s there a chart I can use to know how to time
my insulin injections with my meals?

▼
TIP:

Here is a schedule we provide to our patients with diabetes. The
timing depends on your current blood sugar. In general, rapid-
acting insulin should be taken about 20 minutes before the meal if
your sugar is high and after the meal if your sugar is low. Using this
table should improve your after-meal blood sugar levels.

WHEN TO INJECT

If blood sugar value 45 minutes before meal is:	**Inject Insulin**
<50 mg/dl	at end of meal
50–70 mg/dl	at mealtime
71–120 mg/dl	at mealtime
121–180 mg/dl	at mealtime
>180 mg/dl	15–30 min before meal

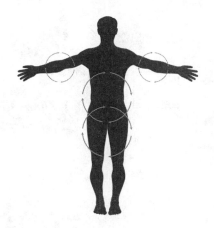

*S*hould I rotate my insulin injection
between my arms, legs, and
abdomen?

▼
TIP:

Maybe not. True, rotating your insulin injections helps you
avoid always injecting into the exact same spot on your body.
You don't want to do that because insulin causes local deposits of fat
under the skin. However, insulin is absorbed at different speeds
when it is injected into different areas of the body. Good blood sugar
levels depend on you knowing how quickly your insulin will act.
That is why we say to rotate your injection sites in one general
area—that is, arms, or legs, or around the abdomen, but not all three.
You could give your morning shots in one area and your evening
shots in another area. This provides you with more predictable
insulin absorption and improved blood sugar control. We suggest
using the abdomen as an injection site because insulin is absorbed
more rapidly in this location. Interestingly, rotation of injection sites
is more important with regular insulin than with lispro insulin. In
fact, site rotation has been proved to have little or no effect on the
absorption of lispro insulin.

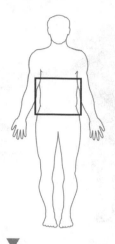

Where should I inject my regular insulin to get the most consistent absorption?

▼
TIP:

We recommend that you use your abdomen. Insulin injected into the abdomen is absorbed quickly and predictably so you know how it will affect your blood sugar time after time. In general, there are three places to inject insulin—the abdomen, the arms, and the legs. Several factors affect the way your body absorbs insulin. If you exercise the muscles of your arms or legs vigorously after an injection, more insulin will be absorbed more quickly. It will be difficult for you to predict how this insulin will affect your blood sugar. Warm temperatures also increase the speed at which insulin is absorbed. Because your abdomen is usually covered by clothing and stays warm, insulin is absorbed more rapidly from this area.

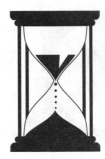

*H*ow long will my injection of regular insulin last?

▼
TIP:

Regular insulin generally lasts from 3 to 6 hours. However, the length of time that regular insulin lasts depends on the number of units that you inject. It also depends on how sensitive you are to insulin in your blood. The more regular insulin you inject, the longer its action lasts. One unit of insulin may last only 1 hour, whereas 10 units of insulin may last 5 hours or more. If you take a small dose of regular insulin before breakfast and your blood sugar starts to rise before lunch, you probably need to increase your regular insulin dose before breakfast. The same concept applies to lispro and aspart insulin, which generally last 2–3 hours. With normal doses of lispro insulin, your blood sugar will begin to rise after 4 hours unless you also take a background insulin such as NPH or ultralente.

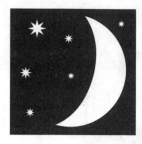

What can I do about low blood sugars at 3:00 A.M. if I take my last dose of regular and NPH insulin before supper?

TIP:

An easy answer is to move your NPH injection to right before bedtime. You may also need to eat a late-night snack before you go to bed. Another successful approach is to change to ultra-lente insulin. Human NPH insulin usually has a maximum effect 8–10 hours after you take it. If you take your insulin at dinnertime (6:00 P.M.), its peak of activity will be at about 4:00 A.M. Because you have also used up the food you ate at dinner by this time, you will probably have low blood sugar (hypoglycemia) at 3:00 A.M. When you have made adjustments to your regimen, get up at 3:00 A.M. and check your blood sugar level to be sure things are going as you planned.

*I*f I mix my regular insulin with my
NPH or ultralente, will this reduce
the effectiveness of my regular
insulin?

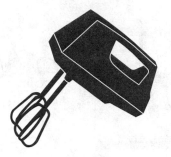

▼
TIP:

No and yes. You can mix regular insulin with NPH insulin without altering the effect of your regular insulin. But, you cannot mix regular insulin with lente or ultralente insulin without risking some loss of the regular insulin's effect. The reason for this loss is that both lente and ultralente insulins contain excess zinc, which binds to the regular insulin and slows its absorption. If you do choose to mix regular and lente (or ultralente), you will need to inject it immediately after mixing up the dose, so the zinc does not have time to bind to the regular insulin. It is best to take separate injections (although inconvenient) if your schedule includes regular insulin plus one of the lente insulins.

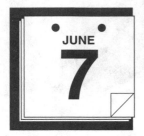

How often should I adjust the dose of my intermediate- or long-acting insulin if my blood sugar is not well controlled?

▼
TIP:

Don't change your dose of intermediate- or long-acting insulin more often than every 3 or 4 days. Many factors besides insulin affect blood sugar levels. Some of these factors are exercise, how much food you eat, what you eat, illness, and the speed at which your injected insulin is absorbed. Until you have looked at these other factors, you should not adjust your intermediate- or long-acting insulin daily. Give your insulin schedule several days to work before trying a new one.

The same is true for regular or rapid-acting insulin. You may make adjustments for a one-time high blood sugar, but changes to your regimen should come only after you've checked all the factors that affect your blood sugar level.

*H*ow can I get my blood sugars
under control when I have to
rotate between night and day shifts
on my job?

▼
TIP:

Clearly, the best option is to negotiate with your employer to stay
on one shift. The Americans with Disabilities Act requires
employers to provide "reasonable accommodation for people with
diabetes." Or you may want to try a more flexible insulin regimen.
Using ultralente with regular insulin or an insulin pump will give
you the flexibility this situation demands. One of your problems is
that your body releases hormones during sleep that make insulin
work less effectively. By rotating shifts, you disturb the normal
release of these hormones. You don't know when the hormones are
being released, so you don't know how your insulin will affect your
blood sugar levels.

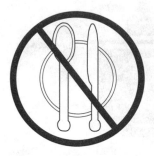

If I am using ultralente plus rapid-acting insulin, do I always need to take rapid-acting insulin at lunch even if I am not going to eat?

TIP:

If you are taking only one injection of ultralente in the evening, taking an injection at lunchtime is almost always necessary because your breakfast injection or rapid-acting insulin will be almost completely gone by lunchtime. If you are splitting your ultra-lente dose to twice a day (as we recommend), you may not need to take any rapid-acting insulin at lunchtime if you do not eat lunch. With experience, you will learn how much rapid-acting insulin to take.

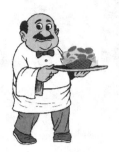

What should I do if dinner is served and it has only been 15 minutes since I took my regular insulin?

▼

TIP:

Foods that are high in carbohydrates (such as bread, starches, fruit, and milk) raise blood sugar rapidly. Protein foods may be partly converted to blood sugar, but the rise in blood sugar will be much later (after the meal). Ideally, you should wait 30–45 minutes before eating for regular insulin to start working. If this is not possible, try eating the foods that won't have much effect on your blood sugar first, such as the salad and meat, or sip on sugar-free drinks like iced tea. Save the starches, such as bread and potatoes, and eat them last so the regular insulin has another 10–15 minutes to work. In the future, you might consider changing to rapid-acting insulin, such as lispro or aspart, which can be taken 0–15 minutes before the meal if your blood sugar is normal.

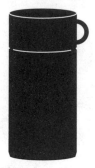

*H*ow should I store my insulin during a long car trip?

▼
TIP:

Your insulin is good at room temperature for at least 1 month. If you keep your insulin cooler than 85°F while traveling, it will be fine. If you are going to leave it in the car while you're out sight-seeing, keep it in a small thermos and maybe even put the thermos in your ice chest. Don't put the bottle of insulin in direct contact with the ice in the cooler because freezing the insulin is just as bad as overheating it. If you are camping out in winter, keep your insulin bottle in your thermos or sleeping bag to prevent it from freezing.

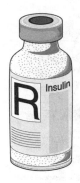

*W*hat causes my regular insulin to get cloudy after several weeks?

▼
TIP:

All insulins have a tendency to change while they are stored. Many factors speed up this change, including warm temperatures and shaking the insulin bottle. For this reason, you should not carry your insulin in your pocket, especially if you are an active person. Keep it in your refrigerator, cupboard, purse, briefcase, or backpack, and protect it from heat and motion. If regular insulin becomes cloudy, throw it away. It has lost its effectiveness. It will not keep your blood sugar from getting too high.

If you inject a mixture of regular and NPH or ultralente insulins, you may be getting NPH or ultralente in the bottle of regular insulin. This will make it cloudy, too. If in doubt, discard the old bottle and replace it with a new bottle.

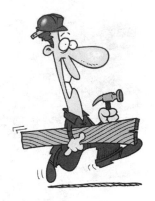

How can I take insulin at lunch when
I'm on a constuction crew and can't
be carrying insulin, syringes, or test
supplies with me?

▼ TIP:

You could look at the blood glucose monitors and injection
devices that are the size and shape of pocket pens. Because you
can carry these instruments in your pocket, they provide a convenient way to monitor your sugar and inject the appropriate amount
of insulin at work. Your diabetes health professional can provide you
with information about these devices. Also, *Diabetes Forecast* magazine reviews the characteristics of these devices and others in the
Resource Guide, which is published as a supplement to *Forecast*
each December.

If I intentionally omit my insulin dose, will I lose weight?

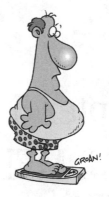

▼
TIP:

Not really. Although recent studies have suggested that some patients do skip an insulin injection to lose weight, we don't recommend it. Skipping an injection is very hard on your system and does not accomplish your goal of fat loss. Omitting an insulin injection lets your blood sugar rise, and you lose proteins, salts, and fluid in your urine. This can make you very ill, perhaps to the point of having to be hospitalized. Do not omit your insulin injection to lose weight.

Chapter 5
ORAL MEDICATION TIPS

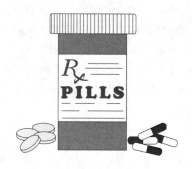

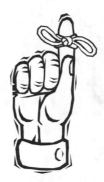

How can I remember to take my diabetes pills to prevent high blood sugars?

▼
TIP:

The best way to remember to take medication is to develop a daily routine. That is, always take the medication at the same time of day and in the same location, such as in the bathroom or at the breakfast table. To further reduce the chance of forgetting to take your medication, use a labeled pill box or pill organizer. These inexpensive boxes are available at drugstores. Set up medications in the pill box a week in advance to make it easy to know whether all your pills have been taken. The more medications you take, and the more complicated your pill-taking schedule is, the greater the likelihood that you will make mistakes. The danger of not taking diabetes medication is that your blood sugar levels will go very high.

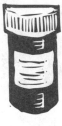

*W*hat should I do if I forget to take my diabetes *pills?*

▼

TIP:

If you forget to take your oral diabetes medication, it is important to know whether to take it when you do remember. The rule is simple. If you are within 3 hours of the time of the dose you missed (and you normally take pills twice per day), go ahead and take your medication. If more than 3 hours have passed, wait for your next scheduled dose. If you are on a long-acting medication that you take once a day, take your medication if you are within 12 hours of missing your dose. Otherwise, wait until the next scheduled time to resume taking your medication.

This plan is appropriate for medications in the classes of sulfonylureas (such as Glucotrol), thiazolidinedione (such as pioglitazone) and biguanides (such as Glucophage). For medications such as acarbose (Precose) or repaglinide (Prandin), wait until your next meal to take them.

What do you suggest that I do when my doctor wants me to take insulin, but I would rather take pills for my diabetes?

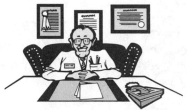

▼
TIP:

If you have type 1 diabetes, pills will not work for you. You will have to take insulin injections. However, if you have type 2 diabetes, then you may respond to pills. Many doctors try pills in patients with type 2 diabetes, because pills are easier to take and have other advantages. Tell your doctor that you would like to try the pills, and if they do not work, then you would be willing to take insulin injections. There is not an absolute "yes or no" blood test to tell how you will respond to pills. The only way to know is to try them for several weeks. Beginning to exercise (or increasing your level of physical activity) will help you gain better control with diabetes pills, too.

If you have type 2 diabetes and are taking insulin, you should talk to your doctor. Many medications, such as metformin, pioglitazone, repaglinide, glyburide, and others, have permitted some people with diabetes to switch to pills and stop their injections. Many new medications for diabetes are currently being tested, so stay in touch with your diabetes health care team.

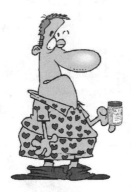

*W*hy does my doctor want me to take insulin at bedtime even though I am already taking pills for diabetes?

▼

TIP:

Your doctor is probably concerned about your fasting (before breakfast) blood sugar being high. When pills are not keeping your fasting blood sugar within the normal range, it is common practice to have you take insulin at night, so that your blood sugar is normal at the start of the day. You'll do much better with pills if your blood sugar level before breakfast is in the normal range. If this program does not work for you, you may have to take insulin both in the morning and at night, even though you have type 2 diabetes.

Chapter 6
SICK-DAY TIPS

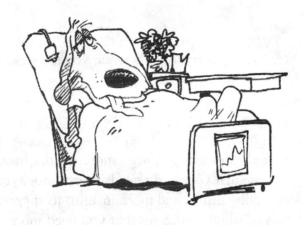

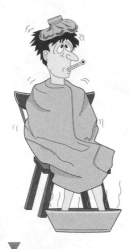

When I am ill with the flu, what should I do to keep my blood sugar from going too high?

▼
TIP:

Monitor three factors every 4 hours when you are sick:

1. Your blood sugar
2. Your urine ketones
3. Your body weight

High blood sugar indicates that you need more regular insulin. High urine ketones indicate that your body needs more carbohydrate intake (sugar-containing drinks and more insulin) to suppress fat breakdown. A loss of weight indicates that you need more fluids. When you cannot get your blood sugar below 250 mg/dl, your urine ketones below 3+, or your body weight close to normal, then you must call your health care team.

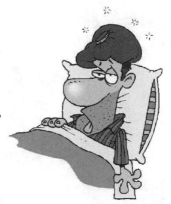

*W*hen I am sick with the flu and
cannot eat food without vomiting,
how do I know how much insulin to take?

▼
TIP:

The guide to how much insulin to take is your current blood
sugar. You need to take enough insulin to keep your blood sugar
below 200 mg/dl, so that you do not become dehydrated because of
excessive urination. For adults, we recommend taking an injection of
at least 5 units of regular insulin every 4 hours and to keep increasing the dose of regular insulin by 1 unit until your blood sugar gets
below 200 mg/dl. This may be more than your usual dose of insulin
even though you are not eating. If you inject regular insulin every 4
hours, you should probably withhold your intermediate- or long-acting insulin until you get well. (Check with your health care
provider.) Of course, if you are relying solely on regular insulin, you
will need to wake up during the night to take an insulin injection. If
you are taking lispro insulin, the dose of the insulin is the same but
you must continue your background intermediate- or long-acting
insulin.

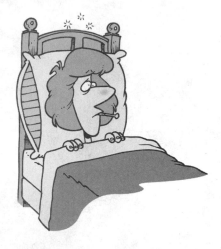

*W*ill fever increase my blood
 sugar and therefore my need
for insulin?

▼
TIP:

Y es. Even mild illness may require you to take a little more
 insulin. And if you develop a fever with chills, muscle
aches, and sweating, you will definitely need increasing doses of
insulin. In fact, your requirements of rapid-acting insulin may
double. Keep a thermometer at home to determine when your
body temperature is above 99°F, because this and frequent blood
sugar checks are the keys to knowing when you need more
insulin. You and your health care team should develop a plan for
what to do if your blood sugar is high when you are sick. Do not
hesitate to call them when you are ill.

*A*t what point must I seek medical
help if I have the flu?

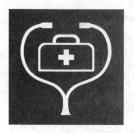

▼
TIP:

You should seek medical help when you cannot keep down liquids. Contrary to popular belief, eating solid food is not essential during short-term illness. Most people have ample body fat stores to provide energy. However, you must be able to drink liquids and, preferably, carbohydrate-containing fluids. If you are unable to hold down any fluids for more than 12 hours, you need to seek medical help immediately. Your body will become dehydrated if you can't ingest salt and water. This can affect you seriously, causing acidosis, unconsciousness, and death. Therefore, if you are vomiting all fluids or are spilling large amounts of ketones in your urine, you should contact your health care team immediately.

Ideally, you should set up a sick-day plan with your health care team before you ever get sick. That way you will have more information about who to call and when.

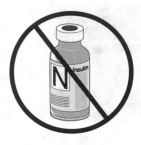

Should I skip my NPH insulin dose in the morning before a dental appointment that prevents me from eating lunch?

▼
TIP:

Not necessarily. You have two options. The first option is to omit the A.M. dose of NPH but take your rapid- or short-acting insulin dose before you eat breakfast. You must take a dose of rapid-acting insulin about 5–6 hours after your morning dose of rapid-acting insulin (this second small dose is to keep your blood sugar under control even though you won't be eating).

The second option is to take your short- or rapid-acting insulin and then to cut your morning NPH dose by about 1/3 (because you won't be eating lunch) and inject that. After the dental procedure (about 6 hours after your morning dose of short- or rapid-acting insulin), check your blood sugar, and if necessary, you can take an additional small dose of regular, aspart, or lispro insulin that should tide you over until dinnertime.

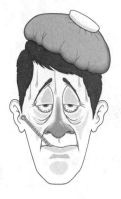

Why are my sugars still high when I had the flu a week ago?

▼
TIP:

Major stresses cause changes in the body that may last for several weeks beyond the time when you get well. Although you may feel better now, these changes (which affect many of the substances in your body that raise blood sugar) are still active. Remember that you may need additional insulin for 1–2 weeks after a major stress (for example, severe flu, surgery, pneumonia, or heart attack) to keep your blood sugar levels in the normal range.

Chapter 7
NUTRITION TIPS

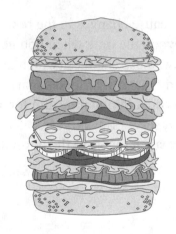

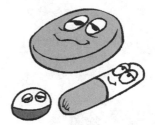

*S*hould I take vitamins or minerals to improve my blood sugar?

▼
TIP:

There is not enough scientific evidence to recommend vitamin or mineral supplements to improve your blood sugar. From time to time, various vitamin and mineral supplements have been popular. Recently, magnesium, chromium, zinc, vanadium, and selenium have been publicized by the media and promoted by health food stores as having a beneficial effect on blood sugar. Nevertheless, eating foods that contain the vitamins and minerals, such as fruits and vegetables, is still the best way to get what your body needs.

In contrast, we strongly recommend that you get pneumonia vaccinations (available all year) and annual flu vaccinations (available in early fall). Vaccinations may prevent (or reduce the severity of) these illnesses, which usually cause high blood sugars. Ask your health care team for their advice.

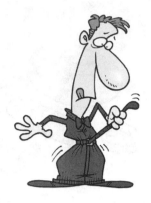

*H*ow can I lose weight when I
hardly eat anything now?

▼
TIP:

I f you are not exercising, you will be surprised at the difference a
daily 30-minute walk can make in both weight loss and blood
sugar control. Walking burns calories and lowers blood sugar. If
exercise becomes a daily habit, you'll need to adjust the amount of
insulin you take and the food you eat.

Another way to lose weight may be as simple as reducing the
food you eat by one slice of bread per day. One slice of bread
contains 80–100 calories, and 30 slices of bread (amount eaten in 1
month) is equal to approximately 1 pound of body weight.
Therefore, if you omit one of your usual slices of bread per day for
1 year, you may possibly lose up to 12 pounds!

Keep a journal of the foods you eat for 3–5 days. Also record
when you eat and the emotion or situation that preceded eating.
Most people are surprised to find that they do eat more than they
realize or that certain situations always trigger overeating. Your
ability to keep a food diary and learn from it will help you lose
weight.

*H*ow will alcohol affect my blood
sugar?

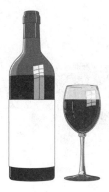

▼
TIP:

Alcohol interferes with your body's ability to produce blood
sugar and causes low blood sugar. Do not drink alcohol if you
are not eating. If you are eating a meal and you drink only a small
quantity of alcohol, then the alcohol should not cause you to have a
severe problem with low blood sugar. You will, however, need to
include the calories that are in the alcohol in your meal plan. In general, one alcoholic beverage substitutes for 1 fat exchange in a meal
plan. Check with your registered dietitian (RD) for help with this.

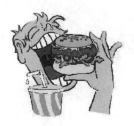

*H*ow can I lose weight and keep eating the
foods that I like?

▼
TIP:

Y ou do not have to give up all the foods that you like. It's the
size of the portion you eat that is important. Some foods are
higher in fat content than other foods. If you cut down on or cut out
high-fat foods altogether, you can lose significant amounts of
weight. To find the fat and caloric content of the foods you eat, look
for paperback books that list this information. These books can be
found at libraries, bookstores, and pharmacies. See how much fat is
in your favorite foods. Eliminating even one high-fat food that you
eat often will result in weight loss. Remember that exercise will
make it even easier to lose weight.

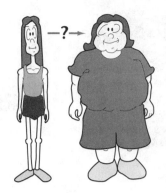

*W*ill I gain weight as I lower my
blood sugar?

▼
TIP:

Not necessarily, especially if you keep track of how much you eat. However, many people do gain weight, and the reasons are complex. One factor is that you are no longer losing large quantities of calories in your urine (in the form of glucose). An equal number of calories (equal to what was being lost in your urine) will need to be deleted from the amount of food you eat. You won't know how many calories this is unless you monitor your weight and what you eat. If you start to gain weight, reduce the amount of food you eat and exercise more. If lowering your blood sugar causes you to have more low blood sugar reactions, then the food that you eat to treat the reactions may add to a weight gain.

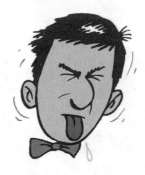

Why don't some sugar-free foods taste very good?

▼
TIP:

While some foods are actually improved by becoming sugar free (canned fruit, for example), other foods are not so successfully converted to sugar free. These are usually foods in which artificial sweeteners (sorbitol, saccharin, or aspartame) are added to taste sweet. But these sweeteners do not cook like sugar, so they don't work well in baked foods and may leave a bitter aftertaste. Also, remember that these foods are not necessarily low in calories. For example, sugar-free pudding made with reduced-fat milk has 90 calories per serving as compared to 140 calories per serving for regular pudding. Although 90 is less than 140, it still isn't calorie free. You don't have to eat only sugar-free cookies. You may have a real cookie—just include it in your meal plan.

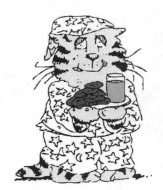

How large a snack should I eat at bedtime?

▼
TIP:

You should eat about 1/7 of your total calories per day before you go to sleep if you have a normal blood sugar level. Your bedtime snack is designed to keep enough glucose in your blood so that your blood sugar does not get too low in the middle of the night. The NPH or ultralente insulin you took before supper can peak during this time and cause low blood sugar. Your health care provider or RD can help you adjust your snack to work with your insulin or medication dose, or adjust your insulin (insulin glargine is peakless), so that your morning blood sugar will be in the normal range.

A snack may not be necessary if your bedtime blood sugar is above 180 mg/dl. If your bedtime blood sugar is lower than 180 mg/dl, you will probably want to have a snack that includes starch and protein, such as peanut butter and crackers or low-fat cheese on toast. You may need to add a glass of fat-free milk or a serving of fruit if your blood sugar is less than 100 mg/dl.

BEDTIME SNACK SUMMARY

Blood Sugar (mg/dl)	Snack Quantity
<100	juice or milk plus usual snack
101–180	usual snack
>181	no snack

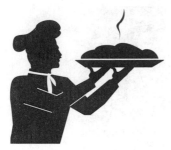

My goal is to be a normal weight with near-normal blood sugars, so how do I reduce fat in a meal when I eat at a restaurant?

▼ TIP:

Meat is the best place to start cutting fat calories. If you order fish that is broiled or baked, it will usually have less than 5 grams of fat per ounce. If you order a meat serving from the menu, look for foods that are grilled or broiled. Also look for a lower-fat meat, such as sirloin, instead of prime rib or filet. Ask the waiter how many ounces are in the serving size. You may even be able to request a particular serving size, such as "only a 4-ounce serving of the sirloin" or request that the meat be prepared with no fat. Other sources of fat are gravies and sauces. You can request that the sauce be served on the side, and check it out before you find your chicken breast swimming in butter. Meats that are processed, such as bratwurst, lunch meats, and sausages, can be very high in fat (as much as 10–15 grams per ounce) and are usually very high in salt as well.

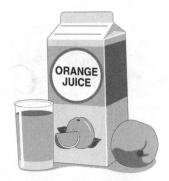

How can I have orange juice for breakfast without risking high blood sugars later?

▼
TIP:

It is better for you to eat the orange (or any other fruit) than to drink the juice from that fruit. If you like the bright wake-up taste of orange juice first thing in the morning, you might try mixing 1/2 juice and 1/2 water. Or you could try a sugar-free citrus-flavored drink mix (and a serving of real fruit later in the day). You will get the tangy orange taste without any sugar! It isn't so much the sugar in the orange but the liquid form that makes orange juice (or any other juice) raise your blood sugar rapidly. Studies comparing juice and sugar-containing soft drinks found that there is no difference in the effect they have on people's blood sugar. We advise people to use juice as "treatment" for low blood sugar, not as food.

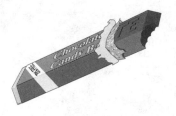

Can I eat candy bars now that the ADA is including table sugar in meal plans?

▼

TIP:

Sometimes. It is true that the most recent dietary guidelines for people with diabetes include foods with sugar, including table sugar. Several studies have shown that table sugar eaten as part of a meal plan does not have any worse effect on blood glucose than rice or potatoes. This does not mean, however, that people with diabetes can eat sweets freely. Sugars must be included as part of your meal plan. And the reason you still want to limit the number of candy bars you eat is that most of the calories in candy bars come from fat. Fat should be limited in everybody's diet! Also, the calories in candy bars are "empty" calories—that is, they don't give you the vitamins or minerals that you need to be healthy.

How can I keep my blood sugar normal during the holidays when high-calorie, high-fat foods are served?

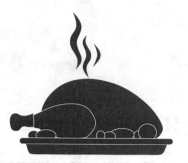

TIP:

Holidays are always difficult because of the change in daily routine and the increased availability of high-calorie, high-fat foods. We recommend several approaches to preventing your A1C from rising during the holidays.

First, a week before the holiday, try to control your blood sugars, so that any indulgences during the holiday will be balanced by these better than usual blood sugar levels.

Second, make it a point never to eat between scheduled meals, even if cakes and cookies are available. Sticking to standard mealtimes will keep your diabetes medications on schedule and prevent high blood sugars.

Third, never accept second portions at any meal, even though they are offered. Simply tell your host that you are full. Don't let the holidays disturb your blood sugar control, and you'll feel better during and after the festivities.

Fourth, exercise more. Take a walk!

Fifth, if you do eat more than usual, adjust your insulin upward.

Chapter 8
EXERCISE TIPS

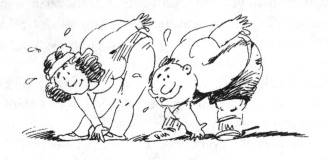

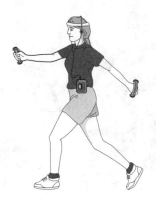

*H*ow can I get the regular exercise
that I need to improve my blood
sugar?

▼
TIP:

Walk. Many people are surprised to learn that walking is an excellent exercise. We recommend walking for everyone. You burn approximately 200 calories in a 1-hour walk. You will lose 1 pound every 3 weeks from this 1 hour of exercise 5 days a week (providing that you don't increase the amount of food you eat). Walk to the shopping center, the supermarket, or the corner drugstore instead of driving. Walking is easy on the muscles and joints and rarely causes low blood sugar. Exercise may make your body more sensitive to insulin, so it can help you achieve a normal body weight and a normal blood sugar level. Start walking today!

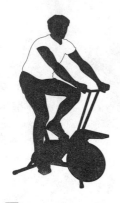

Does exercise raise or lower my blood sugar?

▼
TIP:

Exercise will either raise or lower your blood sugar depending on how much insulin is in your blood. Muscles use glucose, so your blood sugar level gets lower during exercise. This level will go even lower if there is a lot of insulin in your blood. But you must have some insulin circulating in your blood or, in response to exercise, your liver will make more glucose, causing your blood sugar level to rise.

Check your blood sugar before you exercise. If it is low, you can drink a sugar-containing beverage. If it is high, you can take a small dose of regular (or lispro) insulin. If it is higher than 300 mg/dl, we recommend that you delay exercise until the insulin you have taken lowers your glucose to less than 250 mg/dl. The more intense the exercise, the more difficult it is to predict whether your blood sugar will increase or decrease. If you exercise for a long time, recheck your blood sugar halfway through. With experience, you will be able to predict how your exercise will affect your blood sugar levels. You may notice a blood sugar–lowering effect for as long as 24 hours after heavy exercise.

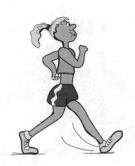

*H*ow much food do I need to eat to
avoid low blood sugars when I
exercise?

▼
TIP:

The amount of food needed to prevent low blood sugar during or
after exercise is different for each person. In general, if your
blood sugar is below 150 mg/dl before exercising, having a snack of
15 grams of carbohydrate is a good idea (one serving of starch, fruit,
or milk). If you have problems with low blood sugars much later
after exercise, have a snack of 15–30 grams of carbohydrate within
30 minutes of finishing the exercise to help your body replace the
glucose normally stored in muscle and to prevent low blood sugar
later. This could be a sandwich, 5–10 saltine crackers, or 4–8 vanilla
wafers or animal cookies. If you are exercising immediately before
or after a meal, you may be able to reduce the insulin used for meal
coverage, because the exercise will reduce your blood sugar, which
normally increases following a meal.

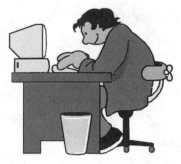

Why do I get low blood sugar when I mow the lawn on Saturday morning but never when I'm at my desk during the week?

▼
TIP:

Muscles use blood glucose to do work, so if you eat the same amount of food and take the same dose of insulin, you can expect your blood sugar to be lower on the day when you are more physically active. You have four choices:

1. Eat more carbohydrate with breakfast.
2. Decrease your morning dose of insulin (about 20–40% less is usually needed to allow for an hour of yard work).
3. Eat a mid-morning snack to prevent the hypoglycemia.
4. Let your grass grow.

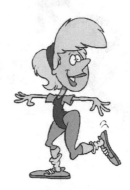

*W*hy does my blood sugar get low in the middle of the night after I exercise during the day?

TIP:

Exercise is good for you, but it can bring on low blood sugar in several ways. Exercise helps you use insulin more efficiently so that a given amount of insulin has more blood sugar–lowering power. These effects of exercise can last for up to 24 hours after the exercise has ended. That's why insulin doses should usually be decreased before and after exercise. Also, you should eat a meal or have a snack before exercising if your blood sugar is normal or low. If you balance your insulin, your food intake, and your exercise, you will have fewer low blood sugars during the night after your daytime exercise.

Why do I always seem to get low blood sugar after having sex?

▼
TIP:

Sex is just as much an exercise as jogging or aerobics. Planning to eat food either immediately before or shortly after sex to cover the glucose that you use is the way to avoid low blood sugar. You may want to check your blood sugar first, even though it may reduce the spontaneity of the moment. You might also consider increasing your snack before going to bed.

Chapter 9
EDUCATIONAL TIPS

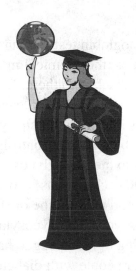

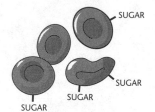

SUGAR

SUGAR

SUGAR

SUGAR

*W*hat is the "glycosylated hemoglobin test"?

▼
TIP:

The glycosylated hemoglobin test measures the percentage of hemoglobin molecules (the chemical in our blood that carries oxygen) that have sugar attached to them. Because this percentage directly reflects the average blood sugar levels over the life of a red blood cell (90 days), this information helps you and your health care team assess your overall blood sugar control. There are several different tests that are used to measure glycosylated hemoglobin (such as a test called A1C), and each test has its own normal range and target values. Ask your doctor what test he or she is using and what the target value should be for you. The glycosylated hemoglobin test, along with self-monitoring of blood sugar, has made good blood sugar control possible for people with diabetes.

*W*here can I find new
information that will help me
with my blood sugar management?

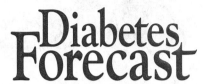

▼
TIP:

There are several ways to find out about new discoveries and products that will help you control your blood sugar levels. You can call the ADA's national center (800) DIABETES (800-342-2383) to ask for information. Or you can call (888) DIABETES, and you will be connected to the ADA office nearest you. They may have information about new products and techniques to treat diabetes. You can subscribe to *Diabetes Forecast*, a magazine for people with diabetes published by the ADA. This magazine has many articles that help you keep up to date. ADA has other books and publications about diabetes that you can buy in bookstores or order over the phone by calling (800) 232-6733. Many health professionals, such as nurses and RDs, specialize in diabetes care and are called certified diabetes educators or CDEs. They have a wealth of information about diabetes. Ask your doctor to recommend a diabetes educator to help you manage your diabetes. For a list of CDEs in your area, call the ADA at (800) DIABETES or the American Association of Diabetes Educators (AADE) at (800) TEAM-UP-4 (800-832-6874).

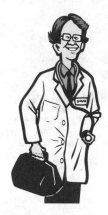

Should I see a diabetes specialist for my diabetes care?

▼
TIP:

In the U.S., 80% of people with diabetes see physicians who are family practice or general practice physicians. If you feel you are getting your blood sugar levels into the goal range and have a good relationship with your doctor, you do not need a diabetes specialist. Sometimes your family doctor will refer you to a specialist for occasional visits or a consultation to get some help with managing your diabetes, but then you can continue your routine care with your family physician. If your primary care doctor can't help you with the daily activities of living with diabetes, you may benefit from diabetes education. Call ADA at (800) DIABETES or AADE at (800) TEAM-UP-4 [(800) 832-6874] to locate a diabetes educator or diabetes education program in your area.

CALENDAR			
JANUARY	FEBRUARY ✔	MARCH	APRIL
MAY ✔	JUNE	JULY	AUGUST ✔
SEPTEMBER	OCTOBER	NOVEMBER ✔	DECEMBER

*H*ow often should I see my
doctor to keep my blood sugar
under control?

▼
TIP:

As you tighten control of your diabetes, you will need to see your
doctor weekly or every 2 weeks, at first. How often you see
your doctor, RD, or diabetes educator will depend on how long you
have had diabetes, your ability to adjust your medication for tight
blood sugar control, and whether you have any diabetic complications or other medical problems that may interfere with your diabetes management. After that, a visit every 3 months may be enough
to reach your target goals.

At a minimum, you should plan on seeing your doctor twice a
year to arrange for necessary eye and kidney checkups and to stay
motivated about good blood sugar control. You should have someone
you can contact on short notice to discuss problems as they arise,
such as unexplained high blood sugars or sudden illness. This person
does not have to be a physician but may be a CDE, RD, nurse practitioner, or nurse case manager.

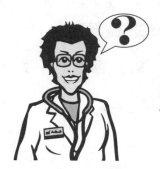

Why does my doctor ask me about the average blood sugar reading on my monitor?

TIP:

You can use the average blood sugar that your meter calculates to improve your blood sugar control. These averages are not a true average of your blood sugar levels but only an average of the times you've actually tested. (If, like most people with diabetes, you measure your blood sugar before meals and at bedtime, this value could more accurately be called your average premeal blood sugar.) People with diabetes with good blood sugar control maintain this average blood sugar below 120 mg/dl. If your average is much higher than this, then you know that you need to adjust your diabetes management program.

*H*ow does the glycosylated
hemoglobin or A1C help
me monitor my blood sugar
control?

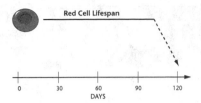

TIP:

These tests tell you how well you are controlling your blood
sugar over a period of several months. Glycosylated hemoglobin
and A1C are names for tests that measure how much glucose (blood
sugar) is attached to your red blood cells. This interaction with glucose occurs slowly and becomes permanent over time. Because a red
blood cell stays in your body 120 days, measuring how much glucose is attached to your red blood cells is a good indication of your
average blood sugar over a 2- to 4-month period. It cannot, however,
tell whether you are having frequent ups and downs in your blood
sugar levels. Studies have shown that the lower your A1C, the less
likely you are to have many of the complications caused by diabetes.

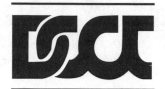

What is the DCCT and how does it affect me?

▼
TIP:

The DCCT is the Diabetes Control and Complications Trial, a long-term diabetes study that proved the complications of diabetes can be delayed or prevented by good blood sugar control. More than 1,400 people with type 1 diabetes were enrolled in this study at centers all across America for a period of 5–8 years. Half of these people received "conventional" diabetes care (1–2 insulin injections per day), and half received "intensive" diabetes management (as many injections as necessary to maintain near-normal blood sugar). People in the intensive therapy group had significantly fewer diabetic complications. As a result of the DCCT, everyone with diabetes (type 1 or 2) should be working to keep his or her blood sugar levels close to normal.

Intensive Therapy Group of the DCCT

Diabetic eye disease	76% decreased risk
Diabetic kidney disease	54% decreased risk
Diabetic nerve disease	60% decreased risk

*H*ow does the health of my teeth *affect my blood sugar control?*

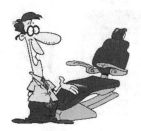

▼

TIP:

Chronic gum disease can be a cause of unexplained high blood sugars. People with diabetes should have their teeth professionally cleaned at least twice a year because they have a much higher risk of developing gum disease than people without diabetes. Gum disease results from the formation of plaque underneath the gum line after eating. Plaque hardens into tartar, which irritates the gums and gradually erodes the underlying bone that holds the teeth in place. Thus, gum disease can lead to the need for dentures. Daily dental care can prevent gum disease from getting started. Brush your teeth at least twice a day with a soft bristle brush and floss daily. Flossing removes food from between the teeth and plaque from the gum line.

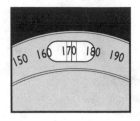

Why have I gained 15 pounds over the 3 years that I have been working to improve my blood sugar control?

TIP:

Some people who practice "intensified management" to keep their diabetes under control gain weight. Because insulin is a hormone that helps your body process the food you eat, one of its many actions is to store fat. It makes sense, then, that injecting insulin to keep your blood sugar down will also result in increased fat storage. The reasons you want good blood sugar control (for example, to decrease your risk of eye and kidney disease) are usually more important than this potential weight gain. The best way to avoid gaining weight is to develop an active lifestyle and follow your health care team's recommended meal plan, limiting fat and total calories.

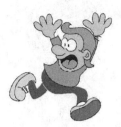

*H*ow can I encourage my child to take
insulin injections if he or she is
scared to death of needles?

TIP:

Try one of the insulin injection devices on the market that do not use needles. They inject insulin by squirting it into the skin at high pressure. Some people with "needle phobia" prefer this method of insulin delivery. Blood sugar control with these devices is as good or better than that achieved with syringe-injected insulin. Although cumbersome and expensive, one of these devices used for a few weeks or months may help your child to become more comfortable with the process so that he or she will be willing to try using the syringe to inject the insulin.

See the tip on inhaled insulin on page 124. You may need to see a mental health professional with your child to help both of you get past this difficulty.

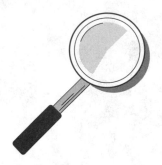

My eyesight is very poor—how can I read the numbers on my glucose meter and then correctly fill my syringe?

▼
TIP:

Many people with diabetes have visual problems. For this reason, there are blood glucose meters that also announce your results. You will be able to check the numbers you can see against the numbers you can hear. To read the numbers on your insulin syringe, you can use a magnifying glass or buy a magnifier that fits on the syringe. You might also consider using a pen-like insulin injector that gives a specific amount of insulin with each click, which you hear as you turn the dial or push the plunger. Your doctor or the ADA can provide you with information on both of these devices.

Chapter 10
NEW TIPS

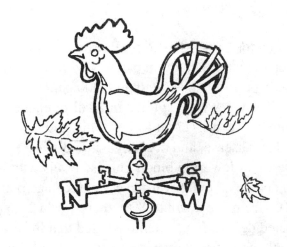

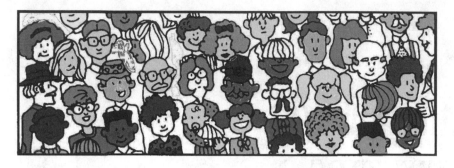

*W*hat is the "UKPDS" study?

▼
TIP:

UKPDS stands for United Kingdom Prospective Diabetes Study, the longest and largest study in patients with type 2 diabetes that has ever been performed. More than 5,000 patients with newly diagnosed type 2 diabetes were studied in 21 different centers in the United Kingdom between 1977 and 1991. This study showed that eye disease, kidney disease, and possibly nerve disease were preventable as a result of lowering blood glucose levels with intensive therapy. It also demonstrated that for every percentage point decrease in A1C (from 9% down to 8%), there was a 25% reduction in diabetes-related deaths. It also demonstrated that lowering blood pressure in people with type 2 diabetes to an average of at least 144/82 mmHg significantly reduced strokes, diabetes-related deaths, heart failure, microvascular (small blood vessel) complications, and loss of vision. This study's results were similar to the DCCT results for people with type 1 diabetes. It emphasizes how important it is for people with type 2 diabetes to bring their blood pressure and blood glucose close to normal levels.

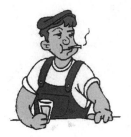

*D*oes smoking affect my glucose control?

▼
TIP:

Yes. Studies have demonstrated that people who smoke have an increased resistance to insulin. This means that whatever insulin you take (or whatever insulin is secreted by your pancreas) does not work as well. Thus, getting your blood glucose close to normal is much more difficult. There are actually many reasons that people with diabetes should not smoke. The primary reason is that smoking is definitely a risk factor for heart disease. People with diabetes already have one strike against them as far as heart disease is concerned. Smoking also has many detrimental health effects, such as causing cancer, lung disease, and early aging. It would be wise to quit.

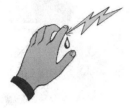

*I*s there a better way than using lancets to get blood from my finger for home blood glucose monitoring?

▼
TIP:

Yes. Although there is not yet a glucose meter available that will allow you to measure your blood sugar without drawing blood, there have been other advances in the field. Specifically, one company has developed a skin perforator that draws a drop of blood from your finger using a low-power laser beam. This device, called the Lasette, produces a small hole in your skin by vaporizing the outer layers of skin with a brief burst of energy. Studies have shown that this works as well as a stainless steel lancet. More important, most patients with diabetes who used the Lasette felt no pain, and 54% of the patients preferred the Lasette over the lancet. Use of the Lasette reduces medical waste and may reduce the risk of exposure to blood-borne diseases, such as hepatitis B, which can be transmitted through a contaminated puncture wound. The Lasette has been approved for home use by the FDA, but whether or not you should purchase one depends on how much they cost, how often you sample your blood sugar, and how comfortable you are using the stainless steel lancets.

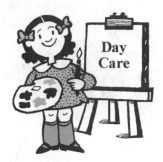

*W*hat should I expect from my child's school or day care regarding his or her diabetes care?

▼
TIP:

The responsibilities for diabetes care should be shared. You provide 1) a treatment plan, 2) all diabetes materials, 3) hypoglycemic treatment foods and snacks, and 4) emergency phone numbers.

The school or day-care center provides 1) immediate treatment for hypoglycemia, 2) an adult to check blood sugar and administer glucagon or insulin, 3) a private area for testing and insulin administration, 4) an adult to oversee the child's meal schedule, 5) access to school medical personnel, 6) permission to eat a snack whenever necessary, 7) permission to miss school for diabetes care with a note from the health care provider, 8) access to the bathroom and drinking water, and 9) storage for diabetes supplies.

The child is expected to 1) cooperate with diabetes tasks [age 8 or older], 2) perform blood glucose testing [7th grade and above], and 3) administer his or her own insulin [high school]. Finally, all children are expected to ask for help whenever necessary.

Discuss these points with the day-care center or school before enrolling your child.

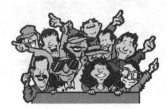

Who should be screened for diabetes?

▼
TIP:

All people above the age of 45 should have a fasting morning blood sugar level test to see if they have diabetes. A fasting morning blood sugar level higher than 126 mg/dl on two occasions indicates diabetes. If they do not have diabetes, then the test should be repeated every 3 years. People who have specific risk factors for diabetes, even though they are younger than age 45, should probably be tested once a year. Such people include

1. Individuals who weigh more than 120% of their ideal body weight
2. People with a parent or sibling who has diabetes
3. Members of certain high-risk ethnic groups (African, Hispanic, and American Indians)
4. Women who have delivered a baby weighing more than 9 pounds or who had gestational diabetes during a previous pregnancy
5. People with very low levels of HDL cholesterol (less than 35 mg/dl) or very high triglyceride levels (above 250 mg/dl)
6. People who have previously been diagnosed with impaired glucose tolerance (a pre-diabetic condition)

It is hoped that increased screening for diabetes will allow diagnosis at an earlier stage and so prevent the complications of the disease.

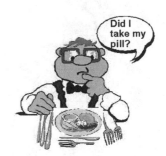

*W*ill the new medication Prandin help
my diabetes?

▼
TIP:

That depends on the type of diabetes you have and your current
diabetes therapy. Prandin (repaglinide) stimulates your pancreas
to produce insulin, much as sulfonylureas do. However, repaglinide
is not a sulfonylurea and is not related structurally to any other medications currently on the market. The advantage of Prandin is that it
works very quickly, so that it is taken with meals or up to 30 minutes
prior to meals and reaches its peak effectiveness within 1 hour. It is
gone from your bloodstream within 3–4 hours. Its primary action is
to raise circulating insulin levels, primarily after meals, when glucose levels are high. Prandin can be used alone or in combination
with some diabetes medications such as metformin (Glucophage).
Side effects of Prandin are similar to those that occur with sulfonylurea treatment, such as weight gain and an occasional low blood
sugar. However, it is generally safe in people who are elderly and
people who have mild kidney and liver problems. The drawback of
Prandin is the need to take it with each meal and, perhaps, the cost.
If you would like to try this medication, discuss it with your health
care team.

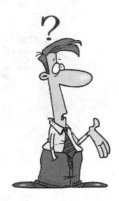

What is the best way to lower my blood sugar if my glyburide isn't working anymore?

▼

TIP:

Glyburide (Micronase, Diabeta) and related medicines like glipizide (Glucotrol) and glimepiride (Amaryl) belong to a class of drugs called sulfonylureas, which work by causing your pancreas to release insulin. These medicines commonly lose their effectiveness after several years. In the past, adding insulin or switching to insulin were your only options. Currently, however, there are a number of other options, including adding a medication such as metformin (Glucophage), pioglitazone (Actos), or acarbose (Precose) to the medicine you are already taking. Because these new medicines work differently from sulfonylureas, they often result in additional blood sugar lowering. All of these drugs reduce A1C by 1–2% when they are added to a sulfonylurea. Talk to your diabetes care team about the pros and cons of adding an additional diabetes medicine to your schedule, and try one for 3–6 months to see whether it works for you.

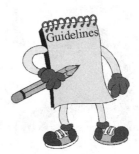

Should I be concerned with glucose control if I have type 2 diabetes?

▼
TIP:

Yes, but maybe not "tight" control. The older you were when you got diabetes, the less benefit you will get from achieving excellent glucose control. This change in benefit level means that your individual risk needs to be refigured before you decide what your target A1C should be. The Veterans' Health Administration (VA) has developed guidelines that you can use depending on the age at which you developed type 2 diabetes. These guidelines are now used in all VA clinics. A patient with type 2 diabetes who developed diabetes at an elderly age may have a target A1C of about 9%, whereas younger patients may benefit from a lower A1C of 7%. If you would like details of these guidelines and what your target A1C should probably be, you can obtain them on the Internet at *http://www.va.gov/health/diabetes/default.htm* or ask your health provider for information on this subject.

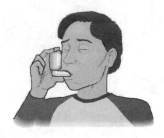

Can I inhale insulin, so that I no longer have to take insulin shots?

▼
TIP:

If all goes well, you can expect to see inhaled insulin available to you very soon. Powdered insulin is inhaled through the mouth and absorbed by the lungs, using an inhaler similar to the device used by patients with asthma. The insulin that is inhaled is very rapidly absorbed into the body. Inhaled insulin is taken before each meal, and intermediate-acting insulin is injected at bedtime. In one recent study in people with type 1 diabetes, 70 individuals used the inhaler and did as well as people taking insulin injections. In patients with type 2 diabetes, a similar result was observed in a study involving 51 participants. Additional studies are planned, and if successful, the results will be submitted to the FDA for approval. This type of insulin administration may be particularly advantageous for children and anyone else who may fear insulin injections.

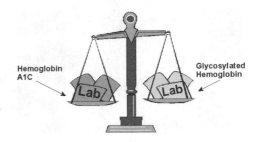

*W*hat is the difference between *glycosylated hemoglobin and A1C?*

▼
TIP:

These are both laboratory tests to measure how much sugar is stuck to the red blood cells that carry oxygen in your blood. Health care providers use these tests to estimate the level of diabetes control during the prior 3 months. Unfortunately, people often use the two terms interchangeably. There are several different kinds of hemoglobin in human red blood cells, and the glycosylated hemoglobin test measures how much sugar is stuck to all of them. The A1C test, on the other hand, measures only how much sugar is stuck to a particular kind of hemoglobin—hemoglobin A_1. Both tests are accurate and reliable, but the normal levels differ, with A1C levels typically being about 2% lower than total glycosylated hemoglobin levels. When your diabetes care team orders a glycosylated hemoglobin or A1C test for you, ask what the normal (nondiabetic) level is so that you can interpret the test. In general, you should aim to keep your glycosylated hemoglobin or A1C level close to the high end of the normal level. Ask your doctor about your level of glycosylated hemoglobin.

101 TIPS FOR STAYING HEALTHY WITH DIABETES (& AVOIDING COMPLICATIONS)

▲

A project of the
American Diabetes Association

▼

Written by

the University of New Mexico
Diabetes Care Team

David S. Schade, MD, *Editor in Chief*
Patrick J. Boyle, MD
Mark R. Burge, MD
Dena Robinson, RN, CDE
Virginia Valentine, RN, MS, CDE

101 TIPS FOR STAYING HEALTHY WITH DIABETES
(& AVOIDING COMPLICATIONS)

▼

TABLE OF CONTENTS

Chapter 1
GENERAL INFORMATION

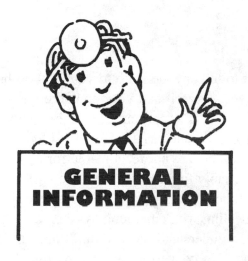

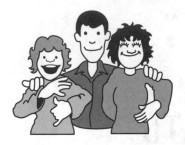

*S*hould I tell my boss and coworkers *that I have diabetes?*

▼
TIP:

Whether or not to tell anyone is up to you. You do have a responsibility to yourself and your coworkers to keep the work environment safe. It is important to have a system in place for managing emergencies, such as a severe low blood sugar or a sick day. Your coworkers are not responsible for taking care of you, but you will probably find that they will be very understanding and want to help you stay healthy. Most people feel more comfortable dealing with emergencies when they have some preparation and understanding. You don't have to make diabetes the daily topic of conversation, and you may feel uncomfortable letting people at work become the "control patrol." This is a personal choice that requires consideration on your part, but you will find that your life is easier if you allow others to support you in managing your diabetes and staying healthy.

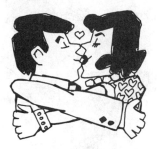

Can I catch diabetes from someone else?

▼
TIP:

No, you cannot. Diabetes is not like a cold or the flu. There are many causes of diabetes, but both types 1 and 2 have never been shown to be infectious or contagious (catchable). You cannot catch diabetes from another person, even by kissing them. Most diabetes develops from an inherited tendency to get it. If you have inherited this gene, you may develop type 1 diabetes when you are exposed to something in the environment. This unknown factor triggers the onset of diabetes. You may develop type 2 diabetes if (in addition to the gene) you gain weight and don't exercise regularly. There are also less common causes of diabetes, such as prolonged, excessive drinking of alcohol or having too much iron in your blood. Thus, there are many causes of diabetes, but catching it from another person is not one of them.

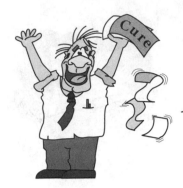

How close are we to a cure for diabetes?

▼
TIP:

It depends on what you mean by "cure." Diabetes is not really one disease. It probably has many causes and, therefore, many cures. Much progress has been made in the last few years toward prevention of diabetes and treatment of the disease once it occurs. These advances are important until cures are available. The ultimate cure for diabetes would probably be a replacement of the cells of the pancreas that make insulin. This could be done by inserting a remote-controlled insulin pump that is automatically regulated by a glucose sensor. The implantable pump has already been developed and tested in more than 400 people worldwide. Glucose sensors are under development and should be available soon.

Another approach is to transplant insulin-producing cells into the person with diabetes. This approach has already been done successfully in animals with diabetes. It has been more difficult in humans, because our body sees these cells as foreign material and tends to kill them off. Many researchers are trying to overcome these problems. What we can say is that we expect a cure for some types of diabetes within the next ten years.

D oes diabetes put me at risk for developing thyroid problems?

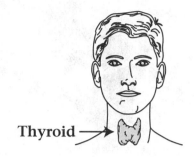

Thyroid ➞

▼
TIP:

Perhaps. The thyroid gland in your neck secretes thyroid hormone. Low levels of thyroid hormone (thyroid failure) are common in individuals with type 1 diabetes. Thyroid hormone gives you energy and helps maintain other organ systems in your body. We recommend that you get a blood test for thyroid hormone once a year, particularly if you feel more tired than usual or have other symptoms such as constipation, dry skin, and feeling cold most of the time. Treatment is easy and inexpensive. This is important, because when low thyroid hormone goes untreated, it can lead to many medical problems. Do not hesitate to ask your doctor periodically to check your blood thyroid hormone level. Remember that other medical problems can occur in people with diabetes that are not directly related to high blood sugar levels.

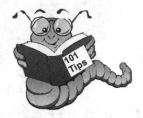

*H*ow can I make the most
of my visit with my
health care team?

▼
TIP:

First, plan ahead. Write down on paper all the questions that you want to ask the team. It is too easy to forget your questions if you don't write them down. Also bring along a pencil or pen to write down the answers. If you're prepared, the visit is more likely to meet your needs. Second, show up for your appointment on time. If you are late, your health care team may not be able to spend enough time with you to solve your problems. (For waiting room reading, you could bring this book or our first book, *101 Tips for Improving Your Blood Sugar*, and review the tips that apply to you.) Third, always bring in all your current medications, so that the health care team can check them. This will ensure that you don't run out of medication and that the pharmacy gives you the medication that your doctor prescribes. Fourth, be sure and bring in records of your recent blood sugars, weight, blood pressure, and exercise schedule. These records help you and the team see your progress in meeting your goals. If you don't have a logbook, bring your blood glucose meter.

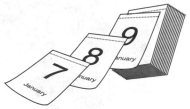

*H*ow often should I plan on seeing
my doctor to be as healthy as I
can be?

▼
TIP:

The frequency of medical visits required for your diabetes
will vary according to how long you've had diabetes, your
ability to adjust your treatment regimen effectively to maintain
good blood sugar control, and whether you have diabetic complications or other medical problems that may interfere with
your diabetes management.

At a minimum, all patients with diabetes should plan on
seeing a doctor twice a year. Recharging your motivation to
achieve good blood sugar control is an important part of every
visit. You should have an A1C test done then, or if you are on
insulin, you should have the test done quarterly to see how your
blood glucose control is doing.

In addition, every patient with diabetes should have someone
he or she can contact on short notice to discuss problems as they
arise, such as unexplained high blood sugars or sudden illness.
This person need not be a physician but may be a certified
diabetes educator (CDE), registered dietitian (RD), nurse
practitioner, or nurse case manager.

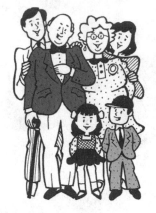

*S*hould members of my family
read this book?

▼
TIP:

Y es! There are several good reasons for each member of your
family to read this book. First, there are many tips that
apply equally well to people without diabetes. Anyone who
wants to stay in good health will benefit from these tips. Second,
your family members can support you better when they understand what is needed. For example, a change to eating healthier
meals is easier if all family members make the same commitment. There are outdated ideas of what is good for a person with
diabetes. Keeping up-to-date makes it easier to plan family out-
ings, picnics, and parties with you in mind. Each family member
should be able to recognize the signs and symptoms of low
blood sugar. Third, family members of people with diabetes have
a higher risk of developing diabetes themselves. By changing to
a healthier lifestyle, you and your family members, we believe,
will prevent or significantly delay the onset of diabetes.

D oes getting diabetes when I am pregnant mean that I am more likely to get permanent diabetes later?

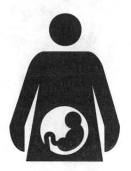

▼

TIP:

Y es. The fact that you get high blood sugars during pregnancy indicates that your pancreas cannot make enough extra insulin to cover the increased needs caused by pregnancy. This suggests that you might develop diabetes even if you never get pregnant again. Approximately 5% of women like you will develop diabetes each year if they don't make efforts to improve their lifestyles. Women gain weight during pregnancy but do not always lose all of it after delivery. With several pregnancies, a woman may gain quite a bit of weight. Therefore, if you develop high blood sugars during pregnancy, it is most important that you lose all of the weight you gained during your pregnancy. Eat healthy meals and exercise daily. This is the best approach you can take to prevent permanent diabetes from occurring.

If you decide to breastfeed, do not begin a weight loss program without medical advice. To breastfeed, you need the same amount of calories that you needed during the last 3 months of your pregnancy. When you stop breastfeeding, then you can focus on losing any extra weight that you still have.

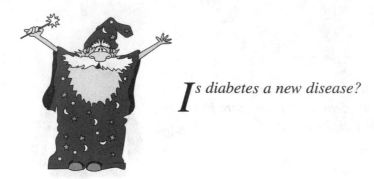

Is diabetes a new disease?

▼
TIP:

No. Diabetes was known 2,000 years ago when Aretaeus of Cappadocia, the Greek physician, named it. However, very little progress was made in understanding or treating the disease until 1869 when Paul Langerhans described small islands (islets) in the pancreas. However, he did not know their function. Things progressed more rapidly when Oskar Minkowski realized that removing the pancreas from a dog caused the dog to urinate frequently. He also found sugar in the dog's urine. In 1909, the Belgian scientist Jean de Meyer used the term "insulin" for a hypothetical substance in the pancreas that controls blood sugar even though insulin had not yet been discovered. Finally in 1921, after a series of experiments, J.J.R. Macleod, Charles Best, Frederick Banting, and James Collip succeeded in purifying insulin and successfully treating a diabetes patient with it. This discovery saved many people from dying in a coma due to high blood sugars. Diabetes has been around a long time, but we still need new and better therapies.

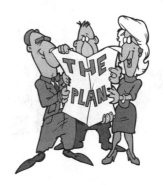

*W*hat is my "health care team" and
how can I find these health
providers?

▼
TIP:

In addition to your doctor, you need someone trained to help
you with the day-to-day challenges of living with diabetes.
Diabetes educator nurses and dietitians, plus your doctor, are the
core members of your health care team. A certified diabetes educator (CDE) is a health professional (registered nurse [RN], registered dietitian [RD], pharmacist, physician, etc.) who has been
trained and "certified" as an expert in diabetes education and
management. If you cannot find a CDE, you may find a nurse or
RD interested in diabetes and willing to help you. Ask your doctor if he or she knows someone with diabetes experience. You
can locate a CDE in your area by calling the American Association of Diabetes Educators (AADE) Awareness Hotline at (800)
TEAM-UP-4. They will ask for your zip code and help you find
a CDE near you. You may also want to look for a diabetes-edu-
cation program that offers individual or group classes. The
American Diabetes Association has a list of "recognized" diabetes programs in your area. Call (800) DIABETES for this
information. If there isn't a recognized diabetes center near you,
call your local hospital and ask about a diabetes education program or diabetes educators on staff.

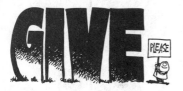

*W*hat can I do to help cure
diabetes?

TIP:

You can do a lot! Most people don't realize how important
their effort can be in helping to cure diabetes. The main
reason that so much progress has been made in the last 50 years
is the work of individuals like you supporting organizations
searching for the cure for diabetes. One of these organizations is
the American Diabetes Association (ADA).

At the local level, you can encourage friends and neighbors
to support fundraising efforts by your local diabetes chapters,
such as walking events. Donations support new research in
diabetes and are deductible from your income tax. Joining will
connect you to up-to-date information on better diabetes
management and keep you informed of important legislation
concerning diabetes in the U.S. Congress. Your letters to your
local and state representatives (congressmen and senators) can
definitely help make state and national monies available for
diabetes research and treatment. Your local ADA office, (888)-
DIABETES, can provide you with their names and addresses.
Remember, you really can make a difference.

*I*s diabetes a dangerous disease?

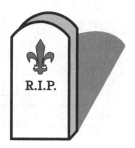

▼
TIP:

Y es, it is. There are statistics to prove that diabetes causes much suffering and loss of time from work. For example, it is the leading cause of kidney failure in this country. In addition, 15,000–30,000 people each year lose their eyesight because of diabetes. This year, 160,000 individuals will die from diabetes-related causes in the United States. In fact, according to experts, during the last 20 years, diabetes has caused more deaths than all of the wars throughout the world in the last century. Unfortunately, the situation is getting worse, not better, because of the increasing number of people developing diabetes. We all need to do our best to prevent and to treat this disease in the U.S. and throughout the world.

The results of the Diabetes Control and Complications Trial (DCCT) and the United Kingdom Prospective Diabetes Study (UKPDS) show that we can live healthier lives with diabetes by keeping blood glucose levels near normal. Modern advances in self-testing and treatment make this possible.

		D	E	M	E	T	R	I	U	S
		I								
S	U	G	A	R		U				
		B				R				
		M	E	L	L	I	T	U	S	
		T				N		W		
W	A	T	E	R		E		E		
		S						L		
								L		

What does the name diabetes mellitus mean?

▼

TIP:

The names "diabetes" and "mellitus" come from two different places. The first name, diabetes, is usually attributed to the Greek physician Aretaeus, who lived in 200 BC. He used the term diabetes, meaning siphon or to flow through, for a disease in which the water that a person drinks runs rapidly through his or her body. His patients sucked up water at one end and emptied it at the other. It was not until the end of the 18th century that the term mellitus was added to diabetes. An Englishman, John Rollo, and a German, Johann Peter Frank, first used the term mellitus (which means sweet as honey) in the medical literature to describe the sweet taste of the urine. So, to answer your question, the name diabetes mellitus means a medical condition in which the patient drinks too much water and urinates frequently. The urine is sweet because it contains sugar.

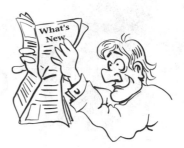

*H*ow can I know whether a new
diabetes product is right for me?

▼
TIP:

This is one time when being a skeptic is a good idea. Many
times, news releases make a product sound like it will work
for everyone, but in fact it may only be useful for specific conditions. In the United States, we have many regulations to protect
us from unproved (and possibly dangerous) new treatments. The
Food and Drug Administration (FDA) has strict guidelines
regarding the research and testing that must be done on a new
drug or therapy before it can be sold to the public. Many times
you will read reports about a new product or drug, but it is still
in the early phases of testing. Testing takes several years. If safety problems or side effects are found during the testing, the product will not be marketed. Your health care team may have
information on new products, so you should check with them
when something new is available. They will help you make a
decision as to whether the new product is right for you.

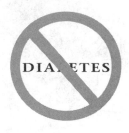

*C*an diabetes be prevented?

▼

TIP:

Many scientists believe that the answer is "yes." Because the causes of type 1 and type 2 diabetes are different, approaches to preventing each form of diabetes are different.

Type 1 diabetes is thought to be caused by an allergic-like reaction, probably to insulin, the pancreas, or some substance in the pancreas. If this is true, then it is possible that diabetes could be prevented by giving the susceptible person small injections of insulin, much like allergy shots may prevent hay fever. This approach has been successful in animals who were bred to get diabetes. However, this approach was not successful in an NIH clinical trial. Other approaches, such as oral insulin, are still being investigated.

Type 2 diabetes does not seem to be caused by an allergic reaction. The cause is probably related to a hereditary defect that reduces a person's sensitivity to insulin. New medications used early may prevent type 2 diabetes. Also, lifestyle changes (exercise and weight loss) may reverse this defect and prevent it. The Diabetes Prevention Program has recently shown that diet and exercise prevent the incedence of diabetes by about 60%, with the oral medication metformin preventing about 30%.

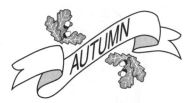

*I*s there a time of year when my family or I am more likely to get diabetes?

▼
TIP:

Yes and no. Many studies have been done to determine when people get diabetes.

Type 1 diabetes (previously called "insulin-dependent diabetes") usually occurs in thin individuals less than 30 years of age. It is more common to develop type 1 diabetes in the fall, which happens to be the season in which many viral infections occur (for example, chicken pox, flu, and measles). The higher rate of type 1 diabetes during the fall months has been used to suggest that type 1 diabetes may be started by a virus that causes an infection. Whether this is true or not has not been found.

Type 2 diabetes (previously called "non-insulin-dependent diabetes") usually occurs in overweight people over the age of 30 years. There does not seem to be a seasonal increase in the development of type 2 diabetes. This difference in the time of year that diabetes develops is one of the many ways the two types of diabetes are not alike.

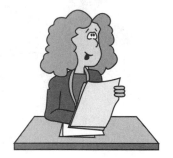

Why do I have a preexisting condition rider attached to my health insurance policy that excludes any coverage for my diabetes for 1 year?

▼
TIP:

Insurance companies separate people into groups depending on their "risk" (the chance that they will cost money to the insurance company). Because diabetes is expensive to manage and because diabetes is associated with other serious diseases, insurance companies feel that they should either charge you more or not cover you for the first year. In this first year with preexisting conditions excluded, you must try to find a way to protect yourself from excessive health care expenses. Before you change jobs, be sure to consider the complete health benefit package of both jobs. Consider the impact your new job may have on your present health benefits package. You may be able to retain insurance coverage from your previous position by selecting your COBRA benefit, which is required by law to allow you to continue your insurance for 18 months. You should also check with your State Insurance Commission to find out if your state has an insurance program for people who are uninsurable because they have a chronic disease. If you are unable to afford insurance or health care costs, many county- or state-supported hospitals have funds that are available to help with medical costs.

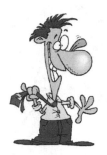

*W*ill Viagra help me if my impotence is
due to diabetes?

▼
TIP:

Maybe. As you are aware, Viagra is the only FDA-approved oral medication for impotence in the United States. This medication has proved safe, and 65–85% of men using it report an improvement in erections. Please note that Viagra does not increase the desire for sex, only the ability to maintain an erection. In one study that focused exclusively on men whose impotence was attributed to diabetes, the men kept diaries throughout the study. These diaries demonstrated that approximately 50% of attempts at sexual intercourse were successful for men taking Viagra, but only about 10% were successful for those taking a placebo. Side effects of Viagra include headaches, facial flushing, and indigestion, but there has been no evidence of an effect on a person's glucose control. No one should take Viagra if he is also taking nitroglycerin or nitrate in any form, because dangerous low blood pressure may result. If you have heart disease or are taking other medications, talk with your health provider about whether this product is safe for you to use.

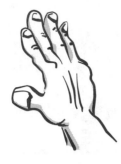

*W*hy are my fingernails thick and pulling
  away from the nail bed?

▼

TIP:

You may have a fungal infection of your fingernails. Fungal infections of the skin, such as "athlete's foot," are more common in people with diabetes. These fungal infections can occasionally involve unusual areas of the body, such as your nails, scalp, or groin. A fungal infection of your fingernails is not a serious threat to your overall health, but it may make your nails brittle and unsightly. You can also spread the infection to other areas of your body, such as your scalp, by scratching with infected nails.

You should see your health care team or a dermatologist to have your infection treated. They can take a sample from under your nails and examine it under the microscope to confirm the diagnosis. Nail infections are difficult to cure, and you will probably require treatment with an oral drug for several months. Because these drugs may damage your liver or bone marrow, you may need to have blood tests every few weeks to monitor your blood cell counts and your liver function. After all of this effort, you may be rewarded with a return of healthy fingernails.

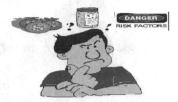

Which type 2 medication should I use?

▼
TIP:

You and your health care provider must discuss this. There are several different classes of medicine for the treament of diabetes, and the one you should use depends on dosing requirements, side effects, hypoglycemia risk, cost, and (most importantly) whether or not it enables you to meet your target blood glucose goals. If you are unable to meet your target goals with only one agent, your health provider may place you on two or more drugs to try to control your diabetes.

Generic Name	Dosing and Side Effects	Hypo-glycemia Risk	Cost
Glypizide (Glucotrol), Glyburide (Micronase, Diabeta) Glimepiride (Amaryl)	1–2 times a day	Medium	Low
Metformin (Glucophage)	1–2 times a day. Causes gas, bloating, or diarrhea in 20–30% of cases	Low	Medium
Repaglinide (Prandin)	3 times a day	Medium	Medium
Pioglitazone (Actos), Rosiglitazone (Avandia)	1 time a day. Causes rare liver problems and requires monthly blood testing	Low	High
Acarbose (Precose)	3 times a day. Causes gas, bloating, or diarrhea in up to 50% of cases	Low	Medium
Insulin injections	1–3 times a day	High	Low

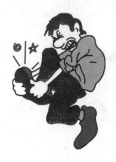

*S*hould I be concerned about a small red blister on my foot from walking in new shoes?

TIP:

Yes! You may look at a small blister and think that it is nothing serious, but it can be. If it breaks, this blister in the skin can allow germs into your foot. These germs can cause not only an infection in your foot, but also in the bone. Infections in the bone are very difficult to treat and often are the cause of amputations. What you should do right now is to wash your feet carefully in gentle soap and water and dry them thoroughly. Then put a small amount of antibiotic ointment on a dressing and cover the wound. Next, call your health care team and let them know that you have a sore on your foot. Your health care team will want to see your foot to decide whether you need to get started on an antibiotic medication. Finally, quit wearing the shoes that caused the blister. Purchasing a comfortable pair of shoes is one of the best investments you can make. The shoes you wear must fit your feet. Careful attention can prevent future problems.

A m I more likely to develop skin infections because I have diabetes?

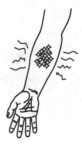

▼
TIP:

Y ou may be. People with diabetes who are overweight or who have high blood sugars most of the time are more likely to develop skin infections than are thin people with normal blood sugars. High blood sugars can interfere with your body's natural defense systems. Once they start, some of these infections can spread rapidly, causing fever, chills, and tiredness. It is very important that you examine your skin each day and promptly take care of any ulcers, redness, or skin breakdowns that may be new. Yeast infections usually occur in warm, moist areas of the body, particularly in the genital region, under breasts, and between folds of skin. Infections of the face, foot, and ear canal may be particularly serious and should be checked by your health care team. Many different types of treatment are available for these skin problems, and you should ask for advice before applying drugstore skin creams. Good skin care is essential for good health.

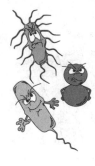

*C*an my diabetes cause diarrhea?

▼
TIP:

Yes. Frequent diarrhea occurs in 5–20% of people with long-standing diabetes. The possible causes include fewer digestive enzymes being released from the pancreas, overuse of magnesium-containing antacids, or too many bacteria in the upper part of the intestine (where they should not normally be). Often, however, the cause is unknown. Damage to the nerves that control movement in the bowel is thought to be a basic cause. Have an evaluation by your health care team. For example, if you don't have enough digestive enzymes, a pill taken with meals may cure the problem. If the cause of your diarrhea remains unknown, there are still treatments that may increase the hardness of your stools and decrease the number of daily bowel movements. Some of these treatments include simple over-the-counter remedies like psyllium (Metamucil) or a kaolin and pectin mixture (Kaopectate). Other people respond to prescription drugs, such as cholesterol-binding resins (cholestyramine), antibiotics (tetracycline or erythromycin), or drugs designed to decrease movement in the bowel, such as loperamide (Lomotil). Whatever the cause of your diarrhea, you deserve a careful medical review of this problem, because chances are good that some of your symptoms can be relieved.

Could I lose my job driving a truck if I start insulin?

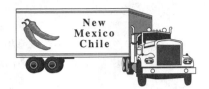

▼
TIP:

If you can prove that your diabetes is in good control with detailed blood glucose records and glycated hemoglobin test (A1C) results, you may be able to continue in the job in your state. Individual state governments have rules for jobs driving automobiles, trucks, or commercial vehicles within that state. Most jobs are reviewed on a case-by-case basis.

However, the U.S. Department of Transportation Federal Highway Administration governs driving commercial vehicles between states. Their policy is that, "A person is physically qualified to drive a motor vehicle if he or she has no established medical history or clinical diagnosis of diabetes mellitus currently requiring insulin for control." This would prevent you from driving a truck across state lines if you are taking insulin. You should contact your state Department of Transportation to see what your state's policy is for various occupations that rely on driving ability within that state.

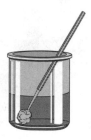

Should I test my urine for glucose and ketones?

▼
TIP:

Sometimes. Urine testing is not an accurate way to measure blood sugar. It is the way to check for ketones when you cannot eat or are ill. A buildup of ketones tells you that you are developing ketoacidosis. Ketones are breakdown products of fat that produce acid in the body. Too much acid can result in you being hospitalized. Therefore, when you are sick with a cold or the flu, you should test your urine for ketones and call your health care team if you detect any. You can buy urine ketone testing strips at the drugstore.

The information about blood glucose that you get from urine testing for sugar is not precise enough to make decisions for treatment. Your kidney does not spill sugar into your urine until your blood sugar is higher than 200 mg/dl. The ADA does not recommend that you use urine sugar testing (especially if you're taking insulin) if you can perform fingerstick blood glucose testing.

*W*here can I find information about
diabetes on the Internet?

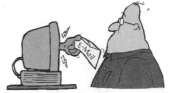

▼
TIP:

There are numerous places to find information about diabetes. The first to consider is the ADA web site (*www.
diabetes.org*). This site gives you information to help you
understand the cause and treatment of diabetes. In addition, the
Centers for Disease Control and Prevention (CDC) home page
(*www.CDC.gov*) offers extensive information about chronic
diseases including diabetes. You can find statistics on the incidence and prevalence of diabetes and its complications and a
patient guide called *Take Charge of Your Diabetes*. This manual can be downloaded free of charge. The CDC site also has a
traveler's health information page, which includes material for
international travelers, geographical health recommendations,
and vaccine information. Diabetes information can also be
found at the NIH web site (*www.nih.gov*), including the home
page for the National Institutes of Diabetes and Digestive and
Kidney Diseases (NIDDK) (*www.niddk.nih.gov*). This web site
offers a nice glossary and definition of many diabetes-related
terms. This site is also linked to *Diabetes in America,* 2nd edition, which contains extensive public information on diabetes
in the United States. These sites should answer most of your
diabetes questions.

Chapter 2
GLUCOSE CONTROL

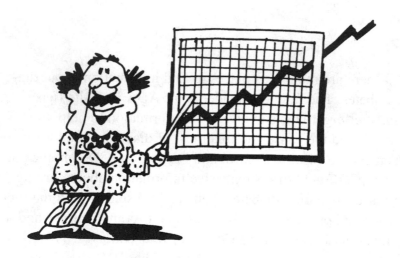

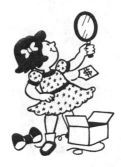

*W*hy can't I get my 8-year-old daughter to help take care of her diabetes?

▼
TIP:

B ecause it is difficult and frustrating for her to do it. Young children usually are unable to assume full responsibility for their diabetes care until they reach the teenage years. In fact, an 8-year-old child cannot understand something as complicated as a chronic disease, and she may actually blame herself for the fact that she has diabetes. She may be more timid than other children her age and worry more than usual when you are apart from her ("separation anxiety").

She has new and challenging tasks every day, like going to school and making new friends, so she may not be interested in caring for her diabetes. She needs to feel secure in her daily activities and let you care for her diabetes for now. It may help her self-confidence if she succeeds at doing some of the basic tasks such as blood glucose checks and keeping her log book. Discuss with your health care team how flexible her schedule can be and the appropriate goals for her diabetes control. You may find that you can loosen up on her control somewhat in the interest of safety and convenience. Remember that the day is coming when your daughter will be able to care for her diabetes herself, and she'll only need your help occasionally. Just don't rush her.

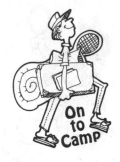

*H*ow can I help my 13-year-old son
cope with his diabetes?

▼

TIP:

This is a hectic period in his life with rapid changes inside
and out, and diabetes care may be low on his priority list.
The onset of puberty can complicate diabetes care. He may
have a dramatic increase in insulin requirements over a short
period of time. Turn over the responsibility for diabetes care to
your son gradually as he is ready to accept it. You will both
need to be flexible to adjust to all the demands on him.

It is possible that your son may be more open to learning
from his peers than from you during the coming years. Help
him get together with other teenagers who have diabetes, so he
can see the various ways they cope with diabetes. Diabetes
summer camp provides an excellent opportunity for this. Your
son will see both healthy and unhealthy behaviors at camp, but
he'll be encouraged to manage his own diabetes with
experience and knowledge. Most states have a diabetes
summer camp with a full medical staff. The friendships that
develop at camp are often strong and can last a lifetime.
Contact the ADA at (888) DIABETES (342-2383) for more
information about a camp in your area.

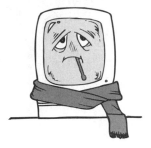

*W*hat can I take for a cold since it seems that all the cold medicines at the drugstore are labeled "not for people with diabetes"?

▼
TIP:

Probably the best thing to do about a cold is to take acetaminophen (Tylenol) for the aches, pains, or fever, get plenty of rest, and drink lots of fluids. Be sure to check your blood sugar often and be ready to respond to a rise in your blood sugar. You and your health care team need to set up a sick-day plan. Then you'll know better what to eat or drink, when to test your blood glucose and ketones, and when to call them for help.

Drugs that help reduce the symptoms of a cold are cough medicines, antihistamines (block allergic reaction), and decongestants (reduce swelling in the nose). The cough medicines and antihistamines tend to make you very sleepy. Chemicals in decongestants work in your swollen sinus tissues by making the blood vessels narrower and thus reducing blood flow. This may help your runny nose, but if you have heart disease or very poor circulation, they can cause serious problems. However, if you have diabetes, the label warns you to talk to your doctor before taking this medicine.

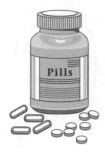

Will the medication I am taking for depression affect my blood sugar?

TIP:

Probably not. Depression is more common in patients with chronic diseases like diabetes—up to 40% of people with diabetes may have depression at some point in their lives. Medications for depression have no major direct impact on how your oral diabetes medications or insulin work to control your blood sugar.

On the other hand, keeping diabetes management at the top of your list of things to deal with can seem impossible if you are depressed. While there are many ways of dealing with depression, sometimes several months of treatment with medication can allow you to get back to being yourself faster. A vicious cycle can develop where high blood sugars make you feel sleepy and as though you don't have enough energy to get out and exercise. The exercise would help bring the blood glucose down and make you feel better physically and mentally. Dealing with depression can break the cycle and put you back on track, eating right and exercising, to help you feel better all the time.

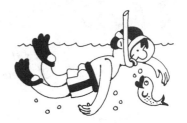

Because I have arthritis in my hips, can you recommend exercises other than walking?

▼

TIP:

Many people with arthritic pain in their hips or knees cannot take the 30- to 60-minute walk that is recommended to improve blood sugar control. You can do armchair aerobics and stretches while sitting. Water aerobics in a swimming pool is another activity that does not put stress on your joints. If you can do them, gentle "standing" exercises such as tai chi or chi kung can give you a no-impact workout. All exercise routines should include a 10-minute warm-up period, 10–30 minutes of exercise, and a 10-minute cooldown period. The exercise must be intense enough to get your heart rate up but not so intense that you can't speak. You may break out in a light sweat (if you're not in a pool).

Weight loss is not the only benefit of exercising. Exercise also increases insulin sensitivity, improves blood flow to the heart and muscles, and helps improve blood sugar control. As with all exercise programs, you should consult your health care team for recommendations about the activity that is right for you. Don't let your arthritis prevent you from exercising.

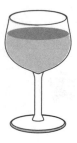

Is it acceptable for me to have a glass of wine with dinner?

▼
TIP:

It may be. The key is the food you are eating. Alcohol can cause severe, life-threatening low blood sugar, even in people who do not have diabetes. That is why we say drink only with food. There is evidence that small amounts of alcohol are okay for people with diabetes if you are not pregnant or do not have a history of alcohol abuse. For example, one recent study shows that moderate alcohol intake (no more than one drink a day) is associated with lower blood sugar levels and improved insulin sensitivity in healthy people who do not have diabetes. Another study shows that blood sugar levels do not differ for 12 hours after a meal between diabetes patients (both types 1 and 2) who drink a shot of vodka before dinner, or a glass of wine with dinner, or a shot of cognac after dinner and those who drink an equal amount of water. Finally, a number of studies have suggested that moderate alcohol intake may have a positive effect on blood cholesterol and lipid levels. Just remember that alcohol calories should be included in your meal plan (one alcoholic drink is 1 fat exchange) and have your one drink with food.

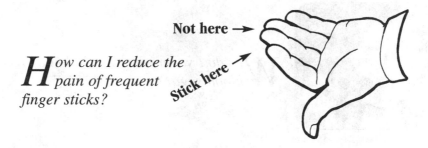

Not here →

*H*ow can I reduce the pain of frequent finger sticks?

Stick here →

▼
TIP:

O ne technique is to stick the side of your finger where there are fewer pain sensors instead of sticking directly into your fingerpad. Another technique is to use an automatic (spring-loaded) lancet holder that can vary how deep the lancet goes. Use the shortest depth that will give you an adequate drop of blood for testing. Since skin thickness varies from person to person, you'll need to try different depths to see what works for you.

Because of the danger of transmitting hepatitis and other blood borne diseases, never "borrow" another person's device. Hopefully, in the next few years, noninvasive blood sugar monitors will become available for you to use. These monitors will sample your glucose level without having to stick your finger at all. In the meantime, there is a new lancet called Lancette that uses a laser to extract the drop of blood for testing. It is reputed to be less painful to use. Talk with your health care team about this device and to get information on others that may be developed.

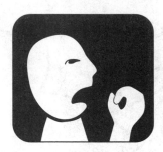

*W*hy do I yawn when I have low
blood sugar?

▼
TIP:

Probably because low blood sugar makes you feel tired. The
classic signs and symptoms of low blood sugar include
sweating, hunger, nervousness, and agitation. However, many
people with diabetes do not have the usual symptoms. Some
people have no symptoms at all!

Other people have unusual symptoms of low blood sugar.
In some people, a change in their personality can occur, so that
they become hostile and combative. Some people simply look
"glassy-eyed," "spacey," or are mildly confused. It is very
important to know what your low blood sugar symptoms are,
so that your friends and family will know when to help you.

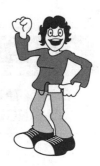

Would an insulin pump help me prevent complications?

▼
TIP:

Maybe. If it helps you keep your blood glucose close to normal levels, yes. But an insulin pump is not for everyone. If you have been unable to get your blood glucose levels into goal range, a pump may be a good choice for you. A pump, also called a "continuous subcutaneous insulin infusion system," can do some things that conventional insulin injection therapy can't. Using a pump requires motivation and a willingness to measure your blood sugar four or more times a day and to make decisions based on the results. A pump cannot "read" your blood sugar, so you have to do blood sugar tests regularly to tell the pump how much insulin you need. The downside is the cost. A pump costs about $5,000 to start and about $75 a month to maintain. You should talk to your health care team and insurance company about whether a pump would be a good idea for you. Newer pumps have more features and are more reliable than older models. More features allow more flexibility of lifestyle to help you stay in good control.

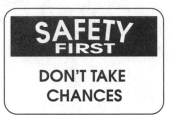

*I*s it safe for me to use birth control pills if I have diabetes?

▼
TIP:

B irth control pills appear to be safe for women with diabetes to take, and they are certainly safer than a pregnancy for which you are unprepared. There is controversy among diabetes specialists about the best form of birth control for women with diabetes. Under certain circumstances, estrogen-containing birth control pills may affect blood sugar and blood cholesterol levels. For this reason, some physicians have not prescribed them for women with diabetes. Studies have shown, however, that blood sugar levels are no different in women who take birth control pills than in women who do not. Similarly, blood cholesterol and lipid levels are no different in women with diabetes who use birth control pills than in those who do not. There are other effective birth control methods, such as a diaphragm, that will not affect blood sugar at all. If you are concerned, talk to your health care team about which method of birth control will work best for you.

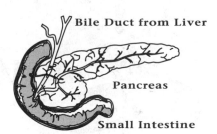

Bile Duct from Liver

Pancreas

Small Intestine

*W*ould a successful
pancreas transplantation
cure my diabetes?

▼
TIP:

Y es, but a pancreas transplantation is not as easy as it
sounds. Only a few hospitals in the United States do pancreas transplantations. The problem with any transplantation is
rejection of the foreign tissue by our own bodies. There are
drugs that suppress the body's rejection efforts, but these make
diabetes control much more difficult. To be considered for a
transplantation, you have to meet criteria that may vary from
center to center:

1. You must have type 1 diabetes.
2. Most centers will only do a pancreas transplantation if you
    also need a kidney transplantation. Anti-rejection drugs are
    expensive and hazardous, and the kidney transplantation
    would automatically require the same anti-rejection drugs
    needed for the pancreas transplantation.
3. You must have insurance or health coverage to pay for the
    transplantation (many insurance programs consider this an
    experimental treatment), the medications, and follow-up
    care needed after the transplantation. A pancreas
    transplantation may cost more than $100,000.

Perhaps new therapies will find a way to replace insulin-
making cells without requiring anti-rejection medications.

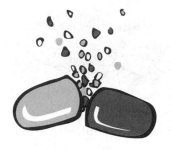

Why are my blood sugars high while I am taking prednisone for my asthma?

▼
TIP:

Prednisone is used for a variety of conditions such as asthma and other lung problems. It acts like a hormone that your body makes called "cortisol." Cortisol and prednisone both cause the body to make glucose when you're not eating (like during the night). They can worsen diabetes control. Cortisol is called a "stress hormone" because the body releases it to deal with stresses like accidents, infections, or burns. That's part of the reason why it takes more insulin to keep blood sugars near normal during an infection. If you have had prednisone prescribed for any reason and you have diabetes, you will need to take more diabetes medication. Prednisone's effect on your blood glucose will go away a day or two after you stop taking it. Your health care team can help you alter your diabetes treatment until you can stop taking the prednisone.

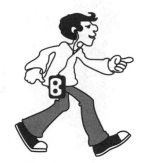

Will my 11-year-old son's diabetes have any long-term effects on his psychological health?

▼
TIP:

Coming to terms with a lifelong, chronic disease like diabetes is a big job for a child. It is not surprising that psychological problems can occur soon after diabetes develops. In general, most children who have family support adapt well and have no long-term psychological problems as a result.

One study has shown that children diagnosed with diabetes between the ages of 8 and 14 were initially more depressed, dependent, and socially withdrawn than other children. By the time a year had passed, most of these problems were gone. By two years after diagnosis, however, children with diabetes again had a higher risk of depression and dependency than children without diabetes.

Children seem to cope with the initial stress of developing diabetes, but as they realize that diabetes is a permanent condition, they may experience a period of depression. It is important for parents to realize this and to contact the health care team if you are concerned that your child might be depressed. In the interim, be supportive of your child and watchful for signs that might signal the onset of depression, such as a change in appetite, lack of interest in activities, or withdrawal from social groups.

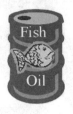

A re there any health benefits to fish oil?

▼
TIP:

Possibly. It is known that people with diabetes typically have elevated levels of fatty particles in their blood known as triglycerides. High levels of triglycerides are considered to be one of the reasons that people with diabetes have an increased risk for heart disease. Oils from a variety of fish, such as sardines, are thought to have beneficial effects on blood triglyceride concentrations in patients with diabetes. A recent review of 26 separate studies concluded that fish oil may be of benefit in people who have diabetes and elevated triglyceride levels. Specifically, 2–5 teaspoons of fish oil were shown to reduce triglyceride levels by an average of 30–50%. Unfortunately, this was accompanied by a small increase in the levels of LDL cholesterol, another fatty particle that has been connected with the development of heart disease. Blood glucose levels may also be slightly increased by the daily use of fish oil. For now, you might consider replacing the red meat in your diet with fish several times a week. If you have high triglyceride levels, ask your doctor about the possibility of including a daily dose of fish oil.

Why should I check my sugar when I can "feel" when it's high or low?

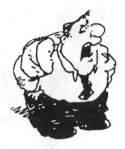

▼
TIP:

Because you can't always feel it. Many people with diabetes believe that they have specific feelings when their sugar is either too high or too low. Although this may occasionally be true, it is unreliable. Studies have been done in people with diabetes in which their blood sugar has been acutely raised or lowered without them knowing which. They were then asked what they thought their blood sugar level was. No individual could accurately predict when his or her blood sugar was high and how high it was. On the other hand, many people could tell when their blood sugar was low or at least dropping rapidly. Unfortunately, when you consistently have high blood sugar, you often feel like your blood sugar is low even when it is still high. Because you make important decisions depending on your blood sugar level, always check your blood sugar before taking insulin, exercising, or driving a car.

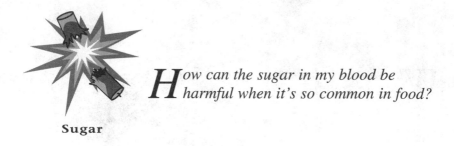

How can the sugar in my blood be harmful when it's so common in food?

Sugar

▼
TIP:

The sugar in food is powerful. It can be thought of as tiny packets of bundled-up energy. Normally, the body does not let the amount of sugar in the blood rise very high because it will react with the wrong tissues. In fact, of all the substances that circulate in your blood, sugar is one the body regulates most carefully. Even in people without diabetes, too much sugar is thought to be responsible for many of the changes that occur with aging. However, when a person has diabetes, his or her body cannot prevent high blood glucose levels from occurring. Over long periods of time, high levels of sugar can cause serious damage to many tissues, especially your eyes, kidneys, and nerves. This damage results in the "complications" of diabetes. These can be avoided or greatly delayed by leading a healthy lifestyle and keeping your blood sugar in your goal range.

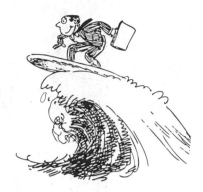

Should I expect my blood sugars to level off after I start a new diabetes medicine?

▼
TIP:

Yes. Blood sugars initially fall in response to the medicine. But there is an effect that has to do with the fact that high blood sugars tend to cause more high blood sugars. If your blood sugar has been high for some time, your pancreas can't immediately readjust. Your body has been using insulin poorly. When you interrupt the cycle and spend more time in the normal blood sugar range, you begin to increase your body's ability to stay there. After several weeks of improved control, many patients find that they need less insulin or oral medication to keep their blood sugars under control. It may take more medication to get your blood sugars to begin to go down, but how much medicine you need may decrease as your overall diabetes control improves.

Some patients with type 2 diabetes who take a diabetes medication and who also start exercising and eating better find that, after a while, they can stop their medication as long as they continue the other activities. Talk to your health care team before stopping any medication. If you get the "go ahead," monitor your blood sugars while you continue with your diet and exercise program. However, at the first sign that your blood sugar levels are going back up, contact your team.

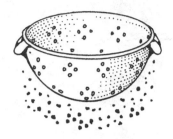

Why did my weight increase after I got my blood sugars under better control?

▼
TIP:

Some oral diabetes medications, such as glipizide and glyburide, and insulin will tend to cause weight gain when you achieve better blood sugar control. You are having a very common experience. When your blood sugars were high, you were losing many calories in your urine. The kidneys can only absorb a limited amount of sugar and then, like a sieve, they let the extra sugar go through into the urine. This loss of sugar in the urine begins at a blood sugar level of about 200 mg/dl. So you waste part of the calories you are eating when your blood sugar exceeds this level. This may sound like a great way to eat too much and also control your weight, but the long-term effect of high sugar is very damaging to many parts of your body. Your body needs insulin to store amino acids (the building blocks of protein in muscle) and to make muscle. So, take your medication as prescribed by your health care team, reduce your food intake, and exercise regularly to control your weight.

Chapter 3
HEALTH FOODS

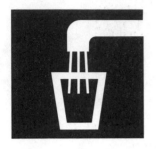

Will chromium help me stay healthy and improve my blood sugar control?

▼
TIP:

Your body does need some chromium to be healthy, but you're probably asking whether you need to take a chromium supplement. Most people do not need these supplements. Chromium is a naturally occurring mineral found in tap water and also present in tiny amounts in our bodies. Whether or not taking chromium will help you has been examined in many research studies. If you're getting enough chromium in your diet, there is no need for additional vitamin and mineral supplementation for most people with diabetes. Adequate diet means that you are getting a normal amount of calories from a variety of foods. Most people get into trouble when they eliminate one or more of the food groups or drastically reduce the calories needed to maintain a reasonable weight. Eat your fruits and vegetables and don't go below 1,200 calories a day.

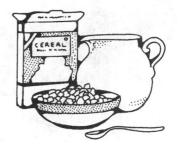

*W*ill fiber in my diet help me?

▼
TIP:

Igh-fiber diets may be beneficial to you, particularly if you have high blood fats or impaired glucose tolerance. Fiber is found primarily in fruits, vegetables, beans, and cereals, such as wheat and oats. Insoluble fibers like cellulose, found in wheat bran and celery, are dense and chewy. Soluble fibers, in whole oats and green peas, are soft and rather gel-like when mixed with water. Most fiber is not absorbed by the body, so it passes out in the stool. Any compounds that are bound by fiber in the intestine are also not absorbed. Many studies have been done to determine whether fiber is beneficial. Most studies show a positive (although limited) effect on blood fats. That's why high-fiber diets usually lower blood cholesterol. Some studies (primarily in type 2 diabetes) have also shown an improvement in blood sugar levels, but this improvement is usually small. You can add high-fiber foods, such as whole grains and beans, to your meals. Another way to increase the fiber in your diet is to take a tablespoon of pseudophilin (Metamucil) before you go to sleep.

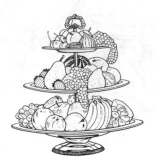

*S*hould I use fructose as a sweetener
when I bake?

▼
TIP:

Fructose is not necessarily better for you than plain sugar.
Fructose is a naturally occurring sweetener like table sugar
(sucrose). It may produce a smaller rise in blood sugar than the
same number of calories of table sugar. This is good for people
with diabetes; however, large amounts of fructose can increase
your total cholesterol and bad cholesterol (LDL) levels. That's
why fructose is really no better for you than other sugars. People with abnormal blood cholesterol levels should avoid consuming large amounts of fructose.

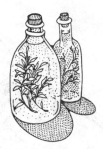

Will ginseng help me control my blood sugar?

▼
TIP:

Ginseng, derived from plants, is a chemical that has been used for many centuries to improve overall health and increase energy and well-being. It is often made into tea and taken with food. It is very popular in the U.S. and in some European and Asian countries. There are very few studies that test its beneficial effects in people with diabetes. Recently, one small short-term study from Finland suggested that individuals with type 2 diabetes who drink ginseng tea daily may have a lower blood sugar than those who do not. Whether or not this effect lasts longer than one year is not known. At this time, ginseng is not a recommended treatment for diabetes, but that recommendation could change. Stay in touch with your health care team for updates.

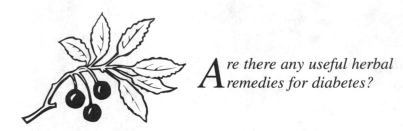

A re there any useful herbal
 remedies for diabetes?

▼
TIP:

W e don't know. Diet or herbal remedies were all we had
  for most of the 2,000 years since diabetes was first
described. Health food stores carry dozens of products designed
for people with diabetes to use, ranging from blueberry leaf and
wild cherry bark to preparations called "Hysugar" and "Losug-
ar." Few of these products have been tested or proven to be safe
and effective. Because herbal remedies are classified as food
supplements, they are not regulated by the FDA. Moreover,
none of these products alone result in adequate blood sugar
control in most people with diabetes. You should discuss any
anti-diabetes health food products with your health care team.
You may find that they are somewhat skeptical, but they will
probably not object to the use of these products in moderation
if you are demonstrating good control of your diabetes and
doing the other things necessary to stay healthy with diabetes.

*W*hat is folic acid?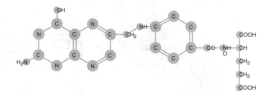

▼
TIP:

Folic acid (or folate) is a member of the B-vitamin family found in green, leafy vegetables. It plays an important role in several chemical processes in your body. Many medical experts are currently recommending that people increase their intake of folic acid because folic acid lowers homocysteine levels in our bodies. Homocysteine is a by-product of the metabolic breakdown of a particular amino acid (the building blocks of proteins) called cysteine. There is a growing amount of scientific evidence suggesting that people with high levels of homocysteine are more likely to suffer from a heart attack or stroke. Although the issue remains to be settled, some studies suggest that people with diabetes have higher than normal amounts of homocysteine in their bodies, and this fact may be related to the increased number of heart attacks and strokes that occur in people with diabetes. Thus, it may be beneficial for people with diabetes to supplement their diet with the Recommended Daily Allowance (RDA) of 180–200 mcg per day for men and women and 400 mcg for pregnant women. This is the amount of folic acid usually found in daily multi-vitamin preparations.

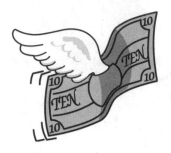

*W*ill magnesium supplements help my diabetes?

▼
TIP:

Probably not. The ADA does not recommend routine blood tests for magnesium levels, nor does it recommend that people take magnesium unless they have been shown to be deficient in this mineral. Magnesium deficiency may play a role in causing insulin resistance, carbohydrate intolerance, and high blood pressure. People who eat a varied diet should not become magnesium deficient because magnesium is found in many foods (including cereals, nuts, and green vegetables).

People at risk of magnesium deficiency are those with congestive heart failure, with potassium or calcium deficiency, and who are pregnant. Others at risk have had heart attacks, ketoacidosis, long-term feeding through the veins, long-term alcohol abuse, or have taken drugs such as diuretics over long periods of time. If a blood test shows these people need magnesium, a supplement may be given by the doctor. People with kidney disease should be very careful not to get too much magnesium and only take it under a doctor's care.

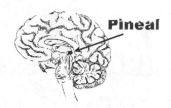

*I*s *the melatonin miracle real?*

▼
TIP:

There is very little scientific proof that taking melatonin supplements is beneficial. Melatonin is a substance that is normally secreted by a small part of the brain called the pineal gland. The exact role that it plays in humans is not clear, but research suggests that it may help regulate your sleep. It has become popular and is sold in health food stores. Many unproven beneficial effects have been attributed to melatonin, including better sleep, elimination of jet lag, reversal of the aging process, enhancement of sex, and protection against disease. Are these claims too good to be true? Yes. If you buy melatonin, you are probably just wasting your money. You may ask, "Is there any harm if I take melatonin for sleep?" The problem is that there are no long-term studies that show melatonin is safe. In fact, some doctors fear permanent damage to your normal sleep patterns if you take melatonin. There may also be other hazards that will become known only after melatonin has been in use several more years. For now, it is wise not to take melatonin supplements until there is better evidence to support its safety and effectiveness.

Chapter 4
DIETARY ADVICE

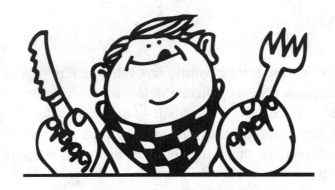

*H*ow can I overcome my craving for chocolate?

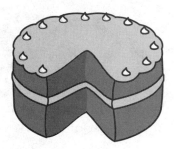

▼
TIP:

G ive in once in a while! By denying your desire for chocolate (or any other particular food), you are setting yourself
up for failure. If you find yourself craving a food and having to
put effort into avoiding it, you may eventually give up and eat
too much of it. Then your blood sugar control suffers, and you
feel guilty and depressed. Think about some healthy ways to
satisfy your craving. For chocolate lovers, dark or bitter chocolate is preferred to milk chocolate, which has higher dairy fat.
We suggest low-fat frozen yogurt. It tastes great, has less than 1
gram of fat, and is inexpensive. Another treat is chocolate graham crackers, which may also be used for making desserts.
Make a fancy dessert with angel food cake, strawberries, and
chocolate syrup. Yes, the syrup has some sugar in it, but it is
almost fat free. Whether you have type 1 or type 2 diabetes, fat
must be a concern for you and is actually the worst part of most
candies. Recent research has shown that sugar has about the
same effect as an equal amount of carbohydrate from potatoes
or rice on your blood sugar. When you must have chocolate,
substitute it into your meal plan for other carbohydrates. You
can also look for some relatively low-fat chocolate foods that fit
into your meal plan.

What diet change must I make to improve my blood pressure?

▼
TIP:

If you are sensitive to sodium, lowering the sodium in your diet may make a big difference in your blood pressure. Less sodium in your body means you will retain less water. There will be less fluid in your blood vessels and less "pressure" in the system. Sodium is a major part of table salt. Sodium is also used as a preservative and flavor enhancer in foods that may not even taste "salty." Try these tips to lower your sodium intake: 1) Always taste your food before reaching for the salt shaker, 2) Use pepper and other seasonings to add flavor before adding salt, 3) Cook with a variety of seasonings, such as onion and garlic, 4) Add a dash of lemon juice to vegetables and salads to brighten the flavor, 5) Avoid "seasoned salt" or garlic salt; use garlic powder or fresh garlic, 6) Try a commercial salt-free seasoning mix and carry a small container with you, 7) Ask for foods to be prepared without salt in restaurants and ask for sauces "on the side," 8) Read the labels on prepared foods and canned goods to find the high-salt items and look for no-salt-added or low-sodium products.

Remember, the closer to nature a food is, the more likely it will be low in salt.

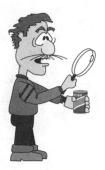

*D*oes reading food labels help me stay
healthy?

▼
TIP:

Yes. Food labels give you important information that can
help you eat healthy meals and snacks. New regulations
by the FDA have increased the information that must be put on
food labels. Food labels must include

1. The standard serving size
2. Calories and calories from fat in each serving
3. A list of nutrients and ingredients
4. The recommended daily amounts of nutrients in the food
5. The relationship between the food and any disease it may
   affect

Try to make a habit of reading the labels of the foods you buy
and become familiar with the amount of calories, fat,
carbohydrate, and sodium in them. For many foods, you will
have a choice of different brand names, and by comparing the
information on the labels, you can choose the brand that is
healthier. Food label information helps you keep track of the
amount of nutrients that you are eating daily. This information
is vital to a healthy diet.

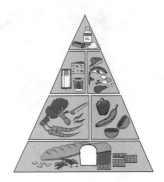

*W*ill the USDA Food Guide Pyramid help me live healthier with diabetes?

TIP:

Yes. The Food Guide Pyramid was developed as a guide to healthy eating for all Americans. It's healthy eating for people with diabetes, too. The pyramid shape tells you how much to eat of different foods. The bottom section—the largest section—is the bread, cereal, rice, and pasta group, and most people should eat 6–11 servings a day. The two sections above starches are vegetables (3–5 servings a day) and fruits (2–4 servings a day). These first three sections together cover more than half of the pyramid. This tells you that half or more of your daily food intake should come from these foods. The next two sections are the dairy group (2–3 servings a day) and the meat, poultry, and fish group (2–3 servings a day). You don't need as much of these foods. Also, they may be high in fat. The small top section contains the fats, oils, and sweets group. You need very little of these foods, which is why they don't have serving suggestions. They can be very high in calories without much nutrition. Following the Food Guide Pyramid can be an easy and healthy way for a person with diabetes to achieve good health and nutrition. ADA developed a Diabetes Food Pyramid that is very similar to the USDA pyramid. Ask your RD for help using these nutrition tools.

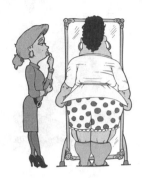

Should I join an expensive diet and weight-reduction program to lose weight?

▼

TIP:

We don't recommend it. You will probably waste your time and your money. Advertisements for these programs usually show "before" and "after" photographs of heavy people who have lost weight. What these advertisements don't show you are the people who never lost a pound. More importantly, long-term studies have shown that almost all of the people who lose weight rapidly over several months gain it all back by the end of 5 years. This has also been the experience of our patients who have tried these programs. Also, very-low-calorie diets can be dangerous, because they can cause serious chemical imbalances and vitamin deficiencies. A much better plan to lose weight is to make small changes in your lifestyle, so that you lose only 1/2–1 pound per month. Over 5 years, this small change equals a 50-pound weight loss! In comparison to expensive diet programs, low-cost weight-reduction programs, such as Weight Watchers or TOPS (Take Off Pounds Sensibly), can provide much support and advice for you. In addition, your health care team can be of great help in suggesting ways of making small but positive changes in your lifestyle to accomplish your weight goals.

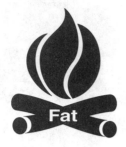

Why do I spill ketones in my urine?

▼
TIP:

Ketones in the urine show that fat is being burned for fuel by your body. This typically occurs when you do not have enough insulin in your body to metabolize sugar as fuel or when you are fasting. Thus, spilling ketones into your urine means either that your body is dangerously low on insulin or that your diet is working. When ketones build up due to a lack of insulin, the condition is called "ketoacidosis," and it can be dangerous. Ketoacidosis is more common in type 1 diabetes, occurring when people are first diagnosed with diabetes, when they stop taking insulin for some reason, or when they are ill. Most people develop symptoms that make them consult a doctor, such as stomach pain, nausea or vomiting, rapid breathing, frequent urination, extreme thirst, or fatigue.

If you are on a diet that does not provide enough calories to your body, then your body burns fat for energy. This is the effect you want from your diet, because burning fat will cause you to lose weight. A by-product of fat metabolism, however, is ketones, and these ketones spill into your urine just as they do in ketoacidosis. If you are feeling fine and controlling your blood sugar, then the ketones in your urine are probably a safe result of your diet.

How can I get my spouse to follow his or her meal plan?

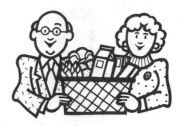

▼

TIP:

We have several suggestions. There are many reasons that your spouse might not follow the prescribed diet. First, he or she may not understand the meal plan. Did he or she see an RD and receive easily understood written instructions describing the meal plan? Second, your spouse may not believe that following it will work. Ask him or her to try the prescribed diet for one month and measure weight and blood sugar daily to see what the effects are. Then she or he can decide whether the diet will help achieve his or her goals. Third, your spouse may not want to eat foods that are "different" from those that the rest of the family eats. It helps if the whole family changes to a healthier diet. (A "diabetic" diet or a meal plan is the same balanced healthy diet that everyone should eat.) The RD can help him or her fit some of his or her favorite foods into the meal plan. Fourth, do you understand the details of the diet? If you select and prepare the food that your spouse eats, you may want to discuss the meal plan with your RD. Finally, remember that changing eating habits will involve a change in lifestyle, which is difficult for anyone. Don't try to change too many things too quickly. Your spouse will need support, understanding, and patience to achieve his or her goals.

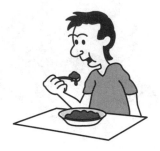

*I*s it a good idea to eat 4 or 5 small
meals during the day instead of 3
large meals?

▼
TIP:

Yes! Scientists have been looking for the ideal frequency of
meals since the beginning of diabetes research. There are
many benefits to eating small amounts of food over the course
of the day instead of larger amounts at mealtimes. These benefits include decreased blood sugar levels after a meal, reduced
insulin requirements over the course of the day, and decreased
blood cholesterol levels. These benefits probably stem from a
slow, continuous absorption of food from your gut, which
spares your body the work of switching over to a "fasting"
state. Also, eating several small meals a day may decrease your
hunger and reduce the number of calories you eat during the
day. Finally, there are diabetes medications available, such as
acarbose, that slow the absorption of food and have much the
same effect as eating your food slowly over the course of the
day. The practice of nibbling is not for everyone; but if it helps
you maintain good blood sugar control and a desirable body
weight when doing it, then continue.

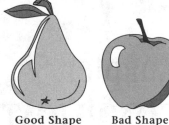 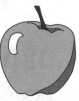

*H*ow can I use the waist/hip
ratio to improve my health?

Good Shape   **Bad Shape**

▼
TIP:

The waist/hip ratio can be used to predict your risk of
developing heart disease in the future. Take a tape measure
and measure the circumference of your body at its largest
diameter at the level of your hips. Next, measure the size of
your waist (your stomach) at its largest diameter. Be honest;
don't pull in your stomach when measuring. Okay, now you
are ready. Divide your waist size in inches by your hip size in
inches. If the answer is less than 1.0 for men (0.85 for
women), then your shape is good. What this means is that your
body is pear shaped rather than apple shaped. If the result is
more than 1.0 for men (0.85 for women), you are at an
increased risk to develop heart disease. The reason for the
increased risk is that you have more fat in the stomach area
than on your hips and thighs. For unknown reasons, fat located
above the hips is a major risk factor for future heart disease. If
you are at an increased risk and overweight, you need to work
on losing weight. After you have lost 5 pounds, remeasure
your waist/hip ratio. Keep reducing your weight until your
waist/hip ratio is below 1.0 if you are a man (0.85 if you are a
woman). All obesity is bad for your health, but obesity above
your hips is especially hazardous.

Chapter 5
COMPLICATIONS—MICRO*

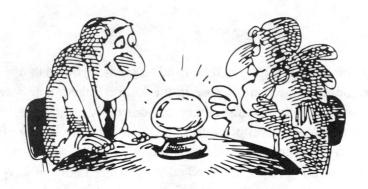

*disease of the small blood vessels

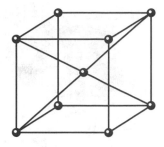

*W*hat does the term AGE mean in reference to diabetes?

▼
TIP:

Good question! AGE is an abbreviation for advanced glyco-sylation end product. This complicated name describes the process of sugar becoming permanently attached to body tissues. The sugar may cause damage, so that the tissues can no longer carry out their normal function.

A common example is glycosylated hemoglobin, which is glucose permanently attached to hemoglobin protein in your red blood cells. However, since new red blood cells are continuously made by your body, little long-term damage results from this attached glucose. In contrast, tissues in your eyes, kidneys, and nerves remain in your body for a long period of time, so the attached sugar can do significant damage.

A new medicine called aminoguanidine can block sugar from permanently attaching to and damaging your body tissues. Hopefully, this medicine will prevent some of the complications of diabetes. This medicine is currently being tested in many medical centers throughout the United States. Studies in animals suggest it should work well in humans. If it does, then many of the complications of diabetes will be preventable.

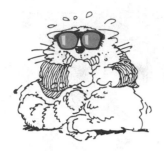

*W*hat kinds of eye problems are
caused by diabetes?

▼
TIP:

Diabetes is the number one cause of blindness in the United States. Fortunately, many eye problems are treatable if they are identified early. One of the most serious eye problems caused by diabetes is retinopathy. In this disease, fragile blood vessels grow in the back of the eye and can bleed easily. Such bleeding can cloud the vision and lead to permanent scarring of the back of the eye (the retina). People with diabetes also have cataracts (a permanent clouding of the lens), "floaters" that temporarily interfere with vision, and a swelling of the eye nerves that can cause permanent damage to your sight (macular edema). Abnormal function of the nerves that control the eye muscles can result in double vision. All people who develop double vision should see an eye doctor as soon as possible to rule out other possible causes, such as a small stroke. Cataracts can be corrected surgically. Laser therapy helps stop retinopathy or macular edema if it is performed before there is too much damage. A yearly eye examination by a doctor who specializes in diabetic eye disease is the best way to detect eye problems in the early stages, and keeping your blood sugar near normal can help reduce your risk of eye disease.

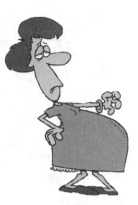

Why would my health care team be concerned about my becoming pregnant if I have high blood pressure and have had laser treatment of my eye problems?

▼
TIP:

Many changes in blood flow and pressure occur during pregnancy that can aggravate eye disease and kidney disease. The number of blood pressure medications that can be used safely during pregnancy and not injure a developing fetus are limited. You should discuss the options and the severity of your complications openly with your health care team as part of your prepregnancy planning process. Existing complications of diabetes can get worse during pregnancy. This is not to say that you should not get pregnant if you have mild diabetic complications. Many women with long-standing diabetes are able to have a normal pregnancy. However, the complications may make the pregnancy more difficult. One means of assessing the risks of pregnancy is called the "White classification" and is used by some obstetricians specializing in patients with diabetes and pregnancy. How long you have had diabetes and the severity of your complications determine the level of risk using the White classification.

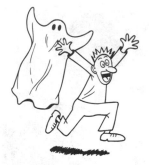

*C*an I ignore the risks of diabetic
complications since the thought of
them scares me?

▼
TIP:

No, because there are some things you can do now to prevent the disabling complications of diabetes. Adjusting
your food, physical activity, and medication (if any) to bring
your blood glucose levels to near-normal ranges can help you
avoid or delay complications. Research has proven that. You
are expressing emotions that most of us go through at some
time in our lives. All of us have fears of growing old or disabled, whether we have diabetes or not. The challenge we all
face is how to live a healthy life. We all want to live well every
day that we live. We want to be fully functional and independent. You can decide to ignore the changes taking place in
your body but that won't make them go away. Or you can take
charge to change the outcome, so that you can live your life
without fear. Your knowledge of the effects of diabetic complications on your body is information that can give you power
over the future!

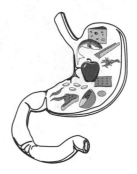

*D*uring a meal, why do I get filled up
before I finish eating?

▼
TIP:

You may have a complication of diabetes causing your
symptoms that is called "diabetic gastroparesis." It means
that the stomach empties very slowly. It is caused by damage
to the nerves that control the pace at which food leaves the
stomach and gets processed in the gut. Some people experience nausea, while others may only note that they can't eat as
much at one time. If the rate of food emptying from your
stomach is too slow and you took insulin before the meal, your
blood sugar may fall before the food has had a chance to be
absorbed. You may have to adjust when you take your insulin
injection to prevent low blood sugars and to match the absorption of your carbohydrate. High-fiber or high-fat foods tend to
make gastroparesis worse. There are some medications that
can help improve gut function. Talk to your health care team
about the best approach for you.

*C*ould *my diabetes cause one of
my eyes to be red and painful?*

▼
TIP:

Perhaps. Allergies to pollens and dust in the air are the most common cause of red eyes, but this rarely causes pain. An eye infection that can cause red eyes is viral conjunctivitis, or "pink eye." Unfortunately, this infection has to run its course because antibiotics cannot help speed recovery. Serious bacterial infections can start on the surface or behind the eye of a person with diabetes and require strong antibiotics to cure. A common complaint of patients with either viral or bacterial infections is that they wake up in the morning with their eyelashes sticking together from the pus that has collected over the night. If your pain is more like a pressure sensation, then you may have glaucoma. Glaucoma is too much pressure in the eye and is more common in people with diabetes. It can be detected during your yearly eye exam. The test involves blowing a small puff of air (which doesn't hurt) at the surface of the eye. Your doctor may prescribe eye drops that lower the pressure in the eye. This condition is definitely worth finding early because it is treatable. Left untreated, glaucoma can result in blindness.

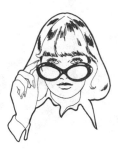

*W*ill my diabetic kidney disease get
worse if I get pregnant?

▼
TIP:

There is about a 30% chance that your kidney function will
worsen during pregnancy, but these changes often improve
after delivery of the infant. Many women with diabetes will
first show signs of abnormal kidney function (spilling protein
into the urine) during pregnancy. If you have kidney disease
before getting pregnant, then there is a chance that it will get
worse during pregnancy.

Moreover, babies born to mothers with diabetic kidney
disease have a higher risk of stillbirth, respiratory distress,
jaundice, and abnormally small body size compared to babies
of mothers with diabetes without kidney problems. Also, about
30% of these babies are born prematurely. You will need to
have tight blood sugar control and careful control of blood
pressure before and during the pregnancy. Thus, it can be
done, but you should know the risk before you get pregnant.

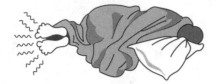

Why do my feet burn at night when I'm trying to go to sleep?

▼
TIP:

The nerves in your feet have been affected by your diabetes. "Painful neuropathy" is a term used to describe diabetic feet that are painful without an obvious cause. People with painful neuropathy usually describe a "pins and needles" sensation or a dull burning in the feet and legs that is more apparent at night (when there are few other things to distract you). You may also experience frequent leg cramps. Because painful neuropathy is difficult to cure once it is established, the best treatment is to prevent it by controlling your blood sugar. These nerve problems occur more frequently in men and in people who have had diabetes for many years, are tall, smoke, or have poor blood sugar control.

If you already have painful neuropathy, there are treatments available that provide some relief for about 50% of people. These treatments include the use of antidepressant medicines, certain heart medications, and creams made from chili peppers (capsaicin). These creams are rubbed on the feet to desensitize them. If you do not get relief from one of these treatments, the good news is that the pain from this neuropathy often lessens over time.

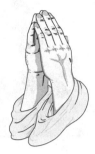

*I*s there a simple test to see whether my
diabetes is causing my hands to be stiff
and rigid?

▼ TIP:

High blood sugars over a long period of time can increase
the stiffness of tissue around your finger joints. This can
eventually cause stiff hands and prevent you from straighten-
ing your fingers. This stiffness may make it difficult to write or
to pick up small items and do other fine movements. An easy
test for this condition is called the "prayer sign," in which you
hold your hands together, one palm facing the other palm, to
see whether your fingers can lie flat against each other. If a
space exists between your right and left hands when you try to
push your hands together (as in the above figure), this is a
"positive" prayer sign. High sugars may be causing this condition. Arthritis can also cause a positive prayer sign. In the near
future, new medications may become available that will reduce
this stiffness. In the meantime, you should try to keep your
blood sugars as close to your goal range as possible.

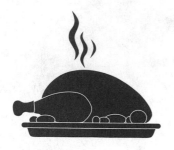

*S*hould I eat more protein to replace the protein I am losing in my urine?

TIP:

U sually the answer is no. The protein that you are losing in your urine (known as "spilling protein") is a sign that the filters in your kidney are showing wear and tear. Normally, the blood in your body goes through your kidneys to remove waste products. Kidneys act like a sieve that retains valuable chemicals but lets water go through. The protein in your blood is supposed to stay in your body, but when the kidney filters are damaged from years of high blood sugar and high blood pressure, they let protein slip through as well. Also, the waste products from protein can be stressful to the kidney.

Reducing the amount of protein in your diet may help the kidneys and slow damage to them. You should talk to your health care provider or RD about reducing protein in your diet. You might not know that many foods such as cereals and grains contain protein. You may need help designing a meal plan that helps you reduce overall protein but gives you the essential types and amounts that you need. Wise food choices and following your meal plan are important parts of keeping your kidneys healthy.

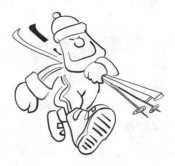

*S*hould I limit my exercise program
for one month after laser therapy
on my eyes?

▼
TIP:

Y es. Diabetic eye disease (retinopathy) is a condition of
overgrowth of fragile blood vessels in the eye that can
cause bleeding, scarring, and loss of vision if they break. Even
though you have had laser therapy, you should still be careful
to avoid situations that can stress these vessels. Avoid exercises
that cause you to strain, such as weight lifting or any exercise
that causes you to hold your breath. Underwater diving can
also cause increased pressure in the eye and should be avoided.
Another consequence of laser therapy is the possibility of a
loss in peripheral vision (the ability to see clearly off to the
side). For this reason, some sports (such as racquetball or tennis) may be hazardous, because they require you to respond to
a ball coming at a high speed from all angles. You should discuss any exercise program with your eye doctor if you have
had laser therapy.

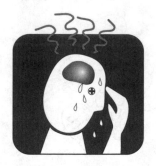

Why have I recently begun to sweat profusely when I sit down and eat food, even though the food does not contain hot, spicy items?

▼
TIP:

A complication of diabetes that is related to nerve damage is called "gustatory sweating." The person with diabetes breaks out in a sweat from chewing food. The cause of this sweating is not known, but it may be related to having high blood sugars for a long time. You may also have increased sweating or flushing of the neck and chest. Cheese or chocolate are the most common foods to cause sweating, but pickles, alcohol, vinegar, fresh fruits, and salty foods may do it, too. Various types of medications have been tried to treat this problem with varying levels of success. Although in some cases it stops by itself, try to keep your blood sugar as normal as possible and avoid specific foods. This may prevent sweating caused by food.

Chapter 6
COMPLICATIONS—MACRO*

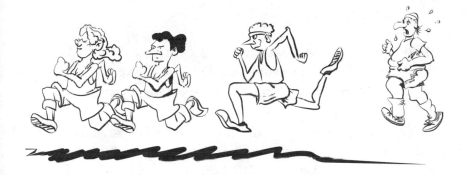

*disease of the large blood vessels

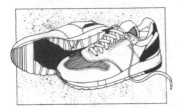

Since I don't want to end up with foot problems, how do I know whether my athletic shoes are okay?

▼
TIP:

It is best to buy shoes from a store that has experienced personnel who know how to measure your feet and fit your shoes correctly. A "certified pedorthist" is a specialist in fitting shoes and inserts for a proper fit with no pressure points. When you get new shoes, wear them for only a few hours, and then check your feet for any red areas or sore places where the shoes might be rubbing. Even well-fitted shoes may have a seam or area that rubs on your foot. Get padded athletic socks that protect your feet from blisters. Athletic shoes have become very high-tech these days and have different features depending on the exercise you are planning to do. It is a good idea to get the ones with extra cushion because this reduces the wear and tear on your joints. Look in the Yellow Pages for stores that specialize in athletic shoes or have a pedorthist on staff.

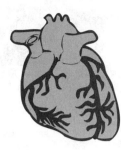

*A*m I at more risk to develop heart
disease because I have diabetes?

▼
TIP:

Yes. For unknown reasons, having diabetes does put you at
an increased risk of heart disease and other diseases that
are caused by blocked arteries. In fact, your risk is the same as
a person without diabetes who has already had one heart
attack. That is why it is very important for you to minimize
your other risk factors by getting plenty of exercise, keeping
your weight normal, avoiding cholesterol and fatty foods (saturated fat), and maintaining normal blood pressure. Walking is a
good exercise and helps in all those areas as well as reducing
stress. Most important (at least in our opinion) is that you do
not smoke cigarettes. If you are already smoking, join a "quit
smoking" support group. These are available in most communities and health care facilities. Nicotine skin patches may
help. Many of the risk factors that cause heart disease can be
greatly reduced with a healthy lifestyle, and this should be
your goal with or without diabetes. However, because you
already have one risk factor for heart disease (diabetes), there
is even more reason to reduce other risk factors.

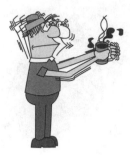

Why do I get dizzy when I stand up?

▼
TIP:

Patients with long-term diabetes can lose the ability to maintain their blood pressure in response to changes in posture. Your blood pressure can drop very low when you stand up and cause dizziness, temporary loss of vision, or fainting spells.

You may be experiencing "postural dizziness," which can be serious. Abnormal function of the nerves that regulate your heart and blood vessels is the most common cause of postural dizziness, but other causes must be ruled out by your health care team. Blood pressure medications, such as diuretics, can cause postural dizziness and so can antidepressants, nitroglycerine, and certain calcium-blocking drugs.

If your postural dizziness is due to diabetes alone, then you will need specific treatment for this problem. Tilting your bed so that the head is 6–9 inches higher than the foot may reduce your dizziness. Other therapies include carefully increasing the salt in your diet, wearing support stockings to prevent blood from pooling in your legs, or taking a hormone pill (Florinef) to help your body retain fluid. These treatments can be dangerous in people who have heart disease, so be sure to consult your health care team before trying any of them.

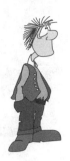

*I*s my 25 years of diabetes to blame for my recent trouble maintaining erections?

▼
TIP:

Maybe, but there are other causes for this condition. Your doctor should begin by checking for psychological and emotional causes. This includes asking you questions about depression, because depression affects sex drive. Other causes may be poor circulation to the penis or hormone levels. Blood flow to the penis may be too low to get or maintain erections. Long-term high blood sugars can affect these blood vessels or the nerves to the penis. If this is the problem, there are devices to aid you in getting an erection. All men have reduced male hormone levels as they get older. Replacing these hormones with monthly injections (or daily skin patches) of testosterone may improve sex drive. There is an oral medication that helps up to 60% of men with diabetes obtain erections (Viagra). This medication has proven very popular but is expensive. Some high blood pressure medications can cause sexual problems as a side effect and switching from one to another may help. Drinking alcohol can affect male hormone levels and can depress your brain's ability to get sexually aroused. There are many causes and many treatments for impotence. See your health care team for an evaluation or referral to a specialist.

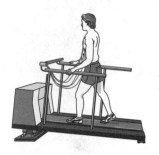

*S*hould I have a yearly test to see if
I have heart disease?

▼
TIP:

Ask your diabetes care team each year if you have any
health complaints that would indicate that a heart test is
necessary. Heart disease is the cause of death in about 80% of
people with diabetes. People with diabetes do not always
develop symptoms (such as chest pain) when they are having
heart stress or even a heart attack, and heart disease can occur
at a young age. Testing is required to diagnose heart disease at
a stage when it is treatable. If you have had diabetes for many
years, ask your health care team whether a screening test for
silent heart disease is necessary—especially if you plan to start
an exercise program or you have multiple risks for developing
heart disease. Your health care team will probably refer you to
a heart doctor (cardiologist) for these tests, and the type of test
may vary. Some cardiologists prefer a simple exercise treadmill test, in which your heart is monitored while you walk
uphill on a treadmill. Many cardiologists now prefer to stress
your heart with a medication instead of exercise. A test, called
a dipyridamole stress test, shows how your heart functions
when it works hard and may reveal areas of heart damage.
This damage may then be treated with medications or surgery.

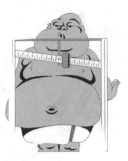

Since I can't reach or see my toes very well, how can I adequately care for my feet?

▼
TIP:

Many people with diabetes have difficulty seeing their feet well and trimming their toenails. The reasons for this problem are many, including poor eyesight, obesity, arthritis, back pain, and other medical conditions that may prevent you from leaning over toward the floor. Have a member of your family examine your feet once a day for sores and nail problems. We strongly recommend that most people with diabetes do not try to cut their own toenails, but go regularly to a podiatrist for routine foot care. Podiatrists are trained to provide good foot hygiene and nail care. They can be located in the Yellow Pages under Physicians & Surgeons, DPM (Podiatric), or ask your health care team for a referral. Good foot care is extremely important to your good health. It may save your feet.

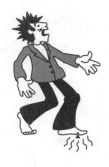

*D*o I need to have special foot care if my feet don't hurt?

TIP:

Yes. If you have had diabetes for many years, it is common not to feel pain in your feet. Thus, you may not notice sores and blisters that would normally cause you to avoid walking. Even if you don't have any sores, corns, callouses, or thickened toenails, you should still check your feet daily and use a moisturizing lotion after bathing—but not between your toes. Going barefoot is not recommended because of possible injuries to your bare feet. Always take off your shoes and socks during your quarterly visit to the health care team as a reminder to have your feet checked. The team will test to see whether you can feel a soft touch or little changes of direction in your toes, and examine your reflexes and your ability to feel a tuning fork vibration. They will look for areas of skin breakdown on the bottom of your feet and between your toes and will check to be sure that you do not have an ingrown toenail. Ingrown nails easily become infected and require special care. You should see a podiatrist if you have a tendency to develop ingrown toenails. A podiatrist will also remove any calluses that you have. Many of the infections that end in leg amputation started out as tiny, nonpainful foot sores that didn't heal.

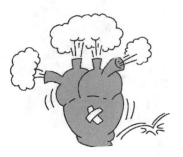

Why did my doctor start me on a cholesterol-lowering drug even though my cholesterol levels are only borderline high?

▼

TIP:

Because your doctor wants to prevent or delay heart disease. Heart disease is the number one cause of death in people with diabetes. Blood lipid (fat) levels are one of the most important ways to determine your risk for developing heart disease. People with diabetes tend to develop heart disease with lower lipid levels than nondiabetic patients, so some doctors try early on to lower blood lipid levels in their patients with diabetes. This is probably a good idea, especially if you are a person who has several other risk factors for the development of heart disease. These risk factors include smoking, high blood pressure, and a history of heart disease at a young age among your close family members.

Because the risk of heart disease is high among all people with diabetes, they should stop smoking, eat a low-fat, low-cholesterol diet, avoid weight gain, and exercise regularly. If these measures fail, then drug therapy is usually considered.

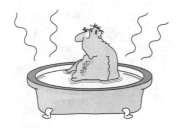

If I am on insulin, is it all right for me to sit in a hot tub?

▼
TIP:

Under certain conditions. People with diabetes should be careful with hot tubs or saunas. Excessive heat can make your heart beat faster and if you have an underlying heart problem (like angina), you may end up with serious heart damage. When your whole body gets overheated, your heart tries to increase the blood flow to your skin to get rid of some of the extra heat you have absorbed from the water or steam. If you use insulin to control your diabetes, you may find that this increased blood flow to the fat (where you inject your insulin) increases the rate at which the insulin is absorbed. So a dose of a longer-acting insulin that is intended to last throughout the night will be absorbed much more rapidly. This causes low blood sugars during the hours after you get out of the tub. We recommend temperatures no higher than 105° and that you stay in the water for no longer than 20 minutes. Discuss your plans with your health care team.

*W*hy do I sometimes leak urine?

▼
TIP:

Approximately 25% of all people with long-term diabetes have some problems with bladder function. Most of these problems result from faulty signals from the nerves that control the bladder. Some of these problems are minor, such as an inability to empty your bladder completely when you urinate, a slow rate of urine flow, or an inability to tell when your bladder is full until it is overflowing. When you accidentally leak urine, the problem is usually more advanced and is called "incontinence." The most common cause of incontinence is an inability to tell whether your bladder is full, so the bladder becomes too full and overflows. Men with incontinence often have an enlarged prostate gland pressing on the bladder, and this can be treated with medicine or corrected by surgery. All men with diabetes over the age of 40 should have a prostate exam every year. If you have overflow incontinence, you may be able to manage the problem by reminding yourself to urinate on a schedule every day. You may strengthen the muscles around the bladder by doing "kegel" exercises (tensing and relaxing) or stopping the flow of urine several times. If you continue to have trouble, seek help from a bladder specialist (a urologist).

Will lowering the fat in my diet reduce my risk for heart disease?

Type of fat	Effect on your body	In summary...
Saturated fat: animal fats, lard	increases cholesterol increases heart disease	☹

Monounsaturated fat:
  olive oil, canola oil,
  nuts, avocado
	lowers cholesterol
	no effect on HDL
	(good cholesterol)
		☺

Polyunsaturated fat: corn oil, safflower oil	lowers cholesterol positive and negative effect on HDL	☺

TIP:

In most cases, yes. You will especially lower your risk if you lower the saturated fats. Fats fall into one of three groups.
Saturated fats: Increase cholesterol in your blood and the risk of heart disease. They are usually solid at room temperature and are found in animal fats (meat, butter, lard, bacon, cheese); coconut, palm, and palm kernel oils; dairy fats; and hydrogenated vegetable fats (such as vegetable shortening and stick margarine).
Monounsaturated fats: Lower total cholesterol, do not affect HDL levels, and may reduce triglyceride levels. Food sources are olive oil, peanut oil, canola oil, olives, avocados, and nuts (except walnuts, which are polyunsaturated).
Polyunsaturated fats: Lower cholesterol levels but may also lower HDL levels. Food sources are vegetable oils such as corn, safflower, soybean, sunflower, and cottonseed.

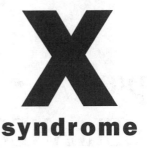

syndrome

*I*s my high blood pressure related to my diabetes?

▼
TIP:

Probably. People with diabetes are more likely to have high blood pressure. And people with the following symptoms are more likely to develop diabetes or heart disease. The combination of high blood pressure, high blood fat levels (triglycerides), obesity (primarily around and above the waist), and insulin resistance is commonly called "syndrome X," or the metabolic syndrome. It is not a specific disease but a group of related risk factors that often exist together. The person with syndrome X is at a higher risk of developing diabetes and heart disease. Syndrome X is very common and may affect up to 25% of all middle-aged American males (and less commonly, females). So, to answer your question, high blood pressure and diabetes are related and often occur in the same individual. The important health message is that a person with syndrome X should immediately seek medical advice to reduce his or her weight and blood pressure. You should not wait until you develop diabetes or heart disease to change to a healthier lifestyle.

Chapter 7
MISCELLANEOUS

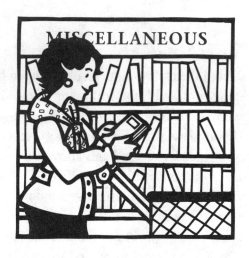

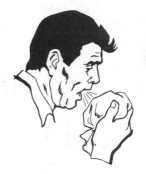

*W*hat can I take for a cough that is caused by my ACE inhibitor medication?

▼
TIP:

M any people with diabetes have problems with high blood pressure. Angiotensin-converting enzyme (ACE) inhibitors are ideal for this problem. One of their side benefits is to reduce blood pressure in the kidneys and to protect them from damage. Studies have shown that these medications actually reduce the rate of kidney damage caused by diabetes. Unfortunately, these drugs also affect the lungs, and about 20% of people treated with them develop an annoying cough. Although this cough is not dangerous, some patients have to stop taking their ACE inhibitor medication because they can't tolerate the cough. Losartan (Cozaar), a new type of ACE inhibitor, blocks the actions of angiotensin at its cellular receptor. This drug and other drugs like it have many of the benefits of the other ACE inhibitors on your blood pressure and kidneys, but they do not cause a cough. Ask your health care team whether this might be a good medication for you.

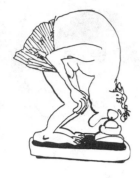

Why do I gain weight as I get older?

▼

TIP:

Unfortunately, most people do gain weight as they get older. There are several reasons. As you get older, your activity level changes to less strenuous exercise. For example, in the 20- to 30-year-old age-group, many people jog, play tennis, work out at health clubs, etc. In later years, people change activities to include golf, bowling, and watching television. As your activities change, you burn fewer calories. If you're still eating the same amount of food that you always have, weight gain will follow. In addition, recent studies have suggested that older people are actually more efficient at storing food as fat. This means that for the same amount of food eaten, more exercise is needed to use it up. You should gradually decrease the amount of food that you eat as you get older to keep your body weight normal. In general, the leaner you are, the longer you will live.

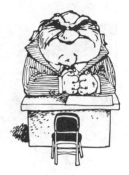

*C*an my diabetes cause constipation?

▼
TIP:

Yes. Constipation is the most common gastrointestinal disorder in people with diabetes, affecting about one in four patients. Your chances of having constipation increase to 50% if you have nerve problems due to diabetes. Most constipation in people with diabetes is caused by failure of the nerves that control the muscles of the bowel or large intestine to work properly. Other possible causes include blockage by a large amount of hard, dry stool; low levels of thyroid hormone; or an undiagnosed tumor. If you have frequent problems, you should ask your health care team for a complete evaluation of your bowel, including thyroid hormone tests. This evaluation may include a diagnostic test called a barium enema or a procedure where a stomach and intestinal specialist (gastroenterologist) inspects your bowel with a fiber-optic viewing device (a colonoscope). If it turns out that your constipation is caused by diabetes alone, then you may get relief by adding fiber to your diet (psyllium colloid) or a gentle laxative, such as docusate.

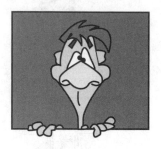

S hould I be concerned about a blood pressure of 128/86 mmHg?

▼
TIP:

The most recent American Diabetes Association guidelines suggest that diastolic blood pressure (the bottom number) above 80 puts you at increased risk. Even mild elevations in blood pressure like yours increase the risk of complications such as retinopathy, nephropathy, and heart disease. You should discuss these readings with your health care team. If your blood pressure readings are consistently high, you may need to start on blood pressure medication. Your doctor may ask you to check your blood pressure many times and in different settings to determine whether your blood pressure is high all the time or goes up only at specific times. If you haven't tried exercise and diet to decrease your blood pressure, it's time to start a walking program and to decrease the sodium in your diet. The recommended amount of sodium is 2,400 mg per day or less. Start by taking the salt shaker off the table. Read labels on foods to identify (and then reduce) the high-sodium foods in your diet. Canned goods and processed foods may be high in sodium. Drinking alcohol can also raise your blood pressure.

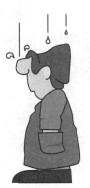

*H*ow do I handle the depression of having
had diabetes for 25 years?

▼
TIP:

Depression is a common condition in people with chronic
diseases like diabetes. Recognizing the symptoms of
depression and making the diagnosis are keys to treating it. A
lack of energy, changes in eating habits, changes in sleep patterns (sleep disturbances that may lead to daytime drowsiness),
and loss of interest in activities that you previously enjoyed are
all symptoms pointing to depression. You may lose interest in
your diabetes management activities when you are depressed.
It is important to talk to your health care team about these
feelings and changes in your life. Your physician may be able
to recommend counselling or temporarily prescribe a medication that can help you enjoy life again.

*I*s there a list of tests and other things I am supposed to be
doing to stay healthy?

Diabetes Checklist		
Care Activities	Frequency	Date
Diabetes Control	Review BG log quarterly A1C goal _____	
Ophthalmology	Annual dilated exam Glaucoma, cataract check	
Renal	Proteinuria/microalbuminuria screen BUN/Creatinine annual	
Neuropathy/Feet	Feet and legs quarterly Podiatry referral as needed	
Cardiovascular Exam	BP quarterly Lipids: annual screen fasting Get a baseline EKG	
Hypoglycemia/ Hyperglycemia	Review management plan Glucagon on hand?	
Vaccinations	Flu: annual Pneumovax	
Diabetes Education	Initial & annual review	
Other:	Hospitalizations: Dates reason:	

▼

TIP:

Yes. The ADA publishes "Standards of Medical Care for
Patients with Diabetes Mellitus" to provide guidelines for
health professionals to manage diabetes and prevent complications. We use a chart based on those standards to help our
patients keep track of all that needs to be done. Some tests come
every 3 months and some yearly. For instance, you should have
your eyes checked by an ophthalmologist and your urine checked
for microalbuminuria (small amounts of protein) yearly. With
these two tests, your doctor can detect eye and kidney problems
early and start treatment. You may want to keep track on your
own flow sheet to be sure you get the tests done at the right time
and to be able to share these results with your health care team.
Talk with them about which of these tests you need and when
you should have each one done.

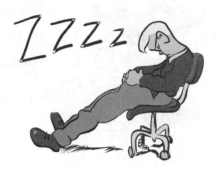

*W*hy do I sleep all the time
and yet never feel rested?

▼
TIP:

There are a number of reasons for someone to feel tired and want to sleep all the time. If your blood sugar is too high, it may make you very sleepy and lack energy. You may get very sleepy after eating a meal, a feeling that might be caused by an increase in your blood sugar. Your tiredness may be a side effect from your medications. Medicines associated with making you feel tired are some ulcer medications, antihistamines, blood pressure medications, treatment for stomach emptying problems (gastroparesis), and most antidepressants. Ask your pharmacist or physician whether any of your medications could be causing your tiredness. You may have a thyroid problem that shows up as tiredness. Finally, you may be depressed and not realize it. Many people with depression sleep excessive numbers of hours and yet never feel rested. Other symptoms of depression include loss of appetite, disinterest in activities that you once enjoyed, and frequent crying spells. Talk to your health care team about these symptoms. There are simple ways to identify depression and good treatments available.

*W*hy does a doctor have to
sign my driver's license
application?*

▼
TIP:

This is so doctors can identify people who should not be
driving for medical reasons. People with diabetes may
endanger themselves and others if their eyesight is badly
impaired due to diabetic eye disease. They may also suffer from
frequent and severe low blood sugars that may interfere with their
ability to operate an automobile. This risk is low, however, with
only one out of every 10,000 automobile accidents being attribut-
able to low blood sugar (a rate that is 1,000 times less than the
risk of an alcohol-related accident). The best general approach to
renewing your driver's license is to establish a relationship with
your health care team, so they know how well you manage your
diabetes. In most cases, your physician will review your files and
sign the form, agreeing that your license should be renewed. If
there is a question about your eyesight, you may be sent to an eye
doctor for evaluation. If your doctor feels that your blood sugar
control is too erratic for you to operate an automobile safely, you
may need to learn more about managing your diabetes responsi-
bly. The potential loss of your driver's license may become the
motivator you need to take charge of your diabetes!

*This is not required in all states.

Why does it hurt when my husband and I have sex?

TIP:

Although men with diabetes more commonly have sexual problems, women may also experience sexual difficulties caused by the disease. These problems may include a decrease in sexual desire, vaginal dryness and pain with intercourse, or inability to achieve orgasm. Complaints such as these are not unique to people with diabetes but tend to occur more often in women with diabetes, especially those who are past menopause. Loss of sexual desire may be a symptom of depression. It frequently responds to medication or a few visits with a therapist. Some women have an increase in sexual desire after treatment with low-dose testosterone (a hormone). Your pain during intercourse, however, most likely is caused by vaginal dryness and failure of your sex organs to adequately prepare for the sex act. If you are entering or past menopause, this problem may improve with estrogen replacement therapy or an estrogen cream that you put into the vagina. The use of sexual lubricants may also greatly improve your enjoyment of sex. Talking about your concern with your health care team may help you resume a fulfilling and mutually satisfying sex life with your husband.

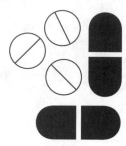

Is there any birth control method that is preferred because I have diabetes?

▼
TIP:

You and your health care team need to decide which birth control method will work best for you. You should use some kind of birth control if you are sexually active and don't want to get pregnant. Birth control pills contain very low levels of estrogen (a hormone), and you can use them. You may need more insulin, because the hormones in the birth control pills might make you a bit more insulin resistant. A combination pill with norgestinate and a synthetic estrogen is the best one for women with diabetes. Foam, condoms, or a diaphragm work well as long as you use them every time. Condoms also provide the extra benefit of protection from sexually transmitted diseases, such as AIDS. If you want a birth control method that requires little effort, there are hormone "implants" and injections. These provide birth control over a longer period of time, but they do affect your diabetes control. Another option for some women is the IUD (intrauterine device), which is a small plastic device placed inside the uterus that prevents implantation of fertilized eggs. Because they can increase your chances of developing an infection, IUDs are not recommended for women with diabetes.

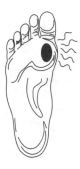

If my feet don't hurt, should I still check them every day?

▼

TIP:

Yes!! You should examine your feet at the end of each day to be certain that there are no sores, cuts, or areas where your shoe is rubbing against your foot. People with diabetes may lose pain sensation in their feet, so they may develop ulcers and open sores and not notice it because they can't feel the pain. Without medical attention, sores may continue to be irritated and not heal properly. Although your health care team should examine your feet at each visit, you need to be on the lookout for any small areas of redness or bleeding. It is essential that your shoes are comfortable and fit well. Special shoes can be made for you if your feet are difficult to fit. Always wear socks or stockings to provide padding between your feet and your shoes. The longer a patient has diabetes, the more common foot problems are. Preventing foot sores is much easier than trying to heal them.

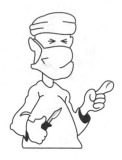

My doctor says that I should have my gallbladder removed, but isn't there a high risk of surgical complications because of my diabetes?

▼
TIP:

Patients with diabetes are at a higher risk of complications during and after a surgical procedure, but many such patients
undergo successful surgery every day. Assuming that your surgery
is necessary, then it is most important that your surgeon and your
diabetes doctor work together before the surgery is performed to
prevent problems. You should have a thorough medical checkup of
your heart and kidneys, and you should make sure that your blood
sugar control is good over the weeks prior to surgery. You should
also be sure that you have had plenty of fluids to drink before
reporting to the hospital. During the surgery, your doctors may
control your blood sugar with intravenous insulin and glucose.
Your diabetes doctor may even wish to be present during the
surgery. After surgery, tight blood sugar control helps you reduce
the risk of postoperative infections. By taking these precautions,
you will have the best chances for a successful operation.

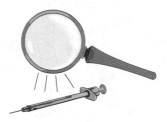

How can I accurately measure 1/2-unit doses of insulin for my 2-year-old son who has diabetes?

▼
TIP:

It is helpful to use low-dose (50-unit) or very-low-dose (30-unit) syringes when measuring small amounts of insulin because these syringes are narrower and have an expanded scale on the barrel. Syringe attachments that magnify and make it easier to read the scale are also available in many pharmacies. In addition, insulin manufacturers will provide diluting fluid if necessary for more accurate measurement.

Many children are extremely sensitive to insulin, and it is not unusual for doctors to prescribe 1/2-unit doses of insulin for such patients. One recent study determined how accurately the parents (caretakers) of young children with diabetes were able to prepare very small doses of insulin. The results of this study suggest that people do not measure insulin very accurately in 1/2-unit doses. Interestingly, the study also found that people tend to overestimate the dose and deliver more insulin than they are supposed to. The good news is that each person tends to overestimate by the same amount nearly every time. So small children with diabetes may need to have only one caretaker who prepares their insulin injections to keep measurements consistent.

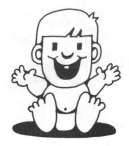

What are the risks to my baby during my pregnancy?

▼
TIP:

Pregnancy in diabetes carries risks for both you and your baby. Babies born to mothers with diabetes have higher rates of birth defects and stillbirth. They can also be abnormally large, which complicates the delivery. You can avoid many of these problems by achieving near-normal blood sugar control before and during pregnancy. For example, infants born to mothers with diabetes have about a 10% chance of being born with a birth defect, compared with only 2% of babies born to nondiabetic mothers. These birth defects typically involve the spinal cord, the kidneys, and the heart. This risk of birth defects can be greatly reduced, however, by achieving normal blood sugar control before pregnancy even occurs. In fact, blood sugar control is most important during the first 12 weeks of pregnancy because this is the time when all of the infant's major organs are formed. To be safe, you should plan on achieving a glycosylated hemoglobin (A1C) level within 1% of normal before you start trying to get pregnant. If successful, you will give your baby the best chance for a healthy start in life, and you will also decrease the chances of delivering a very large baby. This will improve your chances of staying healthy, too.

If I am hospitalized, what should I expect regarding my diabetes care?

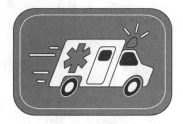

▼
TIP:

Your blood sugar control may worsen in the hospital because of varying content and timing of meals, inactivity, stress of being in the hospital, and changes in your insulin dose. The physician might not know your diabetes as well as you do. Stay involved in your diabetes care (assuming that you feel well enough). Measure your blood sugar yourself and keep a record by your bedside, so you can discuss your blood sugar levels with your doctor. Your blood sugar should be measured at least four times a day. Your doctor should establish a target range for you, usually less than 200 mg/dl. Expect your insulin or oral diabetes medication at a reasonable time (always before meals). If you feel that you are not getting enough food, ask for more and tell your doctor. If you are unable to eat, expect your diabetes to be controlled by insulin given in your IV. This will require frequent monitoring of your blood sugar to ensure that it does not go too low or too high. You should also expect the doctor to check your urine ketones more frequently in the hospital than you do at home, because fasting and stress can both lead to ketoacidosis. Taking an active role in your own diabetes care in the hospital will increase your chances of staying healthy.

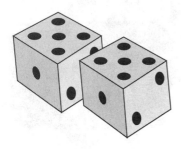

If I have "impaired glucose tolerance," what are my chances of getting diabetes later in life?

▼
TIP:

Impaired glucose tolerance (IGT) is a dangerous pre-diabetic condition. Reversing it with diet and exercise may prevent you from getting diabetes. IGT is a gray area between having normal blood sugar and having diabetes. If you have IGT, your pre-breakfast blood sugar values are slightly elevated, usually above 110 mg/dl. This level is not high enough to qualify for a diagnosis of diabetes, which is above 126 mg/dl. Although you don't have diabetes, 5% of people with IGT do develop diabetes every year. This means that if you have had IGT for five years, your chances for getting diabetes increase to about 25%. People with IGT are usually overweight, don't get much exercise, and often have relatives who have type 2 diabetes. Most doctors believe that if people with IGT improve their health by losing weight and getting more exercise, their chance for developing diabetes will be much lower. Also, eating a low-fat and high-fiber diet may help. You should get your blood sugar level checked at least once a year and if it is high, go to work on getting it into the normal range and keeping it there.

Chapter 8
NEW TIPS

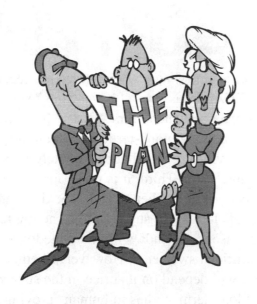

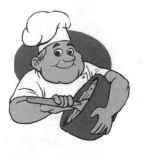

Should I use the new artificial sweetener Splenda instead of the other available sweeteners?

▼
TIP:

Splenda (sucralose) is a new, noncaloric sweetener recently approved by the FDA. It has several advantages over previously approved artificial sweeteners. First, to date it has shown no toxicity in humans, although long-term studies are not yet available. Second, it is noncaloric and approximately five times sweeter than table sugar. Third, it is much more stable than either Nutrasweet or Equal when used in cooking and baking. Fourth, Splenda tastes like sugar and has no unpleasant aftertaste. For these reasons, Splenda will undoubtedly become very popular as an artificial sweetener. However, whether or not you should use it will depend on its price in the supermarket and concern that long-term studies in humans proving its safety are not yet available. However, to date, animals given high doses of Splenda have shown no adverse effects.

Should I take an aspirin daily if I have diabetes?

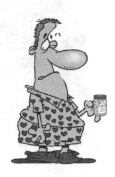

▼
TIP:

Probably. Diabetes increases your risk of dying from complications of heart and cardiovascular disease, so this is a reasonable question to ask. In November 1997, the ADA concluded that low-dose aspirin therapy should be prescribed, not only in patients with diabetes who have had heart attacks but also in patients with diabetes who are at a high risk for future heart and artery disease. This includes both men and women. The reason that people with diabetes may be at greater risk is that their platelets (parts of cells circulating around in the blood that clump and prevent bleeding) may clump more spontaneously than in people who do not have diabetes. Aspirin prevents this clumping and, therefore, may prevent heart attacks. Taking aspirin, however, is not without risk. It can cause stomach and intestinal bleeding. That's why people with bleeding ulcers shouldn't take aspirin. However, this risk is greatly reduced if you take enteric-coated aspirin of 81–325 mg a day. In fact, the lower dose (81 mg) of enteric-coated aspirin has been shown to be just as effective as any higher doses in preventing platelets from clumping. You should discuss the use of aspirin with your physician to make sure that it's safe for you.

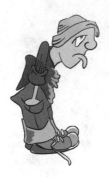

How can my adolescent son or daughter learn to be happy in spite of having diabetes?

▼
TIP:

Studies have shown that adolescents with diabetes have lower "quality of life" scores and are more prone to depression than teenagers who don't have diabetes. As you can imagine, the prospect of living the rest of your life with a disease that requires constant attention can be overwhelming. One recent study, however, suggests that a brief period of training in "coping skills" can improve both an adolescent's quality of life score and his or her diabetes control. Such training involves unlearning bad coping skills (such as eating too much or denying the problem) that everyone uses to deal with stressful circumstances. The adolescent then learns new skills that give him or her healthier, more productive ways to react to stress. These skills were taught by trained professionals in 4–8 90-minute sessions over one month. Adolescents who received the coping skills training showed improvement in scores that measured their confidence in managing diabetes, tendency to depression, and overall quality of life. Teenagers who received training in coping skills also had lower blood sugar levels than those who did not. Ask your son or daughter's diabetes care provider how your child can receive coping skills training.

What will help heal the ulcers on my feet?

▼
TIP:

Healing requires good foot care from your health provider including antibiotics and removal of the dead tissue. You do your part by not walking on the foot, keeping it clean and dry, and following your health care team's guidance.

A new medication called Regranex gel (becaplermin) has recently been approved by the FDA for use on foot ulcers that have adequate blood vessels going to them. This medication enhances new blood vessel formation and healing of your ulcer. It is made by recombinant gene technology and not directly from blood products and, therefore, is probably safer than if it were made directly from blood. If you use this medication, there are several steps you should consider. First, before applying the gel, your ulcer must be clean and all nonliving tissue removed by your physician or podiatrist. Healing may begin within 2 weeks and be completed in 10 weeks. Studies in patients with diabetes show that Regranex is better than using good ulcer care alone. Regranex healed approximately 50% of the ulcers compared to 30–40% healed with standard care alone. Unfortunately, this medication is very expensive. Hopefully, the price will drop in the future. This medication may give you the extra assist you need, but your foot still requires careful care and close follow-up with your physician.

How high is my risk for heart attack with type 2 diabetes?

▼ TIP:

Higher than you might think! In people who don't have diabetes, one of the strongest predictors for the development of a heart attack is a previous heart attack. A recent study has shown that people with type 2 diabetes who have not had a heart attack still have as high a risk for a future heart attack as a person without diabetes who has already had a heart attack. In other words, your risk for a future heart attack is as high as the risk for a person without diabetes who has known heart disease. This finding suggests that risk factors for heart disease, such as smoking, high blood pressure, and high blood cholesterol levels, should be treated very aggressively in people with diabetes. Some experts even feel that people with type 2 diabetes should be treated with medication as if they already have heart disease. So if your diabetes care team suggests specific treatment to lower your risk of heart attack, you should strongly consider giving it a try.

Is insulin resistance important to my diabetes? What can I do about it?

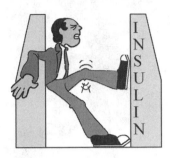

▼
TIP:

Yes, insulin resistance makes diabetes worse. We don't know why people with diabetes have insulin resistance. Physicians recommend several ways to reduce insulin resistance to make your own insulin more effective and better able to control your blood sugar. The nondrug ways to reduce insulin resistance are a low-calorie diet, weight loss, and regular and vigorous exercise. In other words, a healthy lifestyle can help you reduce insulin resistance. Many medications have been approved by the FDA for type 2 diabetes, but three drugs also reduce insulin resistance and, therefore, improve diabetes control. Metformin (Glucophage) acts on your liver and, to a lesser extent, on your muscles to reduce insulin resistance. Pioglitazone (Actos) and rosiglitazone (Avandia) have been shown to act in the liver, muscles, and fat tissue to reduce insulin resistance. These medications are widely used in the management of type 2 diabetes and have been shown to be very effective. If you have type 2 diabetes, discuss with your health provider which approaches are best for you to reduce the insulin resistance in your body.

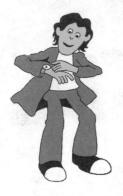

When should I take my lispro insulin injection if my blood sugar is high before a meal?

▼

TIP:

Lispro (Humalog) is a rapid-acting insulin, so it is recommended that you take lispro 0–15 minutes before eating a meal. However, this advice may not apply if you have high blood sugars. You may need to inject and wait for your blood sugar to come down before eating. This will ensure lower blood sugars after eating. A recent study examined the effect of varying the timing of the lispro insulin injection before breakfast in people who had blood sugars of 180 mg/dl. This study showed that for 5 hours after breakfast, blood sugars remained lower when the lispro insulin was injected 15 or 30 minutes before eating compared to an injection right at mealtime. Lispro insulin is a significant advance in insulin therapy and allows you to correct high blood sugars much more rapidly than if you use regular insulin. However, it is good to be aware of the need for proper timing of the lispro insulin injection if you have high blood sugars before mealtime.

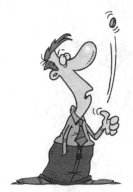

*C*an diabetic complications be
  predicted?

▼
TIP:

Sometimes. We know that certain factors, such as having consistently high blood sugar levels, predict the development of more diabetic complications, but we cannot predict who will get which complications. Still, research studies on complications can be useful and informative. For example, one recent study attempted to determine the most important predictors for eye disease, kidney disease, and amputation among 2,774 patients with diabetes. This study showed that older individuals and people who had less education were more likely to suffer complications. But other factors were also important. In people with type 1 diabetes, the combination of high blood pressure and smoking were the most powerful predictors of diabetic complications. For people with type 2 diabetes, failure to seek regular diabetes care was the most powerful predictor of diabetic complications. Although we can never be absolutely certain that you will not develop diabetic complications, we do know that you can minimize your risk by carefully controlling your blood sugar, controlling your blood pressure, avoiding smoking, and working with your diabetes care team to be as healthy as you can be.

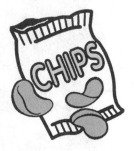

What are "fat replacers"?

▼
TIP:

Fat replacers are ingredients that manufacturers put in food to play the role of some of the fat in that food. These "replacers" can be made of carbohydrate, protein, or fat. The reason that fat replacers may be advantageous to your diet is the simple fact that fat contains 9 calories per gram of food, a very high energy content for a small amount of food. (Carbohydrate and protein have only 4 calories per gram.) On the other hand, many fat replacers, particularly if they are carbohydate- and protein-based, contain only 5 calories per gram of food. So, if you eat the same weight of food, you actually get half as many calories and might, therefore, lose weight. The problem is that many people assume that fat-free foods are so much lower in calories that they can eat larger servings of them. This is not the case; fat free does not mean calorie free. Also, watch for fat replacers that are made of carbohydrate because they will have an effect on your blood sugar level.

How should I manage my diabetes during a prolonged fast such as for Ramadan?

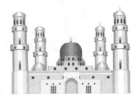

▼
TIP:

Ramadan is a month-long fast observed by the Muslim religion. Whether or not you should participate is a subject of controversy among diabetes care providers, but we recognize that many patients will participate. First of all, recognize that food intake is not totally prohibited during Ramadan. It is only prohibited during daylight hours. Many patients with type 2 diabetes may be able to develop a schedule to meet these requirements, although dosages of certain diabetes medications may have to be decreased or stopped during this period. Prolonged fasting represents a more difficult problem for people with type 1 diabetes. Insulin doses will probably have to be greatly reduced to avoid hypoglycemia, and frequent blood sugar monitoring is essential. Ketones are produced with fasting and insulin deficiency, so check urine ketones once or twice a day to avoid developing dangerous ketoacidosis. Ask your doctor what you do if ketones appear in your urine but you don't have high blood sugar. Finally, develop a plan for treating hypoglycemia while you are fasting. The Muslim religion exempts people who are ill from strict fasting, so it may be reasonable to decide to eat something if your blood sugar drops below some predetermined threshold, such as 60 mg/dl.

101 FOOT CARE TIPS

FOR PEOPLE WITH DIABETES

▲

A project of the
American Diabetes Association

▼

Written by

Jesse H. Ahroni, PhD, ARNP, CDE

101 FOOT CARE TIPS FOR PEOPLE WITH DIABETES

▼

TABLE OF CONTENTS

Chapter 1
GENERAL TIPS

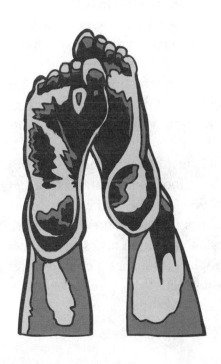

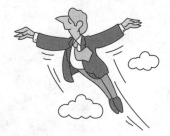

W^{*hy is it important for me to take*} *special care of my feet?*

▼
TIP:

I f you want to be active and independent all of your life—whether or not you have diabetes—you need to have healthy feet. Most people take their feet for granted, but people with diabetes really cannot do that. You are challenged by two complications of diabetes that can affect the nerves and blood vessels of the feet—diabetic nerve damage and poor circulation. These complications make it easier for you to get a foot ulcer that will not heal. Nonhealing ulcers lead to amputation, which will severely limit what you can do for yourself.

The good news is that by taking good care of your feet, you can often prevent diabetic foot complications. If you take care of your feet every day and get good medical care as soon as you even suspect you might need it, you're much more likely to avoid getting the infections that make amputation necessary. In fact, at least 50% of amputations in people with diabetes could be prevented this way. You can protect your feet.

*W*hat foot problems do people with diabetes experience?

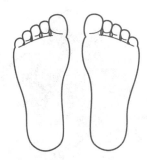

TIP:

People with diabetes have the same foot problems that people without diabetes experience—corns, calluses, bunions, ingrown toenails, arthritis, and broken bones. However, these ordinary foot problems can be more serious in people with diabetes if they also have diabetic nerve disease or poor circulation.

People with diabetic nerve damage cannot feel with their feet normally, so they may not notice an injury, sores, or even high-pressure areas on their feet. They may continue to walk on an injury or high-pressure spot that would cause pain in a person without nerve damage. This continued walking might cause a wound or ulcer. Once the skin is broken, the ulcer can become infected. The blood supply carries oxygen, white blood cells that attack bacteria, and healing nutrients to wounds. It also carries any antibiotics that you take. But if you don't have enough blood supply to the foot, an ulcer can be difficult or impossible to heal. If not treated, some of these foot infections will lead to amputation.

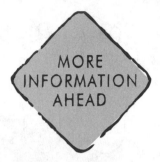

MORE
INFORMATION
AHEAD

*A*m *I more likely to get an infection just because I have diabetes?*

▼
TIP:

Yes. People with diabetes who have high blood sugars most of the time are more likely to develop infections than people with normal blood sugars. High blood sugars can interfere with your body's natural defense systems so infections are harder to heal, too.

Healthy skin is your main defense against infection, and diabetes can make your skin dry and more susceptible to cracking. Once the skin is broken, germs can enter. Fungal diseases that appear in folds of skin and on your feet need sugar and moisture to grow, and they like high blood glucose levels. The damage they do to your skin can allow infection to begin.

*H*ow *common are diabetic foot problems?*

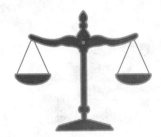

▼

TIP:

The short answer is way too common. About half of the people who have diabetes for 10 years will have some degree of nerve damage. The older you are and the longer you have had diabetes, the more likely you are to have nerve damage—but not everybody gets it. Recent studies show that people who maintain good blood sugar control are less likely to develop nerve damage or poor blood circulation.

It is estimated that 15–25% of people with diabetes will have a foot ulcer at least once. About 70% of these ulcers will heal with good basic foot care. Up to 10% of people with diabetes will have an amputation at some time in their lives. Toe and partial foot amputations are the most common, followed by below-the-knee amputations. Amputation rates are greater with increasing age, in males compared with females, and among African Americans and Hispanic Americans. Experts believe that at least half of these amputations could be prevented by good blood sugar control, better preventive foot care, and better care of foot ulcers.

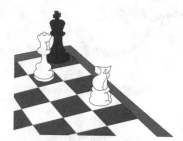

Who is at greatest risk for diabetic foot problems?

▼
TIP:

The people most at risk have diabetic nerve damage and poor circulation; have limited joint mobility, deformity, or thick nails; have already had a foot ulcer or amputation; or have other complications of diabetes, such as eye disease (retinopathy) or kidney disease (nephropathy). Once you have a foot ulcer or amputation, you are likely to get another one. This is because you have serious damage to the nerves and blood vessels of your feet, not because you do not take care of your feet. Most people with diabetes who have had foot problems take better than average care of their feet, but good foot care alone may not be enough to prevent foot problems once they are already established.

Newly diagnosed young people with type 1 diabetes who do not have other complications of diabetes or other foot problems have little risk. The American Diabetes Association (ADA) recommends that annual foot risk screening begin 5 years after the diagnosis of diabetes, but it is never too early to develop good foot care habits.

Older people who are recently diagnosed with type 2 diabetes may actually have had diabetes for years before they find out about it and already have complications. If you have type 2 diabetes, start good foot care right away.

*The thought of complications scares me.
Why can't I just ignore this until later?*

▼
TIP:

Because there are things that you can do right now to lower your risk and prevent the complications of diabetes. Adjusting your food, physical activity, and medications to control your blood sugar may help you avoid or delay complications. Taking good care of your feet will help you keep them. Ignoring your diabetes won't do you any good and is likely to be harmful.

All of us have fears of growing old or disabled. It is normal and appropriate to express these emotions. The challenge is to choose to live well every day. Give yourself the best chance to remain fully functional and independent throughout your life.

Deciding to ignore diabetes and its complications does not stop them or make them go away. Learning about diabetes and your body gives you the power to take charge and direct the outcome so you can live life without fear.

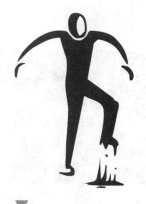

*W*hat can I do to prevent diabetic foot problems?

▼
TIP:

Look at and touch your feet every day: tops, bottoms, backs, sides, and between the toes. Get prompt medical attention for any problems.

Keep your feet clean and dry.

Cut or file toenails with the shape of the toe, smoothing all sharp edges.

Moisturize dry skin with a good lotion.

Avoid injury to your feet. Have corns, calluses, or ingrown toenails treated by a professional.

Wear well-fitting socks, without a thick toe seam, made of a material that wicks moisture away from the skin, such as an acrylic and cotton or wool blend.

Wear well-fitting soft leather or fabric shoes, such as running shoes. Wear house shoes at home.

Check shoes daily for cracks, pebbles, or other things that might damage your feet.

Get your blood glucose under control.

Have surgery to fix deformities such as bunions and hammertoes.

*D*oes my weight affect my feet?

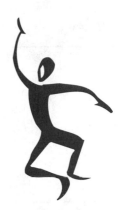

▼

TIP:

Absolutely. This is just common sense. The more we weigh the more stress is transmitted through our knees, ankles, and feet. Many people with foot pain can get relief just by losing weight. Heel pain is one example of a pain that is often weight related. Arthritis pain in the knees and feet is frequently worse in people who are overweight.

People who are obese have a different gait from those who are not. Their feet are placed wider than normal because their thighs hold the legs outward. This places the body weight more towards the inner part of the foot, changing the mechanics of walking completely. There is increased stress on the tendons, ligaments, and joints of the feet.

If you have diabetic neuropathy, your weight is even more important. The stress of additional pounds on numb feet increases the likelihood of your developing ulcers and Charcot deformities.

If you become pregnant, your feet may change shape and size during the pregnancy and for about 6 months after the baby is born. Sometimes they remain permanently larger. Be aware of this and try to wear comfortable, supportive shoes, such as running shoes. High heels are not really a good idea for anyone, but especially not for a pregnant woman.

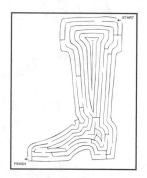

*W*hat does blood sugar control have to do with feet?

TIP:

If you control your blood sugar, you increase your chances of not getting diabetic complications. If you already have complications, you may keep them from getting worse or slow down their progression. With good blood sugar control, you are less likely to develop nerve damage or poor circulation, and you'll heal faster.

Results from the two largest studies of blood sugar control, the Diabetes Control and Complications Trial (DCCT) and the United Kingdom Prospective Diabetes Study (UKPDS), support this. The DCCT studied 1,400 people with type 1 diabetes. Half of the people received "conventional" care (1–2 insulin injections a day), and the other half received "intensive" care (as many injections as needed to keep blood sugar close to the normal range). Patients with near-normal blood sugar levels had a 40–70% reduction in the complications of diabetes. This improvement was gained regardless of the patients' age, sex, or length of time they'd had diabetes.

The UKPDS studied the effects of near-normal blood sugar levels in 5,200 people with type 2 diabetes by placing them in conventional (diet and exercise) or intensive (oral medications or insulin) care groups. The results were dramatic and showed the same strong benefits of near-normal blood sugar levels in preventing or slowing down diabetic complications.

*W*hich health care providers should help *me take care of my feet?*

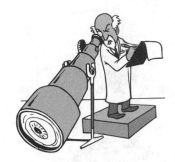

▼
TIP:

The first person to ask about taking care of your feet is your podiatrist or foot care specialist. If you need a referral, ask your primary care or diabetes care provider. At some point, you should see a diabetes educator, usually a nurse, physician's assistant, dietitian, pharmacist, or other health care professional, to learn how to take care of your feet. Sometimes physical therapists are trained to help people with diabetic foot problems. Any of these health professionals may be a certified diabetes educator (CDE) and can help you learn about diabetes and proper care of your feet.

Podiatrists are specially trained to take care of feet and can help you with everything from routine care to foot surgery. Orthopedic surgeons specialize in bone surgery, and some specialize in surgery of the foot and ankle. Vascular surgeons specialize in surgery on the blood vessels, and some specialize in surgery on the blood vessels of the legs and feet. They can help restore circulation to the feet. You would be more likely to see a surgeon if you have problems with an ulcer that won't heal.

Pedorthists are professional shoe fitters who make and fit shoes and insoles for people with foot problems. They can be of great assistance to you, especially if you have lost feeling in your feet.

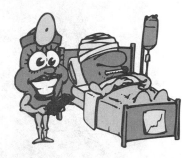

Do I need to see a podiatrist or an orthopedic surgeon?

▼
TIP:

Ask your health care provider. You can see a podiatrist for routine foot care if you cannot see well or reach your feet. Podiatrists are doctors of podiatric medicine (DPM) and, in most states, diagnose and treat conditions of the feet. They perform routine foot care, such as toenail trimming, callus removal, and treatment for ingrown toenails, and perform foot surgery on bones and soft tissue, such as bunion or hammertoe surgery. They can study how your feet and legs work when you move and walk (biomechanics). They can pinpoint bones that are out of place and that put unusual pressure on the skin of your feet. They can design arch supports to help your feet work normally and order special footwear if you need it.

Orthopedic surgeons are medical doctors (MD) who perform surgery on the bones. Some specialize in foot and ankle problems. Orthopedic surgeons do not usually provide routine services such as toenail trimming and removing ingrown toenails. They may perform foot surgery. They too can order arch supports and special footwear if you need it.

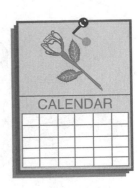

*H*ow *often should I have a doctor take care of
my feet?*

TIP:

*H*ave your feet checked at least once a year, usually at a regular
visit. Your health care provider will look for any changes in
shape (deformity) that change the way you walk and bear weight on
the foot. He'll also check for loss of feeling by pressing a thin
plastic wire called a monofilament against the soles of your feet or by
holding a vibrating tuning fork against the base of your big toe. The
provider will also check your circulation and examine the skin,
especially between your toes and under metatarsal heads (bones in
the ball of your foot).

If you can't examine your own feet or if you have foot problems
or nerve damage, have your feet checked more often, probably at
every visit.

The following are warning signs to have your feet checked:

Redness, swelling, or increased warmth
A change in the size or shape of the foot or ankle
Pain in the legs at rest or while walking
Open sores with or without drainage, no matter how small
Nonhealing wounds
Ingrown toenails
Corns or calluses with skin discoloration
Unexplained high blood sugar levels

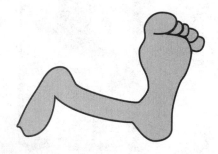

My doctor is busy. How do I get him or her to check my feet?

▼
TIP:

Take off your shoes and socks. If you have trouble doing this, ask the doctor's nurse or assistant to help you. Studies have shown that health care professionals are much more likely to examine the feet of a person with diabetes if the shoes and socks have already been removed when the health care provider comes into the examining room.

Another way to get your feet examined is to ask. Most health care professionals will readily check your feet whenever they are asked.

Finally, if you do not feel that you are getting enough attention to your feet through the regular medical care system, you could go to a podiatrist or orthopedic doctor who specializes in taking care of feet.

I cannot see my feet very well. How can I take care of them?

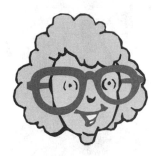

▼
TIP:

Sit down and pull your foot up on your knee or rest your foot on a footstool to get it closer to your eyes. Wear your glasses if you need to, and pick a place with good lighting. Use a mirror or magnifying mirror to examine the bottom of your feet. Medical supply stores and large drugstores have mirrors with long handles.

Be sure to run your hands over your feet. People with poor vision can learn what their feet feel like and can pick up changes in their feet by feeling them. If none of these suggestions works and a podiatrist is not available, you might ask a friend or family member for help or get a professional pedicure at a beauty shop.

Do not cut your toenails or do any kind of corn or callus removal if you cannot see well. Your health care provider, a nurse or assistant, or a home care nurse may be able to help you with foot care. In some communities, foot care is available at senior centers. Another option is to see a professional who specializes in taking care of feet, such as a podiatrist.

TYPES 1&2

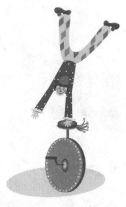

I cannot reach my feet very well. How can I
take care of them?

TIP:

Get a bath bench for your shower or tub in a drugstore or
medical supply store. Have grab bars installed in your shower
or tub. Get a long-handled bath brush or sponge on a handle, so you
can wash your feet while sitting down or holding onto the grab bar.
Rinse your feet before you stand up because soapy feet are slippery.

You can leave one end of the towel on the floor and rub your foot
over the towel to dry it. Dry as well as you can between the toes.
You can also use the sponge on a handle to apply lotion to your feet,
but you need two sponges: one for bathing and one for lotion. Keep
the lotion sponge in a plastic bag.

Most people who have trouble reaching their feet wear slip-on
shoes or shoes with Velcro fasteners. You can also try elastic laces,
found in shoe repair shops. A long-handled shoehorn also comes in
handy, as does a "sock-puller."

You might ask for a referral to an occupational therapist. An
occupational therapist can help you find and use devices like sock-
pullers and long-handled shoehorns. If flexibility is part of your
problem, ask for help learning stretching exercises or yoga postures.

270

1,001 Tips for Living Well with Diabetes

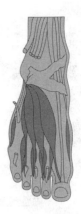

*W*hat changes in the foot are due to
normal aging?

▼
TIP:

Changes can occur in our hardworking feet as we age, especially
joint diseases like arthritis. Bones can shift out of position,
rubbing against shoes and causing pain and the protective buildup of
calluses or corns. We lose some of the fat pad that cushions the ball
of the foot—and people with diabetes may lose it all—causing a
callus to grow as a way to relieve the sharp pressure of bones on the
soles of our feet. This and other changes can make us unsteady, and
our gait or walking pattern may change. Our feet tend to get longer,
wider, and flatter, which affects how our shoes fit.

You can offset some of the effects of aging. Always wear shoes
that fit well. Sometimes changes in the shape of your feet occur so
gradually that you do not notice how poorly your shoes fit, especially
if you have nerve damage and cannot feel your feet. Don't wear
shoes that you have saved for years for special occasions.

An unsteady gait can be a sign of another type of medical
problem, so talk to your provider about it. It may just be time to get
a cane. Your provider or physical therapist can give you tips on
getting a cane of proper length and how to walk with it.

One of the best ways to keep your muscles, bones, and joints
young is to stay active. This is also good for your diabetes. If you've
never been active, you can begin by exercising sitting down.

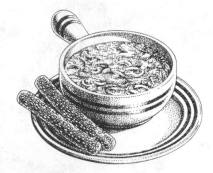

*D*oes a meal plan have anything to do with my feet?

▼
TIP:

Yes. You know that achieving near-normal blood glucose levels can improve your chances of not having nerve damage or circulation problems. Part of managing your blood glucose is following a meal plan, along with daily exercise and diabetes medication if you need it. In addition, we know that what you eat affects your health including your skin, muscles, and bones. A meal plan that is unbalanced with too many processed foods (white flour, sugars, and fats) and too few vegetables and fruits leaves you with fewer weapons to use against bacteria and fungus on the skin. That is why healthy eating for people with diabetes is the same way everyone should eat. Especially important are the vitamins and the minerals that you can get from vegetables and fruits. You also want to be sure that you are getting enough calcium and magnesium for your bones. Ask for a referral to a registered dietitian (RD) if you need help designing or changing your meal plan to meet your needs and to get your blood glucose under control.

What you eat also affects your blood fats and plays an important part in circulation and peripheral vascular disease (see pages 352–358).

Chapter 2
SKIN CARE TIPS

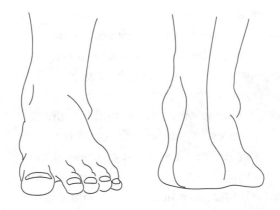

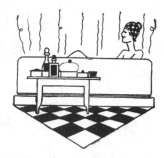

What is the best way for me to wash my feet?

▼ TIP:

The best way to wash your feet is in the bathtub or shower. Wash your feet just like you wash the rest of your body. Make sure the water temperature is not too hot. Check the temperature with your elbow, not with your toes! You can use any good soap. If you have dry skin, you might want to try soap with moisturizer to combat dryness. Soap that is not milled is more moisturizing. (Milling removes glycerin to make the soap harder and easier to shape.)

If you prefer, or if you have to, you can wash your feet in a pan of water. Take the same precautions and be sure that the water is not too hot. It is not necessary to buy a special footbath. If you cannot use the bathtub or shower, any plastic or metal tub the size of a dishpan will work. You may have seen special footbaths in advertisements. Some have heating and vibrating features. If you have one, and you want to use it, you certainly can, but there are no special benefits to be gained.

Be sure to rinse your feet well and be sure to dry very well, especially between the toes. Use a soft fluffy towel to gently pat your feet dry.

*S*hould I soak my feet?

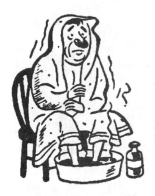

▼
TIP:

It is not necessary to soak your feet. In fact, prolonged soaking opens small cracks in your skin where germs can get in. That's how infections get started. Soaking also removes your natural skin oils. Repeatedly wetting and drying your feet can worsen dry skin problems, especially if you don't use a moisturizing lotion afterwards. For these reasons, soaking is not recommended.

If soaking your feet feels good, and you don't have any wounds on your feet, and the water is not too hot, and you don't stay in the footbath too long, and you use a moisturizing lotion afterwards, and you don't have any dry skin problems, you can probably get away with soaking your feet. However, from a health point of view, the risks of soaking your feet outweigh the benefits.

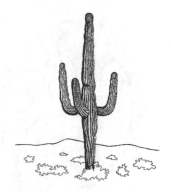

*W*hy do I have such dry skin on my feet?

TIP:

A s we age, skin may become thinner and dryer, so your dry skin may be from normal aging. People tend to have more dry skin in winter because of heating systems blowing dry air. Bathing with very hot water can also contribute to dry skin because it washes away natural skin oils. Harsh soaps and detergents also remove these oils.

People with diabetes can get a type of nerve damage called autonomic neuropathy. The autonomic nerves control blood flow, sweating, and skin moisture. People who have autonomic neuropathy may notice that their feet sweat less or not at all. This can cause severe dry skin.

Several other problems can cause dry skin of the feet. If your dry skin problem is not helped by regularly using a hand or body lotion, seek the advice of your health care provider.

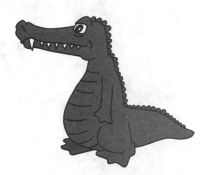

*D*o *I need to use skin lotions? What kind should I use and how often?*

▼
TIP:

Yes, you need to moisturize dry skin to prevent itching and cracking, which keeps germs out. Moisturizers are packaged as creams, lotions, ointments, and oils. Any good body or hand lotion will do, as long as you remember to use it. Select the kind that you like and will actually use every day.

Avoid lotions with alcohol because it evaporates and takes moisture from the skin, which has a drying effect. Some people are sensitive to chemicals in highly perfumed or colored lotions, but there are lotions with no smell or color. Avoid lotions with lanolin if you are allergic to wool. Lotion with mineral oil as one of the main ingredients may not work as well as lotions containing olive oil, almond oil, jojoba oil, or vegetable oils. Aloe vera gel is another good moisturizer.

Ask your health care provider or pharmacist to recommend a moisturizer. You can get a prescription lotion if you have special problems or severe dry skin.

The best time to apply lotion is after a bath or a shower because it seals in the moisture your body has absorbed. Do not apply moisturizers between your toes. Apply lotion once a day, or if you have severe dry skin, two or three times a day. Keeping lotion in your sock drawer may help you remember to use it. You may prefer to apply lotion before going to bed. You can put on a pair of socks to keep the lotion off the sheets and help it soak in overnight.

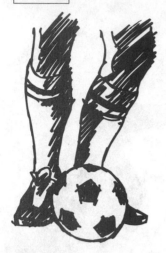

How can I tell whether I have athlete's foot fungus?

▼
TIP:

The only way to tell for sure whether you have athlete's foot fungus is for your health care provider to take a small skin scraping and look at it under a microscope. However, when you have itchy, burning, red, soggy, flaky, cracking, or dry scales between your toes, it is most likely athlete's foot fungus. Therefore, many providers will treat these symptoms as athlete's foot fungus without actually testing for it.

Athlete's foot can also occur on the soles or sides of the feet with many of the same symptoms and problems.

*W*hat should I do if I have athlete's
foot fungus?

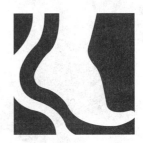

TIP:

You can buy over-the-counter antifungal powders, sprays, and creams. Do not use harsh chemicals like chlorine bleach. Bleach does not kill the fungus and can burn your skin. Apply only a thin layer of medicine. When athlete's foot flares up, apply the medication at least twice a day (morning and night) for at least 4 weeks.

See your provider if you have redness, swelling, or a warm area anywhere on your foot, or if you see any pus. If you have fever or chills or your blood sugar is higher than usual, you may have an infection that needs to be treated.

Your provider can prescribe stronger antifungal creams and pills for severe cases of athlete's foot. Unfortunately, it tends to come back when treatment stops.

Remember to dry well between your toes. You can put on antifungal foot powder. Some people find that lacing a little lamb's wool between the toes helps keep that area dry. Don't use cotton balls or tissues because they pack down and increase pressure between the toes.

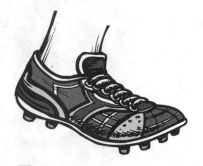

*H*ow can I prevent athlete's
foot fungus?

▼
TIP:

There are several things you can do to prevent athlete's foot fungus from becoming a problem. The main one is to keep your feet clean and dry. Wear socks made of fibers that wick the moisture away from your skin. Put on a clean pair every day. If your feet get wet during the day, change socks more often.

Wear shoes with uppers made of leather or fabric that allow air to pass through. Allow your shoes to dry between wearings. If you have two pairs, alternate between them.

Almost all adults have athlete's foot fungus. There are lots of "normal" germs that just live on your skin, and athlete's foot fungus is one of these. It thrives in dark, warm, moist environments. It is mildly contagious and is passed on by contact in public showers and swimming areas, by sharing towels, or by using soiled bath mats. Wearing sandals at the local shower or pool has not been proven to prevent athlete's foot, but you should wear them to protect your feet from injury.

What should I do about foot odor?

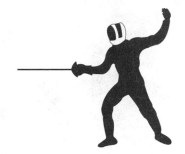

▼
TIP:

Foot odor is caused by the breakdown of bacteria on the skin. Daily bathing, changing socks, and keeping the feet clean and dry can control this. Using an antibacterial soap and a soft brush to gently scrub away dead skin may help. If your feet get wet during the day, you will need to change socks more often.

Always wear socks when you wear shoes. Wear shoes that allow air to circulate, not plastic or synthetic shoes. Dry out your shoes between wearings. Some foot odor problems are more smelly shoes than smelly feet. You may need to get new shoes.

If the problem continues, you might try an antiperspirant for feet or a foot powder designed to control foot odor. Special insoles with activated charcoal and socks that are designed to help control foot odor are available in large drugstores or from a foot care specialist.

Foot odor is sometimes a symptom of a serious problem such as a foot infection or foot ulcer that has gone undetected because of nerve damage. Inspect your feet carefully and if you detect a foot wound, see your provider immediately.

*W*hy do my feet swell?

TIP:

If both feet are swollen, it usually does not have much to do with your feet. If you have too much fluid in your system, it collects at the lowest part of the body due to gravity, and your feet and ankles swell. People with high blood pressure frequently have this kind of swelling. If your heart is too weak to pump blood around the body, the liquid parts of the blood tend to leak out of the blood vessels and collect in the lowest parts of the body. People with congestive heart failure have this kind of swelling. If your kidneys do not function well and you lose protein in your urine, your feet will swell.

Another cause of foot swelling is inactivity. When you are normally active during the day, the muscles in your legs help move blood and fluids back to the heart so they can recirculate. If you are sitting in a car or riding on an airplane all day, your leg muscles will not be working as much and fluid will pool in your feet and legs. That's why it's a good idea to get up and walk around every hour or two on an airplane or stop and walk around at a rest stop when you are in a car for long periods.

What should I do about foot swelling?

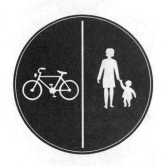

▼
TIP:

Elevate your feet and legs. Put your feet on a footstool, box, or another chair, or sit in a recliner with the footrest up. You can lie down on the couch and put your feet up on a pillow. Try to get your feet above the level of your heart. Any elevation is better than letting your feet hang down.

Another thing you can do is to stay active. Remember, when you are walking, the force of your contracting leg muscles helps blood and fluids return to the heart and keeps them from pooling in your feet and legs.

In some cases, you may be asked to take diuretics, often called "water pills." Water pills make you urinate a lot and leave less fluid in the system. That is how they lower blood pressure and make less work for a weak heart to do. Take your water pills as directed. Most people find it is best to take these pills first thing in the morning because they send you to the bathroom frequently. If you take them too close to bedtime, they might interrupt your sleep.

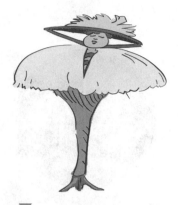

Should I wear support hose to control ankle swelling?

▼
TIP:

Ask your health care provider because support hose should not be worn by people with poor circulation, skin disorders, infections, open wounds, or massive swelling. You must put them on before your feet or ankles swell, usually in the morning before you walk around much. Do not wear them to bed. Fluid will not accumulate in your feet while you are lying in bed.

Support hose come in several styles and colors for men and women and look like regular socks or stockings. Before buying below-the-knee support hose, measure around your calf at the widest part and from the floor to your knee. Do not guess. If you get the wrong size, they will be uncomfortable, and you will not wear them.

Your provider can advise you on how much "squeeze" you need. Hose come in different levels of compression—mild, moderate, and high. Some have high compression in the ankle and low compression in the calf. If they are too loose, they will not help, and if they are too tight, they cut off circulation. They can be custom knit to fit unusual leg shapes and fitted with zippers if you have trouble getting them on.

Chapter 3
NAIL CARE TIPS

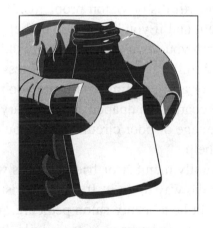

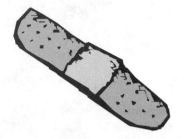

*C*an I cut my own toenails?

▼
TIP:

That depends on whether you can do it safely. Many people have trouble cutting their own toenails safely, especially if they are overweight or have arthritis or vision problems. If you can see and reach your feet well, and if you have good nail clippers, and you are careful, you can trim your own toenails. You could use a large nail file or emery board to file your nails. Filing is less risky than cutting. Nail files for artificial fingernails are good for toenail filing because they have coarser sandpaper than ordinary emery boards. If you have nerve damage or poor circulation or you can't see or reach your feet, ask for help.

If you have a family member or friend who is willing to help you, this might be the way to do it. If no podiatrist is available, another choice might be a beauty salon pedicure. Ask whether your provider has a nurse or assistant to trim toenails. In some communities, foot care is available through senior center programs. Almost all podiatrists will trim toenails. Medicare or health insurance may pay all or part of the cost for a podiatrist to trim your toenails if you have diabetes and meet certain criteria, such as having nerve damage and poor circulation.

What is the proper way to trim toenails when you have diabetes?

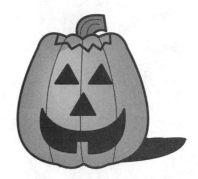

▼
TIP:

You may have seen instructions that say to cut your toenails straight across. However, this often leaves a sharp corner on the nail. It makes more sense to trim your nails with the contour of the toe, being sure all sharp edges are cut or filed smooth. The length of the toenail should be even with the end of the toe.

It is not a good idea to cut into the edges of the toenail or to try to treat ingrown toenails yourself. This sort of "bathroom surgery" is very risky for people with diabetes. The main point of safe toenail trimming is that if you do injure yourself, seek medical attention for any injury that does not heal promptly. If you have nerve damage or poor circulation and you cut yourself, see your provider right away. Do not wait until you develop an infection.

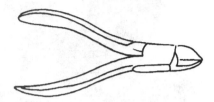

What is the best tool to use to trim my toenails?

▼ TIP:

I prefer the nail clippers that look like a pair of wire cutters or pliers. They are available in large drugstores, beauty supply houses, and cutlery stores. It is not necessary to have a sterile tool, but your toenail clippers should be kept clean, dry, and sharp. When you use a tool that is dull, you have to put more pressure on the clippers, and you can injure yourself if they slip.

Do not use pocketknives, kitchen knives, sewing scissors, or your teeth, or pick at your toenails with your fingers. Once you have diabetes, it is too risky to try to cut your toenails with anything except a good pair of toenail clippers.

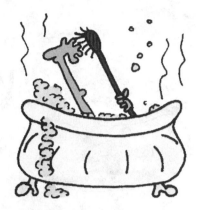

*W*hat should I do if I nick myself while trimming my toenails?

▼
TIP:

If you have nerve damage and poor circulation, go see your health care provider. If you don't, wash the injury with soap and water and pat it dry. It is not necessary to apply antiseptic creams to the wound. You may apply a bandage to keep it clean, but do not wrap the bandage tightly. Make it loose enough so that the circulation is not cut off if the toe or foot swells.

Do not be reassured if the wound does not hurt, because nerve damage may prevent you from feeling it. A wound that does not hurt may still be a serious injury.

Change the bandage and inspect the wound every day. Ask for help if you are having trouble seeing or caring for the injury. If you notice any redness, swelling, pus, or an area of increased warmth on your foot, or if the foot does not heal in a reasonable amount of time, report it to your health care provider right away. If you have an infection, you will need an antibiotic to cure it. The antibiotic creams that are currently available over the counter are not strong enough to cure an infection in a diabetic foot.

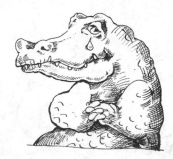

What should I do if I have very thick toenails?

▼
TIP:

A very thick toenail can put lots of pressure on the toe and cause an ulcer, so it is a good idea to have it trimmed down or removed. Whether or not you can trim them yourself depends on how thick they are. Most people need help. It is best to go to a podiatrist or health care provider who is trained to trim thick nails and has special tools to do the job.

A fungus usually causes thick toenails. Creams, oils, and liquid drops are sold over-the-counter to treat fungal toenails. While these products may help soften the nail and retard the fungus somewhat, they usually do not make it go away.

There are prescription pills that may eliminate the fungus on your toenails; however, these medicines may affect your liver. You will need to have a blood test before you start the medicine and about 6 weeks into the 3-month treatment to check on your liver. If it is being damaged, you will have to stop taking the pills. If you want to cure fungal toenails, talk with your provider about these pills. Be aware that the fungus might return after you stop taking the medication.

Some patients report that keeping their glucose levels nearer normal helps with the toenail fungus problem.

What should I do if I have very curved toenails?

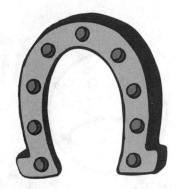

▼ TIP:

If you have deeply curved or ingrown nails, you may need help trimming them. Do not try to cut or dig out the curving toenail. You can injure yourself doing this. In addition, without the right tools it is easy to leave a fragment of the nail that will turn into an ingrown toenail and make the problem worse.

This kind of nail can be challenging even for professionals to cut. It is best to go to a podiatrist or health care provider who is trained to trim them. They have special tools that make it easier to trim very curved toenails.

What should I do if I have ingrown toenails?

▼
TIP:

Ingrown toenails are a common problem for people with and without diabetes. This painful condition results when the nail grows into the skin. You're more likely to get it if you trim the toenails too short and cut down the sides of the toenail. Trim your toenails a bit longer, following the curve of the toe without leaving any sharp corners. If the toenail grows into the skin, it breaks the skin, and infection may develop. If the nail has simply been cut incorrectly, a podiatrist or other health care provider can remove the ingrown portion. He may give you an anesthetic to numb the pain. If you have nerve damage, the ingrown toenail may not hurt, but it certainly needs professional care.

If the problem keeps coming back, the podiatrist will numb the toe and remove a corner of the nail. Sometimes a chemical is put into the corner to keep the ingrown portion from coming back. Sometimes the whole toenail will have to be removed, and then a more normal toenail will usually grow back.

Chapter 4
SHOES AND SOCKS TIPS

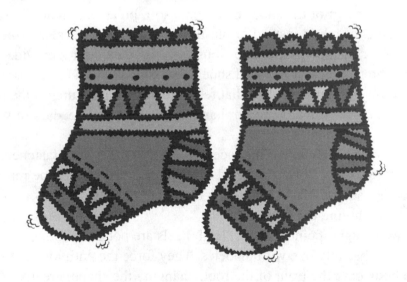

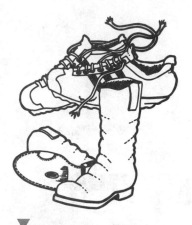

What are the best shoes to wear when you have diabetes?

▼

TIP:

Good quality athletic shoes or walking shoes are excellent choices. A lace-up shoe with a high rounded toe box is ideal. The upper part of the shoe should be a soft, breathable material such as leather or fabric instead of plastic or synthetic materials. Avoid sandals, clogs, thongs, or flip-flops, because they do not provide the same protection that a closed shoe does. If you have a callus or deformity, you need a shoe that redistributes the pressure on the sole of your foot. With a bunion or hammertoe, you may need extra-wide or extra-depth shoes.

If you have trouble tying laces, try shoes with Velcro fasteners. Most tie shoes can be converted to Velcro fasteners at a shoe repair shop. Elastic shoelaces allow you to get your shoes off and on without untying the laces.

Avoid tight, pointed shoes. High heels are not good for any foot—especially one with diabetes. They force the entire weight of the body onto the front of the foot, changing the shape, greatly increasing pressure, and causing ulcers. Look for a shoe that is shaped like a foot. While this sounds reasonable, it can be a challenging task, especially for women. It's worth the effort.

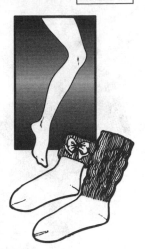

I have wall-to-wall carpeting; can I walk around bare foot or in my stocking feet?

▼
TIP:

No! Carpeting does not prevent you from stepping on pins, tacks, toys, dog bones, and whatever the cat brought in. Get a good pair of house shoes or slippers to protect your feet. The only time to go without shoes is when you are in bed or bathing. Even in the summer at a beach or pool, viruses, bacteria, and foreign bodies are lurking, just waiting for your bare feet. Always wear protective footgear.

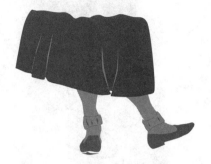

*H*ow can I tell whether my shoes fit?

▼
TIP:

One way is to purchase them from a trained shoe fitter (pedorthist). Have **both** feet measured every time you buy shoes, and shop for shoes in the afternoon or evening when your feet may be swollen. Your shoes need to fit all day. When you try on shoes, check that the ball of the foot rests in the widest part of the shoe. Walk a few steps, looking for signs of a poor fit, like the foot rolling over the sole, too much space between the heel and the back of the shoe, and notice that the shoe bends where your foot does. Be sure there is plenty of room for your toes. There should be a half-inch space between the longest toe and the end of the toe box, but the shoes should not slip. (The longest toe is not always the big toe.) Be sure the toe box is high enough and does not press on your toes.

Trace your foot, cut out the tracing, and place it on the sole of the shoe. Or put the sole of the shoe against the bottom of your foot. These can help you see whether the shape of the shoe matches the shape of your foot. If you have foot deformities or have had an ulcer that is now healed, you should have shoes prescribed and fitted or custom-made by a podiatrist, orthopedic surgeon, or pedorthist. If you have nerve damage, your properly fitted new shoes may feel too big. Also remember that people's feet tend to get longer, wider, and flatter as years go by. You will not always wear the same size.

My feet are different sizes; do I have to buy two pairs of shoes?

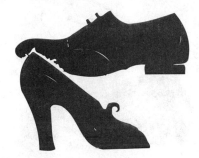

▼ TIP:

It is very common for one foot to be slightly larger or wider than the other. If you need two different-sized shoes or if you have only one foot, you might want to contact NOSE (the National Odd Shoe Exchange). NOSE helps its members with mismatched or odd-sized feet to find shoes. Some members are matched with another member who has exactly the opposite shoe size problem so that they can share shoe purchases rather than having to buy two different-sized pairs to come up with one wearable pair. Although it is rare, some stores will sell mismatched pairs.

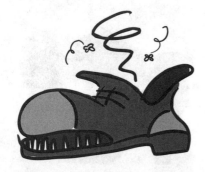

Why should I inspect my shoes every day, and what am I looking for?

TIP:

You are looking for anything that might injure your foot, especially if you have lost feeling in your feet. Look over the top and sole of the shoe, shake it out, and run your hand into it. Look and feel for any pebbles or foreign objects, or nails or tacks that may be coming through the sole. Look for cracked uppers or rough seams that could rub a blister. Replace shoes with worn or loose linings. If heels or soles are worn down, get new shoes or have them resoled so your foot is getting the support it needs.

*W*hat should I do if I need to wear
special shoes for a special occasion?

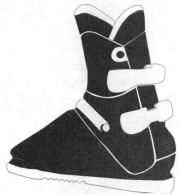

▼
TIP:

The same principles that apply to fitting your everyday shoes
apply to fitting special occasion shoes (see page 296). If you
need to wear golf shoes, rented bowling shoes, ice skates, steel-toed
work boots, ski boots, hiking boots, riding boots, or dress shoes to
match your tuxedo or dress, you'll need to make sure they fit as well
as possible. People prone to diabetes-related foot problems should
not wear a strange pair of shoes for more than an hour or two. After
the first hour, take a break, sit down, and check your feet for redness
or pressure areas. Bring comfortable shoes to change into so you
can avoid developing a blister.

If you need to wear high heels, wear the lowest heel possible
(and no higher than 2 inches) for the shortest time possible. As soon
as you get home or into your car, change into footwear that is more
comfortable.

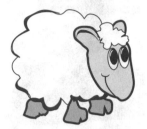

*W*hat are the best socks to wear?

▼
TIP:

Socks or stockings should be of breathable fibers such as cotton or wool, but they should also have acrylic or synthetic material that wicks moisture away from your skin. They should not be too tight or too loose and should fit without folds or wrinkles. Choose socks without seams. Garters or socks that bind may cut off circulation to your feet and legs. If the elastic at the top of your socks is too tight, cut a notch into the cuff of the sock.

Socks shaped like feet are preferable to tube socks, which tend to thin out over the heel and bunch up in the front. Change into clean socks daily. Throw away socks with holes. Repaired socks may have rough patches that can irritate your foot.

You can find extra large socks in big and tall shops, athletic stores, and department stores. Sports stores may have socks that are double knit on the bottom to provide an extra layer of cushioning. Just be sure that they don't make your shoes too tight.

Wear nylon stockings or panty hose for the shortest time possible. Nylon is not a breathable fabric (that's why they make raincoats out of it!). So change into some socks as soon as you can.

*D*o I need custom shoes?

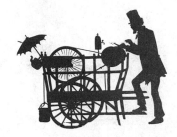

▼
TIP:

Most people with diabetes do not need custom-made shoes.
However, if you are at risk for amputation, you may need a
special shoe—for example, one with extra depth or special inserts.
You are considered to be at risk for an amputation if you have
already had a toe or partial-foot amputation, if you have a foot
deformity, if you have had an ulcer that is now healed, or if you
have diabetes-related foot problems. A podiatrist or other health care
provider who can examine your feet would be the best person to
advise you about this. A referral to a podiatrist may be necessary.

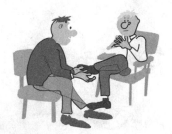

*W*ill Medicare pay for my therapeutic
  shoes?

▼
TIP:

Medicare pays for therapeutic footwear when you meet certain
criteria and fill out the proper forms. This benefit covers
custom-molded shoes, extra-depth shoes, inserts, and some shoe
modifications. Your physician must certify that you are in a plan of
diabetes care, have evidence of foot disease, and need therapeutic
footwear. A podiatrist writes the prescription, and a podiatrist or
pedorthist provides the shoes. You must buy the footwear from a
qualified supplier and file the forms. You can get the forms from the
prescription shoe stores, Medicare, or a podiatrist, or your provider
may help you get them. Usually you have to pay for the shoes, and
Medicare will reimburse up to 80% of the reasonable charge within
limits. Ask about the charge and how much Medicare will pay when
you order the shoes.

Although government programs can be time consuming, prescription
footwear can be an important part of preventing foot problems.

*D*o I need insoles?

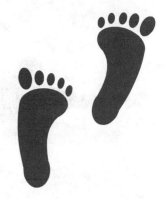

▼

TIP:

Maybe. You can relieve pressure on the soles of your feet by wearing a cushioning layer between your foot and the floor. If you wear thin-soled shoes or if you have high-pressure areas on your feet, it is a good idea to add insoles to your shoes. High-pressure areas are where calluses develop. Most ulcers begin under a callus. So if you can prevent or reduce the size of a callus, you may prevent getting an ulcer in that area, too.

These types of insoles are available in drugstores, grocery stores, sporting goods stores, and running shoe stores for less than $10 a pair. Running shoe stores also have insoles with extra arch support for $15 to $30. Be sure to check with your foot care specialist before buying these. An insole will raise your foot in the shoe, so be sure that you have plenty of room in the toe of the shoes. If your shoes are too tight with the insoles, you would do better with half-insoles that do not go under the toes. You'll need to change your insoles every 3–6 months to prevent foot odor and athlete's foot, and because the cushioning effect wears out.

If you have foot deformities or large calluses on your feet, you may need to have specially made inserts called orthotics to fit your feet (see page 305).

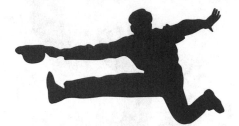

Do magnetic insoles offer any special benefits for people with diabetes?

▼
TIP:

We don't know yet. Although some people will swear that magnets relieve pain, improve circulation, reduce swelling, or provide other health benefits, at this time there are not enough scientific studies to back up these claims. Ordinarily when this is the case and the therapy is not harmful or expensive, health care providers will tell patients to try it and see what they think. However, some magnetic insoles have an uneven surface so they could possibly cause a sore or a foot ulcer in some people with diabetes who have high-pressure areas in their feet. People with diabetic nerve damage might not feel any discomfort from walking on these uneven surfaces and injure their feet. This means that the risks of magnetic insoles appear to outweigh the known benefits, so they are not recommended for people with diabetes to wear at this time. If you are really curious about them, you could try wearing them when you are not walking around, say for about 45 minutes when you are watching television or reading in bed.

What are orthotics?

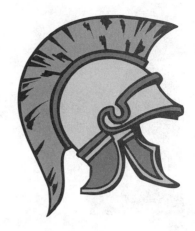

▼
TIP:

Orthotics are specially designed insoles that are worn inside your shoes to control the way your foot moves or to support painful areas of the foot. Often mistakenly called arch supports, they can do much more than that. Additions, top covers, extensions, or wedges can be added to the orthotics to hold your feet in a more stable position inside the shoe. This can help you walk normally, relieve foot pain, avoid calluses and corns, and even help with knee, hip, and lower back pain.

Orthotics are usually custom-made using a plaster model of your foot. They are made of a rigid material, like plastic, but some are made of leather or other soft materials. Graphite orthotics are durable and can be made very thin for comfort. Properly made orthotics are usually comfortable, but some people cannot stand to wear them. Work with your provider to get a pair that you will wear.

Orthotics can be expensive, so check to see whether your health plan will help you pay for them—often they will be covered. One pair may not fit inside all of your shoes, so you may want separate orthotics for dress shoes or sports. Orthotics must be replaced periodically, so ask the person who made them when you'll need new ones.

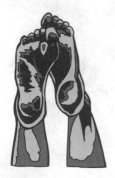

D^o *I need to wear orthotics?*

▼
TIP:

You need orthotics if you have foot pain, a thick callus, or a change in foot shape that prevents you from walking normally. Sometimes people will have knee, hip, or lower back pain because of poor biomechanics in their feet and legs, and they need orthotics, too. If you cannot feel foot pain or whether your foot is in the correct position as you walk, you should have your gait evaluated by a professional. Orthotics are designed to fit the unique shape of your feet and to stabilize them in your shoes so your feet can work normally. If you have a foot deformity and poor sensation or circulation, orthotics can help keep your feet healthy. Discuss your options with a specialist such as an orthopedic foot surgeon or podiatrist. To get medically corrective foot orthotics you must have a prescription from a health care professional.

What is a pedorthist and do I need to see one?

▼
TIP:

A pedorthist is a professional shoe fitter who has been trained in both foot anatomy and shoe construction. Pedorthists fill prescriptions for footwear and orthotics. A custom shoe store may have a pedorthist on staff. A nationally certified pedorthist may use the initials "C. Ped" after his or her name.

If you have a severe foot deformity, you are probably already familiar with people trained in this specialty. If you have trouble getting shoes that fit properly or you need special adjustments to your shoes because your feet are changing shape or you're losing feeling in your feet, it might be a good idea to see a pedorthist.

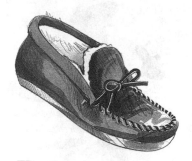

I have had a partial foot amputation. Can I just put padding in my shoes and continue to wear the shoes I wore before the surgery?

▼
TIP:

Maybe. You need to have your foot examined by a podiatrist or an orthopedic surgeon to see where the pressure points are and whether there are any new ones since the surgery. An amputation "creates" a foot deformity, and it is important to fit your shoes properly so that they do not rub a blister or cause a buildup of callus. You may need orthotics or a specially made shoe.

Chapter 5
TREATING
MINOR PROBLEMS

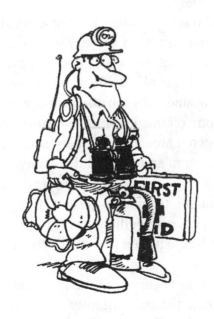

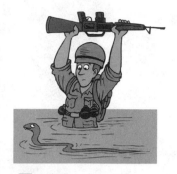

I have a blister on my foot. What should I do?

TIP:

If you have neuropathy or poor circulation, see your health care provider immediately! Don't wait until it gets infected. Then the first thing to do is to stop wearing the offending shoe. Wash the area with warm water and mild soap and dry well. Do not break the blister—this can allow germs to get under the skin. Cover the blister with a dry bandage. If the blister breaks, leave the loose skin as a covering over the wound until it heals. It is not necessary to apply antiseptics, antibiotic ointments, or chemicals to the blister.

Inspect the blistered area daily. If there is redness, tenderness, swelling, pus, or a warm area around the wound after the first day, you may be getting an infection. See your provider to get antibiotics. Over-the-counter antibiotic creams are not strong enough to treat a foot infection in a person with diabetes. If the wound is deep, gets larger, or does not heal within a few days, have it checked immediately.

Don't wear the shoes again until the blister is entirely healed. You might need extra padding, different socks, or something else to keep them from rubbing. Wear the shoes for a short while; then check your feet for signs of another blister. It is better to throw them away than to continue wearing shoes that injure your feet.

I wore well-fitting shoes and cushioned socks, and I still got a blister. How is this possible?

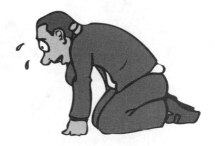

▼
TIP:

A blister is usually a sign of friction. If your shoes do not rub and you are getting blisters on your feet for no apparent reason, check with your health care provider. There is a rare diabetic complication called diabetic bullae. Bulla (bullae is the plural) is the medical term for a fluid-filled blister. The layers of the skin just separate and fill with clear fluid for no apparent reason, usually on the hands and feet. There can be several small blisters, just one, or sometimes a very large blister. There is no special treatment for diabetic bullae, just care for it as you would any other blister.

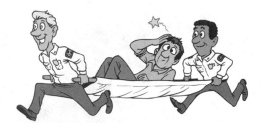

I stubbed my toe, what should I do?

TIP:

Well, that depends on how much you have injured it. While a stubbed toe can be excruciatingly painful, the actual injury can vary from minor to severe. If you don't have peripheral vascular disease, put ice on the injury and elevate it higher than your heart to relieve the swelling and pain. Is the toe in an abnormal position or do you have continued pain, swelling, or an inability to put weight on the foot? Then you need to see your health care provider for an X ray of your foot to make sure that you have not broken any bones. If you neglect a fracture, particularly of the big toe, this can result in a painful deformity. You need early treatment to prevent this from occurring. Sometimes people with nerve damage do not feel pain and can injure a foot or toe quite severely without knowing it. If you have nerve damage, check your feet carefully with your eyes and your hands after any injury to see how bad it is.

If blood accumulates under the toenail, it can put pressure on the toe. You may need to visit your health care provider to have the pressure relieved. Do not try to relieve it yourself by puncturing the nail or performing any other home surgery. When you have diabetes, it is best to have a health care provider treat all foot injuries.

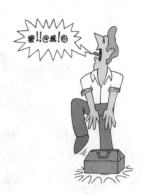

I stepped on a nail. What should I do?

▼
TIP:

If you have neuropathy and poor circulation, see your health care provider right away. Puncture wounds are a serious matter, especially when you have diabetes. Nails and other sharp objects do not have to be rusty to cause lockjaw (tetanus) or to cause an infection in your foot. Punctures through shoes are especially dangerous because sometimes a little rubber from the sole of the shoe is carried into the wound and causes an especially nasty type of infection.

Wash the area with warm water and mild soap and dry well. Cover the wound with a dry bandage. It is not necessary to apply antiseptics or antibiotic ointments. Change the bandage daily. If the bandage sticks when you attempt to remove it, apply a little warm water first. Inspect the wound every day and if you see any redness, swelling, pus, or drainage, or you have unexplained high blood sugar, report it to a health care provider immediately.

All adults should have tetanus booster shots repeated at least every 10 years. If you are not sure when you had your last tetanus booster, it is safe to have another one when you are injured.

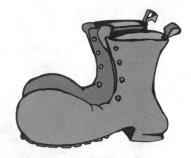

My toenail fell off. What should I do?

▼
TIP:

After a toenail injury, it is very common for the nail to fall off. Sometimes this happens with very thick fungal nails. It will usually grow back within 12–18 months. Keep the area clean and dry while waiting for the new nail to grow back. Protect it from any further damage by not going barefoot and by wearing shoes that have plenty of room for your toes. The nail-growing cells may have been damaged during the injury, so sometimes the new toenail will be a different shape.

What does it mean if my toes curl over?

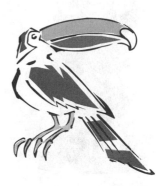

▼
TIP:

It means that you have had a change in the position of the foot bones and have tight tendons in the toe. Toes that are curled or bent are called hammertoes, claw toes, or mallet toes. You may have one or several. A foot deformity like this can set you up for calluses and possibly an ulcer because hard tissue, called a corn, will grow on top of or on the tip of the curving toe. The corn is nature's way of protecting the joint from irritation when it rubs against your shoe. Sometimes toe deformities are very painful. To deal with a toe deformity, you can change shoes, pad the toe, trim the corn, wear orthotics, or have surgery on the foot. If you use corn pads, be sure to buy ones that do not contain any chemicals.

Inspect your feet every day and see your health care provider or podiatrist whenever the corn needs trimming or becomes irritated. Inspect both the top of the toe where the corn develops and the tip of the toe, which can also rub and develop a callus.

Try switching to shoes that have a soft, rounded toe box and a soft insole under the toes to decrease irritation to the toe. Surgery can release the tendons and relax the toe or put the bones in a correct position. But you may also need orthotics to address any biomechanical problem.

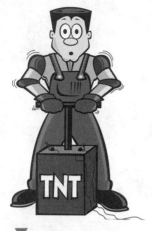

Can I use over-the-counter corn and callus removers?

TIP:

No, you really should not use these products when you have diabetes. Usually the manufacturer will say "not for use by people with diabetes" on the product. Corn and callus removers, corn plasters, and similar products are harsh chemicals, usually acids. They decrease the buildup of hard skin by softening and burning away the corn or callus. If you have diabetic nerve damage, you might not be able to feel it if the chemicals burned too much or got on the surrounding normal skin. It is dangerous for a person with diabetes to get any breaks in the skin because of the risks of infection and difficulty with healing. Therefore, you should avoid putting harsh chemicals on your feet.

You might try a green clay poultice to soften corns and calluses, but you really should try to determine what is causing them. See your regular provider or a podiatrist if you have a corn or callus that needs to be treated.

What should I do about a corn between my toes?

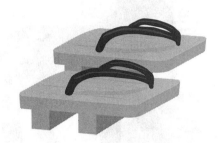

▼
TIP:

Corns between the toes that touch each other are called soft corns or kissing corns. Bones in adjacent toes rubbing together cause these corns. Shoes that squeeze the toes together aggravate soft corns. Sometimes they are very painful.

You can change shoes, add padding, and have surgery for soft corns. Switch to shoes that have a soft and high rounded toe box that does not press your toes together. You can buy special toe separator pads made of soft foam rubber or loosely lace some lamb's wool between the toes to decrease the rubbing. Do not use cotton or tissues between the toes because these materials can pack down and actually increase the pressure. Inspect your feet every day, including between the toes. See your podiatrist or another health care provider if you think the soft corn needs to be trimmed, or if it is irritated or ulcerated.

Early surgery to correct the problem causing the corn is often the best solution to prevent the corn from occurring. Elective foot surgery is often more important for people with diabetes than for the general population. Many foot ulcers begin as a callus or corn.

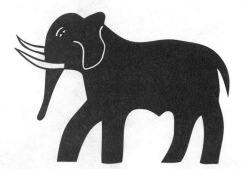

What should I do about a callus on the bottom of my foot?

TIP:

Try to decrease the high pressure on that spot by wearing shoes with a soft insole and a cushioned outer sole. Don't wear house shoes with little cushioning or go barefoot because this will make the callus worse. A hard callus is like having a rock in your shoe. The tissue beneath the callus can become damaged, and most foot ulcers occur there. You need to be evaluated by a professional to see what is causing the callus.

To deal with a callus you can change shoes, get orthotics, moisturize the skin, trim the callus, or have surgery. If it is very thick, you may need orthotics. In any case, moisturizing the callused area with a good lotion keeps it soft. A green clay poultice will also soften it. A callus can be sanded down with an emery board, callus file, or a pumice stone. It may be easier to remove after a bath or shower when the skin is still damp. Go easy and do not injure yourself by scrubbing too hard. Buff the area a little every other day rather than trying to remove the callus all at once. Never try to remove a callus by cutting or trimming it with a razor blade. See your podiatrist or health care provider for ongoing callus care.

*W*hat should I do about a wart on the bottom of my foot?

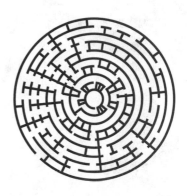

▼

TIP:

Plantar warts are caused by the papilloma virus, which gets under the skin on the bottom of the foot. In some people, plantar warts disappear without any treatment. In others, plantar warts hang around for years even when they are treated.

There are many home remedies for plantar warts, but the best solution is to see your health care provider or a podiatrist. Sometimes it is difficult even for professionals to tell the difference between a plantar wart and a callus. There are several treatments for plantar warts, including leaving them alone if they are not painful. They can be trimmed, padded, or removed with chemicals; burned with liquid nitrogen; or removed by surgery. It is important not to leave a painful scar on the bottom of the foot that can affect walking, so it is best not to try any of these treatments by yourself.

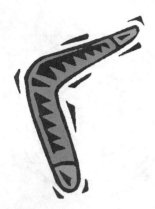

What is a bunion? What should I do if I have one?

▼
TIP:

A bunion is called hallux valgus. Hallux is the medical name for the big toe, and valgus is a word that means turning away from the midline of the body. A bunion is a deformity in the joint of the big toe causing the toe to point away from the arch instead of straight ahead. There is usually an unsightly bump on the inside of the foot. It is believed that uneven weight distribution during walking and stresses in the joints cause bunions and that they tend to run in families. Wearing shoes with pointed toes probably contributes to developing bunions.

If you have a painful bunion or it is difficult to get your shoes to fit, discuss what to do with your health care provider. Don't put it off. You may need special shoes, orthotics, or padding. Some bunions need surgical correction. If you have good circulation, get the surgery done. Early surgery is often the best treatment for people with diabetes. Modern bunion surgery not only removes the bump but also attempts to correct the mechanical problem that caused it so the bunion does not grow back. Bunion surgery can take about 6 weeks to heal, so you will want to have good blood glucose control before and after the surgery to encourage healing.

Chapter 6
EXERCISE TIPS

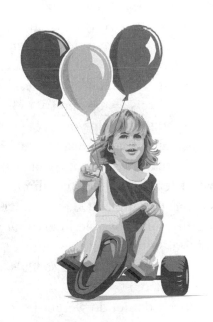

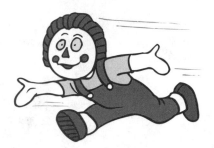

What foot precautions should I follow when walking, running, or jogging?

▼
TIP:

Have a foot exam to discover any deformity, lack of feeling, or poor circulation. Wear clean socks and good-quality walking or running shoes to prevent injury. Always take the time to warm up and do slow stretches to prepare your muscles and tendons—especially your Achilles' tendons. Cool down and stretch after the exercise activity and inspect your feet for redness, blisters, or callus buildup. If you have pain during exercise, stop and try to figure out what is wrong. You may need orthotics to help your feet work normally during physical activity—especially if you are active and have knee pain or pain in the arch or heel area of your foot (plantar fasciitis).

If you have a loss of feeling in your feet, limit repetitive weight-bearing exercises such as jogging and stair climbers because of the high pressure on your feet and possible injury that you wouldn't be able to feel. Be careful of hot sand and pavement around pools and sports courts. Even if you wear thin-soled sandals and water shoes, your feet may still get burned.

If you have a foot ulcer, do not do weight-bearing exercise so it can heal. When the ulcer has healed, try to discover what caused it and take special precautions when exercising to prevent it from coming back.

Drink plenty of water when you are exercising.

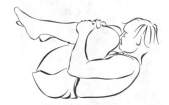

*W*hat forms of exercise are good for people with diabetic foot complications?

TIP:

Short periods of walking can actually improve circulation in your legs and feet by forcing the blood vessels to work harder and expand. In fact, this is the recommended exercise for people with intermittent claudication. Walking is good for your heart and for your diabetes control too. Two 20-minute walks a day is ideal.

If you have lost much of the feeling in your feet, you can participate in non-weight-bearing exercises, such as swimming, bicycling, or rowing, and upper body exercises, such as weight lifting, and range of motion and stretching exercises. You can do yoga. You will achieve your best level of fitness if you do several different types of exercise during the week. For example, you can do aerobic exercise one day, stretching exercises the next, and strength-building exercises the next day. If you row or bicycle on a machine, take care that the foot straps don't injure your feet. In a pool, you may want to wear aqua shoes to protect your feet.

Remember that your household chores, such as vacuuming and gardening, count as aerobic exercise, too.

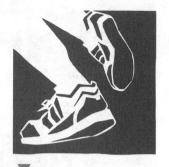

Should I wear special shoes when exercising?

▼
TIP:

Yes, you should always wear good-quality athletic shoes made for the activity you are doing. This means wearing running shoes for running, golfing shoes for golfing, and bowling shoes for bowling. Almost every sport is associated with a special type of shoe appropriate to the particular activity. These shoes are important for preventing injury. And they may help you perform better and enjoy the sport more! If you are in doubt about which shoes to wear, a good running shoe offers support and stability to protect your feet from injury.

Chapter 7
IDENTIFYING
MAJOR PROBLEMS

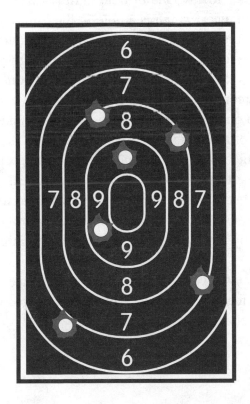

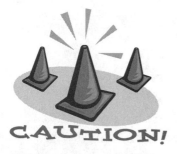

CAUTION!

▼

TIP:

How do I know when I have a foot ulcer?

A foot ulcer is an open sore somewhere on your foot. The term "ulcer" refers to a wound or hole in the skin. We often hear about a stomach ulcer, which is a hole in the lining of the stomach. A foot ulcer is a break in the skin that is usually, but not always, shaped like a crater. Foot ulcers often occur in high-pressure areas, so it is common to find one under a callus or surrounded by callus. The most common foot ulcer locations are on the bottom or side of the big toe and on the ball of the foot, especially under the big toe joint. The ball of the foot under the little toe joint is also a common place for foot ulcers. However, diabetic foot ulcers can occur anywhere on the feet. Be aware that the actual break in the skin can be very small, but a larger ulcer may be hidden from view under the surrounding callus or skin. This is why it is important to have your foot inspected by a professional if you think you might have a foot ulcer.

The only way for you to know whether you have a foot ulcer is by seeing it or feeling it. That is why we ask people with diabetes to inspect their feet carefully every day.

*H*ow do I avoid getting foot ulcers?

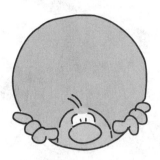

▼
TIP:

You can take two very important steps to protect your feet. Control your blood sugar levels as well as you can. Inspect your feet every day and get regular medical attention at least several times a year. There is no magic to avoiding foot complications. The key is to develop a routine that includes some commonsense everyday attention to your feet.

- Keep your feet clean and dry.
- Wear well-fitting shoes and socks.
- Don't go barefoot.
- Don't soak your feet.
- Don't put lotion between your toes, but put it on the rest of your foot.
- Get monofilament testing at least once a year.
- Treat calluses aggressively by seeing a foot care specialist.
- Get any injury to your foot seen right away!

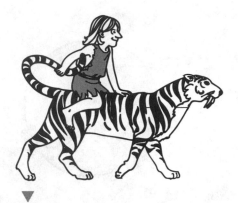

What should I do if I get a foot ulcer?

▼

TIP:

Have any foot ulcer examined by a health care professional, and once you have received treatment, the wound should begin to heal in a week or two. Keep the wound clean and dry and covered with a bandage. Inspect it daily. You must follow the treatment plan. Usually the treatment is to trim or cut away (debride) the dead tissue, to apply a dressing every day, and, if the wound is infected, to take antibiotics. It is likely that you will be asked to change your shoes. You must not walk on an infected foot. Use bed rest, crutches, or a wheelchair, but stay off that foot.

If the wound is not improving after a week or two, let your health care provider know. Be sure that you are doing all you can to follow the treatment plan and help your foot to heal.

This foot ulcer is not getting better. What should I do?

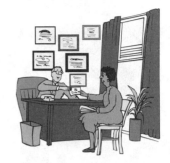

▼
TIP:

If you are following the care plan, taking antibiotics, and not walking on the ulcer but it still isn't healing, ask your health care provider for a referral to a foot care specialist. You may also need to be evaluated by a vascular surgeon to see whether surgery might restore circulation to the foot and help heal the ulcer. As a person with diabetes, you must be in charge of your own health care. Ask for a second opinion or to be referred to a specialist if your wound is not healing. Nonhealing ulcers lead to amputation, so get the help you need.

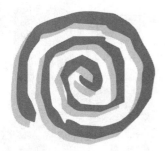

How do I know whether I have an infection?

▼
TIP:

Some signs of infection are

- redness
- swelling
- increased warmth
- pain, tenderness, or limited motion of the affected part
- pus or drainage from the wound

If you have one or two of these signs, have a health care provider check your wound to determine whether you have an infection.

Other signs that an infection has spread beyond the wound are fever, chills, or an unusually high blood sugar. If you have any of these signs, you need to be seen immediately and should go to an emergency room if your regular health care provider cannot see you right away.

Chapter 8
COMPLICATIONS—
NERVE DAMAGE

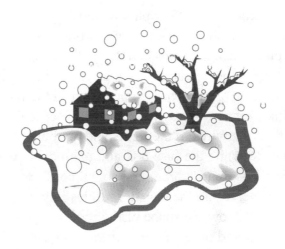

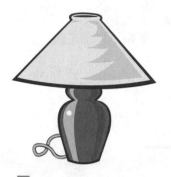

*W*hat is peripheral neuropathy?

▼
TIP:

Peripheral neuropathy is the name for damage to motor and sensory nerves. Motor and sensory nerves help you move and touch the world around you. "Peripheral" means at the edges or away from the center. In this case, the feet are farthest from the center of the body. "Neuro" means nerves and "pathy" means "a disorder of." Because the longest nerves are usually affected first, symptoms such as tingling, burning, or numbness appear first in the feet and hands.

If you think of the nervous system as the electrical system in your house, then the wires to the lights and appliances would be the peripheral nerves, while the fuse box and main cable would be the central nervous system (the brain and spinal cord).

When motor nerves are damaged, muscles in your foot can become weak and allow the shape of the foot to change. Toes can curl up and the fat pad on the bottom of the foot can shift and no longer protect the skin on the bottom of the foot. Those bones can get very close to the skin and can cause calluses. The sensory nerve damage prevents you from feeling pain, so the callus can become an ulcer without you knowing it.

How does diabetes cause nerve damage?

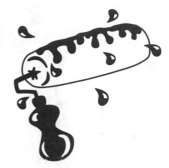

▼
TIP:

Nobody really knows. It is pretty certain that higher than normal blood sugar levels are part of the cause. We do know that keeping your blood sugar in control can lower your chances of getting neuropathy, that people with high blood sugar are more likely to have neuropathy, and that the longer a person has diabetes, the more likely he or she is to have neuropathy.

There are several theories about how blood sugar affects nerves. It is possible that sugar coats the proteins in the nerves and that the sugar-coated proteins no longer function normally. Or, it might be that high blood sugar levels interfere with chemical events in the nerves. Maybe high blood sugar levels damage the insulation layer of cells around the nerves. It might be that high blood sugar levels damage the tiny blood vessels that supply the nerves. Then the nerves would not get enough oxygen and nutrients, and this could cause problems.

Researchers are working to understand the causes of neuropathy and to find treatments to avoid the damage that it does.

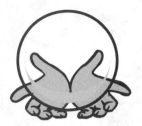

*H*ow do I know whether I have peripheral
neuropathy?

TIP:

If you have had diabetes for more than 10 years and you have not
kept your blood sugar levels close to near-normal levels, you likely
have some symptoms of nerve damage. It affects as many as 75% of
all people with diabetes. Do you have muscle weakness, cramps,
and feelings in your feet and legs such as numbness, tingling, pins
and needles, and burning sensations? Do your feet bother you more
at night? Have you had any episodes of fainting or vomiting or had
a change in bowel habits, bladder control, or sexual functioning?
These systems can be affected by diabetic nerve damage too.

There is no one specific test for diabetic nerve damage. Generally,
if you have two or more symptoms and one of the simple tests for
loss of sensation is positive (you cannot feel the touch of a plastic
wire or a vibrating tuning fork on the bottom of your foot. See
page 336), you will be considered as having neuropathy.

*D*oes diabetes cause more than one kind of
neuropathy?

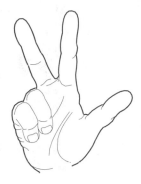

▼
TIP:

Yes, diabetic nerve damage can affect three kinds of nerves in your body: nerves you feel with (sensory neuropathy), nerves that go to the muscles (motor neuropathy), and nerves that control automatic body activities such as blood flow and digestion (autonomic neuropathy). With sensory nerve damage you may not be able to feel heat and cold and may have tingling, pain, or numbness. You may not be able to sense where your feet are and be more likely to fall. With motor nerve damage, muscles are weakened and you are more likely to develop foot deformities such as hammertoes.

Damage to autonomic nerves can affect major systems in your body, such as the heart, stomach, or sexual organs. It can affect heart rate and blood pressure. It can cause gastroparesis and erectile dysfunction. This type of nerve damage can also interfere with the functioning of your bladder, eyes, sweat glands, and hypoglycemia awareness (symptoms of low blood sugar).

The best way to try to prevent nerve damage is to keep your blood sugar levels closer to normal. Getting better blood sugar control can help relieve symptoms of ongoing neuropathy, but you may not be able to reverse extensive damage, such as you find in completely numb feet.

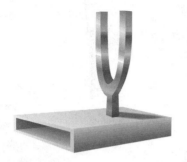

What kinds of tests do I need for peripheral neuropathy?

▼
TIP:

Many people with neuropathy already know that their feet are numb. Most people who have symptoms of neuropathy (pain, numbness, tingling), especially if their symptoms are worse at night, can be considered to have neuropathy. However, you could have neuropathy from a cause other than diabetes, such as vitamin deficiencies, thyroid disease, poisons (alcohol, lead, mercury, or arsenic), and several other diseases. Your provider may want to be sure that you do not have any of these other problems.

One of the most common tests is for the health care provider to touch your feet with a plastic wire called a monofilament. If you cannot feel the wire, you are considered to have nerve damage. Similar tests check whether you can feel a pin prick, a wisp of cotton stroked across the foot, or the vibration of a tuning fork.

If there is confusion about the nerve damage, some people might need a nerve conduction study. On rare occasions, a nerve biopsy in which a small piece of nerve tissue is examined under a microscope is done. If you are asked to have tests for neuropathy, ask your provider to explain the tests to you.

*A*re there any treatments for peripheral
neuropathy?

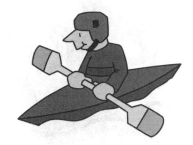

▼
TIP:

T he best treatment is to get your blood sugar levels under control.
Studies show that good blood sugar control can also help
prevent the nerve damage that you already have from getting worse.
Take note that if you should go on insulin or a sulfonylurea and
improve your blood sugar control, the pain may increase for a little
while, until your body becomes accustomed to the lower blood
sugar levels.

Medications such as antidepressants, anticonvulsants (seizure
medicine), muscle relaxants, local anesthetics (such as a lidocaine
patch), anti-inflammatory drugs, vitamins, evening primrose oil, and
capsaicin creams made from hot peppers have been used to treat
neuropathy symptoms. Physical therapy treatments such as
stretching exercises, massage, and electrical nerve stimulation have
also been tried. Although studies of these therapies report some
improvement in painful symptoms for some patients, there is no
single treatment that works for everyone. It may be difficult to get
complete relief. Discuss your symptoms with your provider and try
the treatment you both think might work. If that treatment doesn't
help, let your provider know so you can try another.

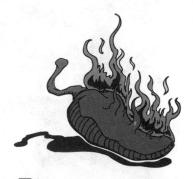

How can capsaicin cream help relieve my neuropathy pain?

▼
TIP:

Capsaicin is a substance found in hot peppers. Capsaicin cream removes a chemical from the nerve ends below your skin and may interrupt your feeling of pain. Apply it lightly several (3–5) times a day. Wash your hands carefully after applying capsaicin—you would not want to get hot pepper cream in your eyes! When you first use capsaicin, you may have a stinging or burning sensation that should disappear in a few days.

Buy only a small amount to try. Do not use capsaicin if you are sensitive or allergic to hot peppers. Capsaicin cannot be used on damaged or irritated skin, wounds, or rashes. Don't put tight clothing or bandages over the cream. Use it 3–4 times a day for 3–4 weeks before deciding whether it is working. Ask your provider or pharmacist if you have questions.

Purchase a product made by a reputable company. Some natural product companies and herbalists make up their own concoctions containing extracts of hot peppers, but the strength and purity of the drug is usually not consistent.

My feet are getting more sensitive, not less. How can this be nerve damage?

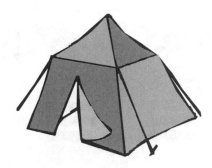

▼
TIP:

When the nerves are in the process of being damaged, many strange signals can be sent up the nerve pathways, including feeling as though your feet are more sensitive than they should be. Some people find it painful for bedsheets to touch their feet. If you experience this, placing a hoop or a box over the end of the bed so that the sheet is kept off your feet might provide you some relief.

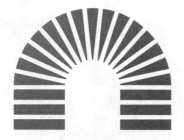

What can I do for the numbness in my feet?

▼
TIP:

This is a very serious condition. The main thing to do about numbness in your feet is to realize that you have it. Most people go to the doctor because their foot hurts. Yours never will. You **must** check your feet by touching them with your hands and by looking at them every day! Controlling your blood sugar as well as possible may help prevent the numbness from getting worse. Get your shoes fitted properly, if necessary by a pedorthist, and find out whether you need special shoes to protect your feet. Check your shoes before each wearing for foreign objects, nails, or anything that would injure your foot. Be sure your socks are not wrinkled or twisted. You may want to switch to socks without a toe seam because the seam can put too much pressure on your toes.

If you find the numbness is uncomfortable, discuss treatments for neuropathy with your health care provider. Whenever there is any injury to your feet or a change in shape or the skin, see your foot care specialist right away. Do **not** wait until an infection develops!

What does it mean if it feels like my feet are burning or tingling, or something is crawling on my feet but nothing is there?

▼
TIP:

Burning, tingling, or crawling sensations on the feet or legs may be a sign that diabetic nerve damage is occurring. The first thing to do is to check to make sure there is no obvious cause for this sensation. If you find this sensation uncomfortable, you may want to talk with your health care provider about possible treatments for neuropathy. You may also want to go over your diabetes care plan to see whether it is helping you keep your blood sugar levels where you want them to be.

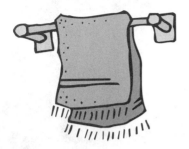

My feet are sweating more. What can I do?

▼
TIP:

An increase in foot sweating can be a sign that diabetic nerve damage is occurring. If you have sweaty feet, wear shoes made of leather or fabric that "breathes." Avoid shoes made of plastic or synthetic materials. Try to change your shoes during the day. If that is not possible, rotate between two pairs of shoes, wearing one on even days and the other on odd days. (Keeping your feet dry helps you avoid fungal infections, but it is also important to avoid excessively dry skin that may crack.)

Wear socks that wick the moisture away from your skin (special acrylic blends). You can find two- and three-layer socks designed to absorb sweat in sports stores. Change socks frequently: at least daily and maybe two or three times a day if necessary. If you have to wear nylon stockings, change into socks as soon as you can. Can you wear cotton tights instead?

You may have to try an antiperspirant containing aluminum chloride, such as "Drysol," which is available with a prescription. An antiperspirant can dry and irritate your skin so use it sparingly and only as a last resort. Follow the directions on the package and stop using the product immediately if you experience any skin irritation.

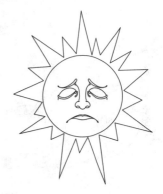

*W*hy *don't my feet sweat anymore?*

▼
TIP:

A decrease in foot sweating can also be a sign that diabetic nerve damage is occurring in the nerves that control sweating. They just don't work normally. However, foot sweating also tends to decrease as we age, especially if we become less active. Wearing different shoes or socks can affect foot sweating, too. You may have recently started wearing shoes that do not hold in moisture, so your feet are drier.

The problem with a decrease in foot sweating, whatever the cause, is that the foot skin tends to become very dry and prone to cracking. It is a good idea to use a moisturizing cream or lotion on your feet (but not between the toes) if you have dry skin.

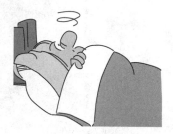

Why do my feet bother me more at night?

▼
TIP:

Nobody really knows the answer to this question. It is thought that the symptoms of diabetic nerve damage (pain, burning, tingling, numbness, etc.) are just more noticeable at night because the nerves of the feet and legs are not getting the other signals that they get during the day when you are up and about and walking more. Also during the day, you get a broad spectrum of sensory signals from things you see, hear, taste, touch, and smell that keep you busy and distracted from the neuropathy symptoms.

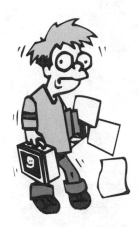

*C*an an unsteady gait be related to diabetic
nerve damage?

▼
TIP:

Yes! When a person has loss of feeling in his or her feet, the
positioning system of the body does not get normal responses
about where the feet are being placed. This can cause the person to
feel unsteady or to trip and stumble. People with nerve damage tend
to walk slower with a wide-based gait compared to how they walked
before having neuropathy. However, an unsteady gait can be a sign
of other problems, too—some of which can be quite serious. If you
are having trouble with your balance or walking, talk with your
provider.

If your trouble is due to nerve damage, it may be time to get a
cane. Your provider or physical therapist can help you get the right
length and give you tips on how to walk with a cane. A physical
therapist can also teach you balance exercises and how to increase
awareness of the position of your feet.

Sometimes diabetes-related muscle weakness can contribute to
unsteadiness in walking. Your provider or physical therapist can
show you muscle strengthening exercises. Some people need a
lightweight brace or ankle support to stabilize the ankles when
muscle weakness is the problem.

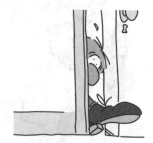

*W*hy does diabetic nerve damage affect the
feet first?

▼
TIP:

Nobody really knows the answer to this question. It is known
that the longest nerves are affected first and the longest nerves
are those traveling to the feet. A nerve has a cell body and then a
long nerve fiber extending from the cell body. It looks a little like a
root from a plant. Some people think that the long nerves are
affected first because the small nerve fibers at the end of long nerves
are the most distant from their cell bodies and are, therefore, the
most easily damaged. Other people think that all the nerves are
affected more or less equally and symptoms appear in the long
nerves first because there are more of these nerves to be damaged.

Chapter 9
COMPLICATIONS—
POOR CIRCULATION

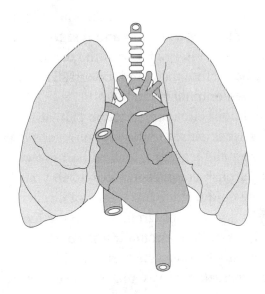

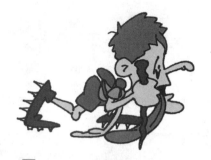

*H*ow do I know when I have poor
circulation in my feet and legs?

▼
TIP:

The hallmark sign of poor circulation is pain or cramping in the
calf or the thigh (usually the calf) that occurs when you walk a
short distance. This pain is a sign that the muscles are not getting
enough oxygen. If you slow or stop and rest for a few minutes, the
oxygen supply usually catches up with the demand and then you can
walk a little further before the pain reoccurs. The medical term for
this condition is "intermittent claudication."

Other signs of poor circulation can be pain at rest, nonhealing
ulcers, absent or weak pulses in the feet or legs, a decrease in blood
pressure in the feet and legs, or a lack of hair growth on the lower
legs. A blue or purplish color, especially when your feet are hanging
down, and having cold feet are also signs of circulation problems.

If you think you have poor circulation to the feet, ask your
provider to evaluate it. Poor circulation is caused by a blockage in
the arteries supplying blood to the feet. The blockage may need to
be removed or bypassed with vascular surgery. A simple treatment is
to walk every day. This exercise can force the blood vessels to
expand and improve the circulation in your feet and legs.

I have varicose veins. Does that mean I have poor circulation?

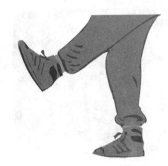

▼
TIP:

Varicose veins are a different type of poor circulation—a poor return of blood to the heart. Your feet are supplied with blood by arteries that carry blood down to them. Veins carry blood from the feet back to the heart. When you stand up, gravity tends to pull blood down towards your feet. Leg veins have valves in them to prevent this from happening. However, if the valves are damaged or too far apart, they do not close properly. This causes varicose veins, which tend to get very full and widen with blood. Varicose veins may look like blue snakes or rivers under the skin. Some of the fluid in the blood leaks out through very small veins (capillaries) and causes swelling. This pooling of blood can cause ulcers on the legs, but these are different from diabetic foot ulcers. Anyone can have varicose veins and leg ulcers.

Wearing support hose and exercise are the two main treatments for varicose veins. Support hose squeeze your legs and prevent blood from pooling in the veins. Exercise also helps keep blood from pooling. When your leg muscles contract, they squeeze nearby veins and help pump blood back to the heart. Surgery is reserved for very severe cases of varicose veins.

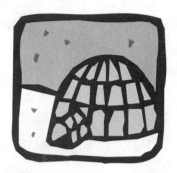

My feet are cold. Does this mean I have poor circulation? How can I warm them?

▼

TIP:

Many things can cause cold feet. It may be a sign of poor circulation, but it is not a reliable sign. If you think you have poor circulation, have your feet evaluated by your health care provider.

The best thing to do for cold feet is to wear one or two pairs of thick socks or warm house slippers. You can try the thin silk socks that are worn under regular socks for added warmth—but check to be sure that your shoes are not too tight. Getting up and walking around or getting regular exercise helps keep your feet warmer, too.

Do not use heating pads or hot water bottles on your feet. Don't sit too close to a space heater, fireplace, or campfire. If you have any diabetic nerve damage, you cannot feel when your feet are too hot or are getting burned, and you could be badly injured.

In addition to making your feet feel cold, nerve damage can affect blood flow and sweating in the feet. People with these problems are not able to release heat from their feet by dilating blood vessels the way someone without nerve damage would. It's best to wear socks and move around from time to time.

*O*ne or both of my feet are red, blue, purple, or darker than they used to be. What do these colors mean?

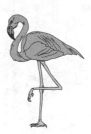

▼
TIP:

Changes in the color of the skin on your feet can mean many things, from having gangrene to having the dye from your socks rub off. Generally, a color change alone does not tell you enough to know whether it is caused by any specific disease.

Your health care provider will want to evaluate the color change along with other signs and symptoms. She or he will look at your skin; check the pulses in your thighs, ankles, and big toes; feel the temperature of your skin, check for infections and broken bones; and evaluate the blood circulation to your feet and legs.

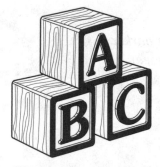

*W*hat *is peripheral vascular disease?*

▼
TIP:

Peripheral vascular disease (PVD) is commonly called "poor circulation" and refers to blockage in the blood supply to the feet. A buildup of plaque inside the arteries that carry blood to the feet causes them to thicken and harden. People without diabetes get this thickening and hardening of the arteries too, but unfortunately these problems can happen sooner and appear to be more severe in people with diabetes. PVD is 20 times more common in people with diabetes than in the general population. Other things that put you at risk of developing PVD are smoking, poor nutrition, lack of exercise, high blood fat levels (including cholesterol), and poor blood sugar control. Women are just as much at risk, and young as well as older people can develop it.

You can help to avoid or limit PVD by stopping smoking and controlling your blood fats levels and blood sugar levels as much as possible. See an RD for help with your meal plan and add more physical activity to your lifestyle.

*H*ow does diabetes cause PVD?

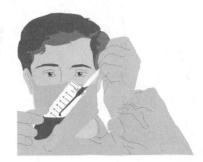

▼
TIP:

The fats in your blood, such as cholesterol and triglycerides, can build up on the walls of your arteries, thickening and hardening them. Diabetes often causes an increase in blood fats, which can lead to the thickening process. This is why your health care provider is concerned about checking your cholesterol and triglyceride levels, two important blood fats. If you have high cholesterol or high triglycerides, you may be asked to change your diet and to try to lose some weight. You may need to take medication to help control high cholesterol or high triglycerides.

It is important to control blood fats because the thickening of the arteries that leads to PVD can also cause heart attacks and strokes. You are at greater risk for these illnesses when you have diabetes.

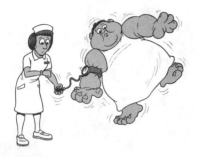

*W*hat does high blood pressure have to do with my feet?

▼
TIP:

High blood pressure (hypertension) damages the blood vessels all over your body and is associated with developing poor circulation. High blood pressure is most related to heart attacks, strokes, and kidney disease, but it also contributes to PVD. If you have diabetes, you need to try to control your blood pressure as well as you can. We know that 35–75% of all diabetic complications result from a combination of high blood pressure and diabetes.

You can help control your blood pressure by changing your meal plan and introducing more physical activity into your lifestyle.

W^{*hat kind of tests do I need for PVD?*}

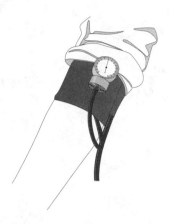

TIP:

Your health care provider will ask questions about your symptoms. He or she will examine your feet and legs and feel for foot and leg pulses, located in the groin, behind the knee, at the ankle, and on top of the foot. You may need to have the blood pressure in your ankle, arm, legs, and toes checked. (The arteries in toes don't get stiff, so measuring blood pressure there may be more accurate.) A Doppler machine may be used, and this test is painless. You may need a test to measure how much oxygen gets to the skin of your feet. If you have an ulcer that won't heal or areas of your foot that break down despite wearing properly fitted shoes, you may need tests such as special X rays and scans. These tests give pictures of the blood flow from your thigh to your toes. For angiogram or arteriogram X rays, you get an intravenous injection of a special solution so the blood vessels show up clearly on the X ray. This solution is called "dye," although it really does not change the color of anything. To keep the dye from causing problems in your kidneys, your provider will give you intravenous fluids before and after the procedure. If you have questions, ask your provider and the people performing the tests to explain things to you.

*W*hat does smoking have to do with my feet?

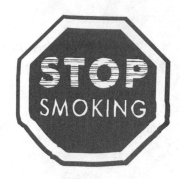

▼
TIP:

S moking is clearly connected to developing vascular (heart and blood vessel) disease. When you smoke, the combustion products of tobacco are absorbed in the bloodstream. These chemicals stimulate the release of other chemicals, which injure the blood vessels and encourage thickening and hardening of the arteries. Smoking also causes your blood vessels to constrict or clamp down, which limits the amount of blood that can circulate.

Smoking and diabetes are a deadly combination for the vascular system. Fortunately, there are many new medications and good programs to help people quit smoking. If you smoke and you're ready to quit, ask your health care provider to refer you to one of these programs to help you do it.

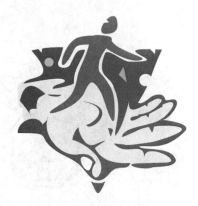

*A*re there any treatments for PVD?

▼
TIP:

Preventing vascular disease is much easier than treating it. That is why your health care provider will stress that you quit smoking, control blood pressure and blood sugar, control cholesterol and triglycerides, lose weight, and stay active. Taking an aspirin a day can help prevent heart attacks and strokes, so some people think this might help prevent PVD, too. Aspirin is not recommended for everyone and can interact with other medications you may be taking, so ask your provider before you start taking aspirin daily.

There are some medications your doctor can prescribe to treat PVD. If you have intermittent claudication (pain in your calves with walking), you might be asked to walk more. Usually you are encouraged to walk to the point of pain, pause, and then walk a little more. Ask your provider to give you instructions. Walking may help stimulate new vessels to grow and this will improve circulation.

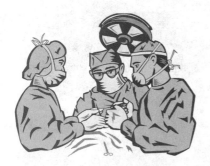

*W*ill I need surgery for PVD?

▼
TIP:

If the tests for PVD show that you have blockage in the larger arteries to your feet or legs, surgeons may try to correct it. One surgery that is not often used for patients with diabetes cleans out the artery that is blocked. Another method called angioplasty involves passing a deflated balloon on a tube to the point where the blockage occurs. Then the balloon is carefully inflated to open the narrowed artery and sometimes a stent (a tiny metal device shaped like a spring) is inserted in the artery to keep it open. This surgery is most successful with a small blockage in a healthy artery. A third surgical method is to bypass the blocked area by using a blood vessel from another part of the body (or an artificial blood vessel). While complicated, this surgery can help save a foot. People with diabetes often have many blockages in the arteries of the lower legs and feet, making it difficult to restore circulation. The relatively new ability to do bypass surgery down to the small arteries of the foot has saved many legs. Not all vascular surgeons do this surgery, so check to be sure that yours can. Your providers will carefully evaluate your condition before recommending surgery. If you must have surgery for PVD, ask your doctors to explain the procedure to you.

Chapter 10
OTHER FOOT PROBLEMS

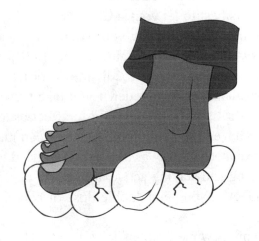

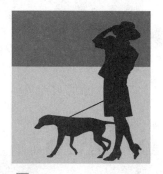

I have arthritis in my foot. How is this going to react with diabetes?

▼
TIP:

Arthritis is a general term that refers to wear and tear on the joints. There are different kinds of arthritis and different treatments for each kind. It is best to let your health care provider diagnose and treat any problems you are having with your joints. Don't assume that any pain, swelling, or stiffness in your foot is "just arthritis." There are many over-the-counter medications for treating arthritis, but consult your health care provider if you take these regularly.

Since both arthritis and diabetes tend to affect us as we get older, it is common to have both conditions. Arthritis can make it difficult for people with diabetes to stay as active as they need to be. However, because exercising and staying active are treatments for both arthritis and diabetes, you get a double dose of benefits whenever you exercise.

There are many new medications for arthritis. The current thinking is that arthritis should be treated more aggressively than it was in years past. Researchers think that starting treatment early could prevent much of the pain and disability associated with arthritis.

Arthritis can limit motion in the big toe joint, which can cause a callus or an ulcer under the big toe.

I have gout in my foot. How is this going to react with diabetes?

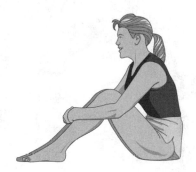

▼
TIP:

G out is a special type of arthritis caused by an excess of uric acid in the blood. Uric acid crystals tend to settle in joints in the lowest part of the body, which is why the big toe is most often affected. These crystals can cause the big toe joint to become extremely painful, red, warm, and swollen. If you have the symptoms of gout, your health care provider may withdraw some joint fluid and examine it under a microscope to look for these crystals. Medications and a special diet to lower the uric acid levels in the body are the main treatments for gout.

Sometimes it is difficult to tell the difference between gout and an infection caused by bacteria. So, if you think you might have gout, it is important to see your health care provider.

Repeated episodes of gout tend to damage the big toe joint and may make it stiff. This can cause a high-pressure spot on your foot that is more prone to developing callus and an ulcer. Be sure to check your feet daily for any signs of redness or ulceration.

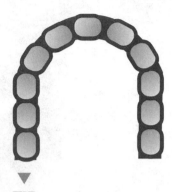

*W*hat is Charcot's joint and how do I recognize it?

▼
TIP:

Charcot's joint or Charcot foot is the term used to describe a severe deformity in a weight-bearing joint. A French physician named J. M. Charcot first described it in the 1860s. Charcot foot refers to the breakdown of the arch and normal foot structure in a person with nerve damage. Because Charcot's joint usually happens to people who have nerve damage, there is not much pain, even though they may have broken bones. There may be redness, swelling, and increased warmth of the foot. Your shoes won't fit. That's when people usually go to see their provider. Stay off that foot. The breakdown may occur fairly quickly. Sometimes it is difficult even for experts to tell the difference between Charcot's joint and infection.

Treatments for Charcot's joint are to immobilize the foot in a cast or special boot and rest the foot so it can heal. Sometimes surgery is done to realign the joints of the foot. If you continue to walk on a foot with Charcot's joint, you will make it much worse. If you can't get your regular shoes on, or if you have any changes in foot shape along with redness, swelling, or warmth, report this immediately to your health care provider.

*W*hat is osteomyelitis and how do I recognize it?

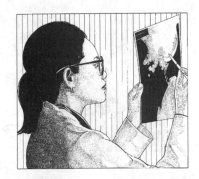

▼
TIP:

Osteomyelitis is the medical name for an infection in the bone. If you have a foot ulcer that is not healing well, your health care provider will want to examine your foot with an X ray or scan to determine whether the nearby bones have been affected. This is important because the treatments for bone infection and for soft tissue infection are different. It is also extremely difficult to heal foot ulcers over infected bone. Sometimes surgery is required to remove bone infections.

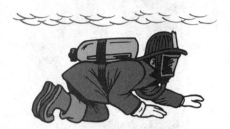

*W*hat is gangrene?
What causes it?

▼
TIP:

G angrene is a term that refers to death of the skin and the underlying tissues. The area of gangrene usually becomes dark brown or black. Once the tissue is dead, it will not grow back.

Severe circulation problems or infection can cause gangrene. Sometimes when a small toe becomes gangrenous, it may be left to just dry up and fall off. Other times the gangrene may be spreading and may need to be removed by surgery. You may need bypass surgery to improve circulation, which will help stop the gangrene from spreading, preserve as much of the toe or foot as possible, and prevent further problems.

I *had to have a toe amputation. Am I*
doomed?

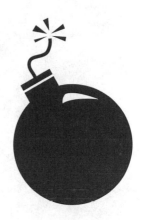

▼
TIP:

No, you are not doomed! However, once you have an amputation, you are at much higher risk for having another one. That is why you need to do everything you can to prevent diabetic foot problems. Check your feet daily, have your provider check your feet at every visit, and try to keep your blood fats and blood sugar levels as close to normal as possible. An amputation can "create" a foot deformity and put unusual pressure on the bones in your foot. You'll need orthotics, padding, or special shoes to be sure that you don't cause another ulcer on this foot. You might need physical therapy to learn how to walk smoothly. You would probably benefit from counseling or joining a support group of other people who have had amputations. You are likely to feel some pretty strong emotions after an experience like this.

Many people who have had a toe, foot, or leg amputation lead full and active lives. Medical science has made excellent breakthroughs in artificial limbs and rehabilitation for people with amputations.

101 MEDICATION TIPS

FOR PEOPLE WITH DIABETES

▲

A project of the
American Diabetes Association

▼

Written by

Betsy A. Carlisle, PharmD, CDE
Lisa A. Kroon, PharmD, CDE

101 MEDICATION TIPS FOR PEOPLE WITH DIABETES

▼

TABLE OF CONTENTS

Chapter 1
GENERAL INFORMATION
ABOUT MEDICATIONS
USED TO TREAT DIABETES

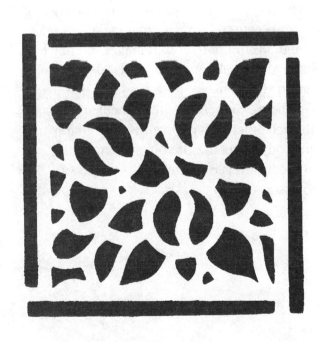

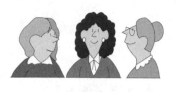

I have many friends and relatives with type 2 diabetes and not one of us is being treated with the same medications. Some of us take no medication at all, others are on a single medication, and even others are taking two or three medications. Two people I know are now using insulin injections. Why are there so many differences in the way we are treated?

▼
TIP:

With type 1 diabetes, the treatment is very straightforward. Because your pancreas no longer produces insulin, you must inject insulin. The treatment of type 2 diabetes is not as simple, because this type of diabetes is caused by many factors: a pancreas that does not produce enough insulin, a liver that makes too much glucose, or muscle cells that are not able to take in the glucose and use it for energy. Different medications are now available that treat these different causes of diabetes. Sometimes these medications are used in combination with each other or with insulin. The goal is to get enough insulin in your body—whether it comes from your pancreas with the help of medications or is injected—to move glucose into your cells to use as energy.

*W*hat medications are available to treat type 2 diabetes?

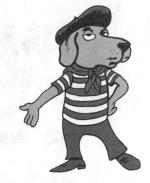

▼
TIP:

A long with insulin, there are five classes of medications available to treat type 2 diabetes. The table below describes the medications in each class. Generally, medications in the same class are not used together because they have the same effect.

Medication Class	Generic Name	Brand Name
Alpha-glucosidase inhibitors	Acarbose	Precose
	Miglitol	Glyset
Biguanides	Metformin*	Glucophage
		Glucophage XR**
Meglitinides	Repaglinide	Prandin
	Nateglinide	Starlix
Sulfonylureas	Glimepiride	Amaryl
	Glipizide*	Glucotrol
		Glucotrol XL***
	Glyburide*	DiaBeta
		Glynase
		Micronase
	Tolbutamide*	Orinase
	Tolazamide*	Tolinase
	Chlorpropamide*	Diabinese
Thiazolidinediones	Pioglitazone	Actos
	Rosiglitazone	Avandia
Combination Products	Rosiglitazone Metformin	Avandamet
	Glyburide Metformin	Glucovance
	Glipizide Metformin	Metaglip

 * Available generically.
 ** An extended version of metformin taken once daily.
*** An extended version of glipizide taken once daily.

101 Medication Tips for People with Diabetes

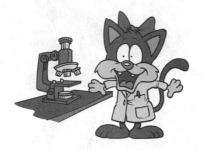

How do the medications listed on page 373 work to lower my blood glucose?

▼
TIP:

All of these medications work differently. Their main site of action in the body and the way in which they lower blood glucose is described in the table below.

Medication Class	Site of Action	Action
Alpha-glucosidase inhibitors (e.g., Acarbose, Miglitol)	Digestive system	Slows the breakdown of starches to glucose. Slows the entry of glucose into the bloodstream after a meal.
Biguanides (e.g., Metformin)	Liver	Decreases glucose production by the liver.
Meglitinides (e.g., Repaglinide, Nateglinide)	Pancreas	Stimulates insulin release by the pancreas in response to a meal.
Sulfonylureas (e.g., Glyburide, Glipizide)	Pancreas	Stimulates insulin release by the pancreas.
Thiazolidinediones (e.g., Pioglitazone, Rosiglitazone)	Muscle	Enhances glucose uptake by the muscle. Improves the body's sensitivity to insulin.

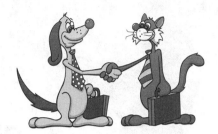

*A*re these oral medications the
same as insulin?

▼
TIP:

No. These medications are used to help your pancreas release
more insulin or help your own body's insulin work better in
lowering your blood glucose. Therefore, you must have a pancreas
that makes and releases insulin for these medications to work (the
exceptions are metformin, pioglitazone, or rosiglitazone, which
work well with insulin). Over time, some people with type 2
diabetes no longer are able to produce any insulin from their own
pancreas and must be treated with insulin injections.

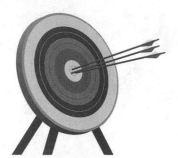

Do all medications used to treat type 2 diabetes work equally well?

▼ TIP:

No. Because the medications used to treat type 2 diabetes differ in the way that they work, they also have different abilities (called potency or strength) to lower your blood glucose. As a general rule, the sulfonylureas, repaglinide, and biguanides are more potent in lowering blood glucose than are the thiazolidinediones or alpha-glucosidase inhibitors when used as single agents.

Medication Class	Decreases Fasting Blood Glucose by*:	Decreases A1C by*:
Alpha-glucosidase Inhibitors (e.g., Acarbose)	10–20 mg/dl	0.5–1.0%
Biguanides (e.g., Metformin)	50–70 mg/dl	1.5–1.7%
Meglitinides		
Repaglinide	60–70 mg/dl	1.5–1.7%
Nateglinide	60–70 mg/dl	1.5–1.7%
Sulfonylureas (e.g., Glipizide or Glyburide)	50–70 mg/dl	1.5–1.7%
Thiazolidinediones (e.g., Pioglitazone, Rosiglitazone)	40 mg/dl	0.8–1.5%

*Each person will respond differently.

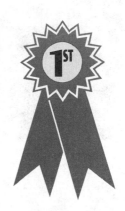

*I*s there a "best" medication to treat
diabetes?

▼

TIP:

S ometimes. There are many factors that help you and your doctor
decide which is the best medication for you. People with type 2
diabetes who are overweight often release adequate amounts of
insulin from their pancreas, but their muscle and fat cells are unable
to respond normally, and their liver manufacturers large amounts of
excess glucose. For these people, metformin (Glucophage) may be a
good choice for initial therapy because it is very effective and
doesn't cause weight gain. Patients who have insufficient amounts of
insulin may respond better to sulfonylureas. Other people may have
problems with their blood glucose rising immediately following
meals. Acarbose (Precose), repaglinide (Prandin), or nateglinide
(Starlix) may be good choices for these people. These factors, along
with your current blood glucose levels and the potency (strength) of
the different medications, help you and your doctor select the most
appropriate medication for you. While there may be several possible
medications to control your blood glucose, other factors, such as the
cost of the medication, the number of times per day you have to take
it, preexisting health problems (called contraindications), and
possible side effects, also help determine which medication is the
best for you.

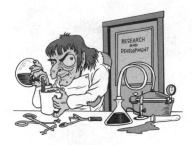

*H*ow will I know if my medication is working?

▼
TIP:

The American Diabetes Association recommends a target plasma glucose level between 80 and 120 milligrams per deciliter (mg/dl). Another measure of overall blood glucose control over a two to three month period is the glycosylated hemoglobin value, or A1C. This value should be less than 7% if the upper normal value at your laboratory is 6% (normal values vary from 4% to 6% at different laboratories). The table below correlates the A1C value with the mean plasma glucose value. It is difficult to tell whether your medication is working without these laboratory tests or without testing your blood glucose values at home. Many people have few or mild symptoms that warn them of high blood glucose concentrations and are surprised when they are told they have diabetes. Some people may notice that their energy levels are increased or that they urinate less after they have been placed on medication.

A1C	Mean Plasma Glucose (mg/dl)
6%	135
7%	170
8%	205
9%	240
10%	275
11%	310
12%	345

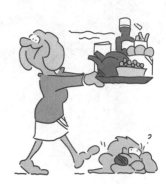

I have controlled my diabetes with diet, but my doctor recently prescribed a medication. Do I still need to follow my diet?

▼
TIP:

Absolutely. The very first step in the treatment of type 2 diabetes is dietary improvement, combined with exercise, to achieve and maintain your desired body weight and lower your blood glucose levels. Medications are added to diet and exercise therapy when your blood glucose levels exceed your recommended goals. Although some patients are able to control their blood glucose and avoid taking medication by following their meal plans and getting regular exercise, most will eventually require the help of medications as well. Typically, a single medication is added to diet and exercise, using the smallest dose that will help you achieve the desired blood glucose range. All medications (including insulin) work best when you follow dietary guidelines designed by a registered dietitian. By following your meal plan, you may be able to control your diabetes with low doses of a single medication. It is worthwhile to keep your medication plan as simple as you can for as long as possible.

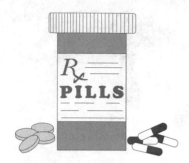

Why am I taking two different medications to treat my diabetes?

TIP:

Two medications (this is called combination therapy) are used to treat type 2 diabetes when the highest dose of a single medication no longer keeps blood glucose values within the desired range. Using two medications that work in different ways to lower your blood glucose often means you can take lower doses of each medication and possibly avoid side effects. Combination therapy can also delay the need for insulin injections for some people.

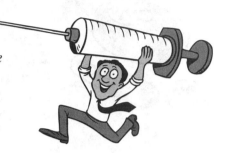

*M*y doctor warned me that I am
taking the highest possible dose
of glyburide and that I may have to
inject insulin in the future. I am
extremely afraid of needles. Is there
any way I can avoid insulin therapy?

▼
TIP:

It depends. There may be other treatment options you can ask for
to delay the need for insulin therapy. Studies show that when you
add a medication that lowers your blood glucose in a different way
to your plan, you might be able to lower your blood glucose further.
Taking a combination of medications and faithfully following your
meal plan and exercise program may help delay the need for insulin
therapy. Over time, however, the pancreas of many people with
type 2 diabetes stops producing insulin. At this point, they must
inject insulin to control their blood glucose levels. Some people
inject a small dose of insulin at bedtime while continuing to take
their medication(s) during the day. While it is normal to be afraid of
needles, you might be surprised to realize that the injections are
relatively painless. You'll inject insulin into the fat layer beneath
your skin (where there are fewer nerve endings) using very short
and thin (referred to as fine gauge) needles. Proper training on
injection techniques will help your anxiety and discomfort and will
help you adapt to insulin therapy quite easily.

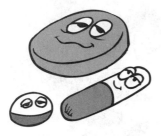

I am now taking two different medications to treat my diabetes, but my blood glucose keeps getting higher. Can I avoid injecting insulin by taking three different pills to treat my diabetes?

▼
TIP:

It's possible. However, the published information about the proper use of three different medications in combination is limited. Also, the cost of the triple therapy and the increased potential for drug side effects and interactions must be considered. You and your doctor must weigh the benefits and risks in deciding whether triple therapy or the addition of a single insulin injection to your current therapy is the best way to treat your diabetes.

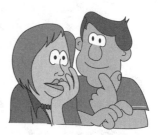

I have a friend with type 2 diabetes who takes insulin injections and tests her blood glucose at home. I am taking a combination of glyburide and metformin. No one ever told me to test my blood glucose. Should I be checking my blood glucose at home, too?

▼
TIP:

Performing blood glucose measurements at home by using a device called a glucose meter will tell you whether or not your diabetes is in good control on a daily basis. Most glucose meters are "plasma referenced," which means the glucose concentrations correlate better to laboratory values. Self-monitoring your blood glucose gives you valuable information on the effect of foods, exercise, stress, or illness on your blood glucose. The results of self-monitored blood glucose testing also help your doctor adjust your current medication regimen. While glucose testing is very useful, insurance plans do vary in their coverage of blood glucose testing supplies such as test strips, lancet devices, and lancets. The bottom line is that all patients who have access to a meter and are capable of obtaining accurate results should self-monitor blood glucose to achieve and maintain good glucose control.

Chapter 2
HOW TO GET THE MOST OUT OF YOUR ORAL MEDICATIONS

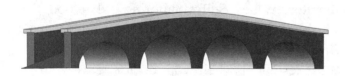

If I forget to take my medication, should I take two pills for the next dose?

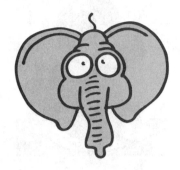

▼
TIP:

As a general rule, you can take a missed dose of any medication as soon as you remember it. However, if you forget to take a dose and it is almost time for your next scheduled dose, skip the missed dose and go back to your regular dosing schedule. Do **not** take a double dose. There are some exceptions to this rule when it comes to medications used to treat your diabetes. If you miss a dose of repaglinide (Prandin) or nateglinide (Starlix), taking the dose between meals could result in a low blood glucose reaction. Therefore, you should not take a missed dose of repaglinide or nateglinide between scheduled mealtimes. These medications are to be taken at mealtime only. If you miss a dose of acarbose (Precose) or miglitol (Glyset), you should resume your usual regimen at the next scheduled meal, since their action relies on slowing the absorption of high-starch foods.

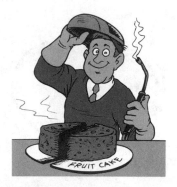

During the holidays when I know I will be eating more, can I increase the amount of medication I am taking to keep my blood glucose under control?

▼
TIP:

Unlike insulin therapy where the amount of insulin can be adjusted to match the carbohydrate portion, it is very difficult to determine how to adjust an oral medication in a similar manner. Trying to increase the dose of your oral diabetes medication during the holidays may result in a low blood glucose reaction. A better idea would be to try to stick to your meal plan as much as possible and increase the frequency of your blood glucose testing to detect any significant elevations in your blood glucose levels.

Should I take my medication on an empty stomach or with food?

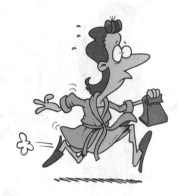

▼
TIP:

Generally, most of the medications used to treat type 2 diabetes can be taken without regard to a full or empty stomach. However, there are some exceptions.

- Acarbose (Precose) should be taken with the first bite of a meal for maximum benefit.
- Metformin (Glucophage) should be taken with meals to minimize stomach upset.
- Replaglinide (Prandin) and nateglinide (Starlix) should be taken within 30 minutes of a meal for maximum benefit and to avoid low blood glucose.

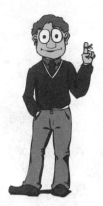

When I refilled my prescription for glipizide, I noticed that the label says to take it 30 minutes before my meals, but sometimes I forget and take it after I eat. Will my medication still work?

▼
TIP:

While some manufacturers suggest taking glipizide 30 minutes before a meal, it has not been proven that this makes any significant difference in the effect of the medication on lowering your blood glucose level. Therefore, you should take your medication as soon as you remember it (see page 385).

*I*s there a best time of the day to take my
medication?

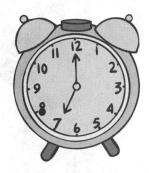

▼
TIP:

This depends on how many times of the day you are supposed to take it. If you take once-daily medications with the same meal each day, you're less likely to forget to take them. It's best to take twice-daily medications with breakfast and your evening meal. Repaglinide (Prandin), nateglinide (Starlix), acarbose (Precose), and miglitol (Glyset) should generally be taken three times daily with meals. Metformin (Glucophage) should be taken with meals, whether taken two or three times daily with the immediate-release form, or once daily with your evening meal for the extended-release form.

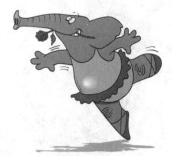

I would like to start an exercise program. Do I need to adjust the dose of my medication if I exercise?

TIP:

During exercise, glucose can enter the muscles without the help of insulin. Because of this, people who exercise vigorously may experience low blood glucose during or immediately following exercise. Exercise also can enhance your body's ability to use glucose. If you inject insulin, you can adjust your insulin dose based on your blood glucose levels before and after exercise. However, there are no such guidelines for adjusting oral medications. Since you are just starting an exercise program, it's important for you to measure your blood glucose levels before and after you exercise. If regular exercise causes a substantial and sustained drop in your daily blood glucose levels or a significant weight loss, the daily dosage of your diabetes medication may need to be decreased by your doctor.

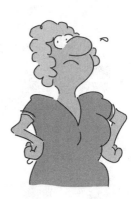

*M*y mother is 70 years old and has just been diagnosed with type 2 diabetes. Her doctor wants to start her on a medication. Is this really necessary at her age?

▼ TIP:

It may be, since diabetes in the elderly can lead to serious complications such as heart disease, stroke, and eye disease if left untreated. Although it may take years for these conditions to develop, your mother may live another 20 years. Diet and exercise are the initial steps in treatment. Her doctor will carefully consider other medical conditions your mother may have before selecting the best medication for her, and will prescribe the smallest effective dose. The doctor will also review any other medications your mother is using to avoid any possible drug interactions. Since kidney and liver function can decline with age, her doctor will order regular blood tests to monitor any need to alter your mother's dose of medication.

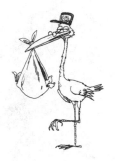

I missed my menstrual cycle and may be pregnant. Will my diabetes medications harm my baby?

▼
TIP:

If you think you may be pregnant, it's important to make an appointment with your doctor immediately so that he or she can evaluate the safety of taking your oral medications. Be sure to tell your doctor if you are planning to become pregnant. Close control of your blood glucose by using insulin injections during your pregnancy reduces the chance of your baby gaining too much weight, having birth defects, or having high or low blood glucose. Once you have delivered your baby and have stopped nursing, you should be able to discontinue insulin therapy and return to taking your oral medications. If you are already using insulin, the amount of insulin you will need to control your blood glucose will change during and after pregnancy. Insulin does not pass into breast milk and will not affect a nursing infant. However, you may need less insulin while breastfeeding than you were using before your pregnancy.

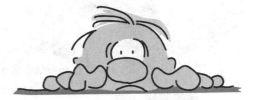

I was told my kidney function is beginning to decline. Will this affect my medication?

▼
TIP:

Your kidneys play an important role in removing medications from your body. Thus, the effect of oral medications or insulin on lowering your blood glucose may be increased because they stay in your bloodstream longer. If this is the case, you may need a smaller dose to control your blood glucose. Laboratory tests such as blood samples and urine collections can be performed to measure how well your kidneys are working. The oral medication of most concern with reduced kidney function is metformin, because of the increased risk for lactic acidosis (high amounts of lactic acid in the blood; see page 406). Certain medications you may be taking for other medical conditions may also slow down the removal of your diabetes medications by your kidneys, so be sure and tell your doctor about anything else you are taking.

I was referred to a heart doctor who gave me a medication called digoxin for heart failure. She told me she would have to change my diabetes medication from metformin to glyburide. Why?

▼
TIP:

Patients with congestive heart failure may be at greater risk for developing lactic acidosis (high amounts of lactic acid in the blood; see page 406) from metformin therapy. The reason for this is that people with heart failure cannot pump blood throughout the body as effectively. This means blood flow to your kidneys is reduced and the amount of metformin in your body may begin to accumulate. Larger amounts of lactic acid may be produced in people who have high amounts of metformin in their bloodstream and also by people who have heart failure. Because rare reports of lactic acidosis in patients with heart failure have been documented, the manufacturer of metformin warns against using this medication in patients with congestive heart failure requiring treatment with medications such as digoxin (Lanoxin), furosemide (Lasix), or captopril (Capoten).

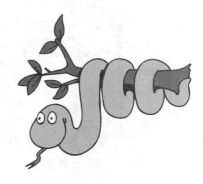

I am allergic to sulfa antibiotics such as Bactrim. Am I more likely to be allergic to any of the medications used to treat diabetes?

▼
TIP:

It's possible that people with allergies to sulfonamide-type medications, such as sulfa antibiotics or thiazide diuretics (water pills), develop allergies when using sulfonylurea medications, such as glyburide. Although cases of cross-reactivity (actually developing an allergy from a sulfonylurea) are rare, if you have a severe allergic reaction (hives, breathing problems, or severe rash), it would be better for you to use a different medication than a sulfonylurea, if you can use one that is as effective. Talk to your doctor to weigh the benefits and risks.

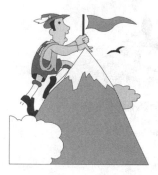

Both my friend and I take glyburide. She takes a 5 mg tablet two times daily and I take two 5 mg tablets once daily in the morning. Which is the better way to take this medication?

TIP:

The number of times a medication is given during the day is based on something called the "half-life" of the medication. This term refers to the amount of time it takes for about one-half of the medication to be removed from your body. When glyburide was first introduced to the market, it was thought that its half-life was only a few hours and that its effect lasted approximately 12 hours. Thus, glyburide was given twice daily. Now that glyburide has been used extensively in many people, it has been determined that its effect lasts 24 hours or longer. That means it can be given once a day. Whether you take glyburide once or twice daily makes no difference on its ability to lower your blood glucose; however, most people find taking glyburide once daily is easier to remember.

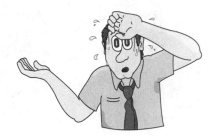

I have been taking 20 mg of glipizide (Glucotrol) two times daily. My doctor just added metformin (Glucophage) to my therapy. I've read that this medication does not cause low blood glucose reactions. Is this true?

▼

TIP:

Yes, but only when metformin is used by itself. You can divide the oral medications currently available to treat type 2 diabetes into two groups: Group #1, hypoglycemic agents such as the sulfonylureas (Glucotrol), repaglinide (Prandin), nateglinide (Starlix) and insulin; and Group #2, antihyperglycemic agents such as metformin (Glucophage), rosiglitazone (Avandia), pioglitazone (Actos), and acarbose (Precose). Group #2 medications lower blood glucose but do not carry a risk for causing low blood glucose reactions (hypoglycemia) when used by themselves. However, when Group #2 medications are used in combination with Group #1 medications, the risk of hypoglycemia increases. Therefore, as your final dose of metformin is determined, you should monitor yourself for symptoms of hypoglycemia (you may sweat, feel nervous, or tremble) and report any of them to your doctor. You should also perform more frequent self-monitoring of blood glucose.

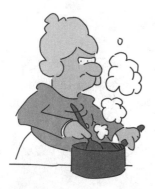

I have been taking 850 mg of metformin twice daily with meals. Now my doctor has added repaglinide (Prandin) to my therapy, and I was told not to take this new medication if I skip a meal. If I do skip a meal, should I also skip my dose of metformin?

▼
TIP:

No. Because repaglinide lowers blood glucose very quickly (usually within 1 hour after taking it), you should only take repaglinide with meals to avoid hypoglycemia. In contrast, metformin does not cause hypoglycemia when taken by itself, so you should still take it.

Chapter 3
COMMON SIDE EFFECTS
OF ORAL MEDICATIONS

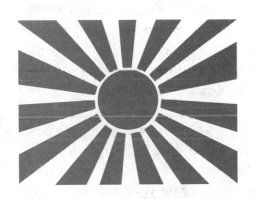

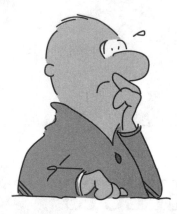

*I am taking acarbose (Precose) and have
been experiencing gas, cramps, and
diarrhea. Could my medication be causing
these symptoms?*

TIP:

Yes. Stomach upset, gas, and diarrhea can occur in people taking
acarbose (Precose) and miglitol (Glyset). This is because these
medications work by slowing the digestion of carbohydrates, and
their presence in your digestive tract causes these symptoms. Your
stomach pain and diarrhea will lessen with time and usually
disappear. However, your symptoms of gas may not go away
entirely. You can minimize these effects by starting with very low
doses of acarbose, such as 25 mg once daily, and increasing the dose
very slowly over several months. The usual dose is 50 mg with each
meal, although up to 100 mg can be used. If you are in a lot of
discomfort, ask your doctor if you can decrease your dose of
acarbose and make any necessary increases more slowly.

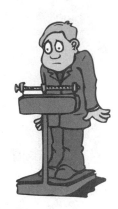

A fter my doctor started me on glyburide, my blood glucose got better, but I have gained 8 pounds. Is this caused by my medication?

▼
TIP:

A long with better glucose control, people taking glyburide or other sulfonylureas often experience weight gain. This is because these medications stimulate insulin release from the pancreas. This means less glucose is lost in the urine. Also, high insulin levels in the bloodstream can stimulate your appetite and promote food storage as fat. You may feel more hungry and ultimately gain weight—sometimes up to 4 to 8 pounds. A significant amount of weight gain can cause you to need a larger dose of medication to control your blood glucose. To avoid this problem, you should continue to follow your prescribed meal plan and exercise, and be alert for any increased appetite or subsequent weight gain.

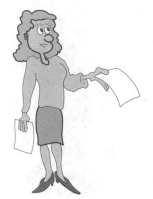

My doctor has given me a prescription for rosiglitazone (Avandia). What are the side effects of this medication?

▼
TIP:

Rosiglitazone (Avandia) is one of the newer medications available for the treatment of type 2 diabetes. It works by improving the ability of your muscle to respond to your body's own insulin or insulin that you may be injecting. Rosiglitazone is usually taken once or twice daily, and is generally well tolerated. Some side effects you may experience include symptoms of hypoglycemia, fluid retention, and weight gain. A drug similar to rosiglitazone (troglitazone or Rezulin) was removed from the market because in rare occasions it was associated with liver problems (see page 405). So far, rosiglitazone and another drug in this class, pioglitazone (Actos), seem safer in this regard. Even so, it is important to watch for liver problems. You can help monitor your liver function in between your periodic blood tests by immediately reporting to your doctor any unusual symptoms of nausea, vomiting, fatigue, or dark urine.

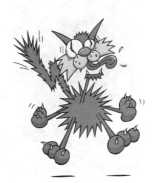

I sometimes feel shaky, nervous, and sweaty. Is this a side effect from my diabetes medication?

▼
TIP:

Possibly, especially if you are taking any medications in the sulfonylurea class, repaglinide (Prandin), nateglinide (Starlix), or insulin. These symptoms are typical warning signals from your body that your blood glucose is dropping below a normal level and you are experiencing hypoglycemia. Because your brain always needs a certain concentration of glucose in your bloodstream to function, these symptoms generally occur when blood glucose values fall below 70 mg/dl. However, the exact concentration at which these warning symptoms occur varies from person to person. While the reason you are having these symptoms could be from taking too much medication, other possible causes include a skipped meal, extra exercise, a drug interaction with your diabetes medication and another medication, or a change in your kidney or liver function. It is very important to recognize what these symptoms mean so that you can appropriately treat your hypoglycemia (see page 404). You also need to figure out what caused the hypoglycemia so you can prevent it next time. If you have frequent hypoglycemia, it is important to notify your health care provider, since your medication dose may have to be reduced.

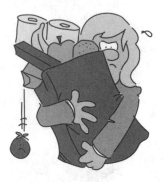

Should I buy glucose tablets to treat my hypoglycemia?

▼
TIP:

Not necessarily. Hypoglycemia should be treated with 10 to 15 grams of a quickly absorbed carbohydrate (glucose or starch). Examples of food sources containing 10 to 15 grams of carbohydrate include 1/2 cup orange juice, 1/3 cup apple juice, two teaspoonfuls of sugar (or 2 cubes), or 5 to 6 pieces of Lifesavers candy. Unfortunately, because hunger is a symptom of hypoglycemia, many people overtreat hypoglycemia by ingesting large amounts of glucose (for example, 1 or 2 candy bars) which results in hyperglycemia (high blood glucose levels). Because glucose tablets are a premeasured source of glucose (5 grams of glucose per tablet), you may find them easier to use. You also may find it convenient to carry glucose tablets with you when you are working or traveling.

*M*y doctor has prescribed
pioglitazone (Actos) for my
diabetes, but told me I will need to
have frequent blood tests to check my
liver's ALT level. What is this?

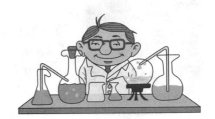

▼
TIP:

U nlike troglitazone (Rezulin), which was removed from the
market due to liver toxicity, pioglitazone (Actos) and
rosiglitazone (Avandia) have not been associated with liver injury.
However, the Food and Drug Administration (FDA) still
recommends periodic measurements of liver function tests for both
drugs. Testing should be performed prior to starting therapy and
then periodically thereafter per the judgement of your health care
professional (e.g., every 6 months). When the liver is damaged by a
medication, a substance called alanine aminotransferase (often
abbreviated as ALT) is released into the bloodstream. In most cases,
ALT levels return to normal when you stop taking the medication.
Therefore, it is very important to keep your appointments to have
your ALT level checked. Any symptoms of nausea, abdominal pain,
fatigue, itching, or yellowing of your skin should also be reported
immediately to your doctor, since these symptoms could also
indicate a problem with your liver.

I read that metformin (Glucophage) could cause lactic acidosis. What is this and how would I know if I had it?

TIP:

L actic acid is a substance that is normally produced by your body in small amounts and removed by your liver and kidneys. Lactic acidosis occurs when this substance builds up in the bloodstream. The risk of developing lactic acidosis is greater if you have other health conditions, such as heart failure and lung, kidney, or liver problems. Your doctor should do a blood test prior to starting metformin to assess your liver and kidney function. If you have any of the above health problems or if you drink alcohol heavily, you probably shouldn't take metformin. Otherwise, you are at a very low risk for developing lactic acidosis from metformin. You should, however, contact your doctor immediately if you suddenly develop diarrhea, fast and shallow breathing, muscle pain or cramping, tiredness, weakness, or unusual sleepiness. These can be symptoms of lactic acidosis. You should also let your doctor know if you get the flu or any illness that results in severe vomiting, diarrhea, and/or fever, or if your intake of fluids becomes significantly reduced. This is because severe dehydration can affect your kidney or liver function and increase your risk of lactic acidosis from metformin.

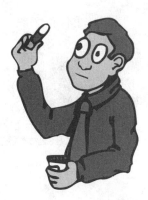

I'm going to have an X-ray of my kidneys and was told to stop taking my metformin. Why?

▼

TIP:

Special X-ray and radiologic tests that require the injection of a dye often cause your kidneys to be temporarily less efficient in clearing lactic acid and other substances from the body. To lessen the risk for lactic acidosis during such a procedure, metformin is stopped before the test and restarted about 48 hours afterwards. Before restarting your metformin, you should have a blood test to make sure that your kidneys are working normally again.

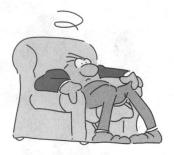

Since I have started taking metformin (Glucophage), I have experienced stomach cramps and diarrhea. Should I stop taking my medication?

▼
TIP:

No. Stomach upset and diarrhea occur commonly during the first two weeks of beginning metformin (Glucophage) therapy and usually disappear after a few weeks. Taking each metformin dose with a meal can help reduce stomach discomfort. However, if you have severe discomfort or these side effects do not go away over time, you should contact your doctor. You may need your current dose of metformin lowered or you may need to stop taking metformin, either temporarily or permanently.

I am taking repaglinide (Prandin) for my diabetes. Does this medication have any side effects?

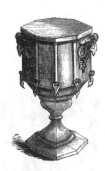

▼
TIP:

The most common side effects reported with the use of repaglinide (Prandin) are hypoglycemia and weight gain. Hypoglycemia can be avoided by taking repaglinide with meals. If you skip a meal, you should skip your dose of repaglinide. Mild weight gain from repaglinide occurs in people being newly treated for diabetes, but usually does not occur in people being switched from a sulfonylurea drug, such as glyburide, to repaglinide therapy.

Chapter 4
GENERAL INFORMATION ABOUT THE USE OF INSULIN IN TYPE 2 DIABETES

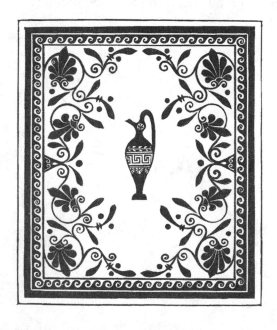

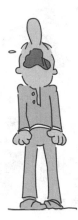

*M*y doctor recently switched me from taking two different medications for my diabetes to insulin therapy. Does this mean my diabetes is getting worse?

▼
TIP:

Not necessarily, but it may be changing. In the early phases of diabetes, the pancreas of a person with type 2 diabetes has a greater ability to make insulin than in the later stages of diabetes. Therefore, medications that stimulate the pancreas to make more insulin work better in people who have had diabetes for fewer than 10 to 15 years. As years go by, insulin levels decline and it becomes necessary to supplement the insulin made by the pancreas with insulin injections. Other possible explanations for rising blood glucose levels include weight gain, a decline in your activity or exercise level, a change in your eating habits, taking your medication irregularly, illness, infection, or emotional stress. Depending on your glucose level and other medical conditions, insulin may be needed, either temporarily or permanently.

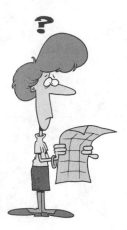

A friend of mine was recently switched from two different oral medications to insulin therapy alone. My doctor added a single injection of insulin at bedtime to my glipizide (Glucotrol). Why didn't my doctor add another kind of medication to my glipizide instead?

▼

TIP:

There are no "recipes" for treating diabetes, because every person's circumstance is unique. When people with type 2 diabetes begin to respond poorly to a combination of oral medications, some diabetes doctors have them discontinue all oral medications and start insulin therapy, because they believe failure to respond to medications means that the pancreas is no longer producing enough insulin. Others choose instead to add a single dose of intermediate to long-acting insulin at bedtime to one or two oral medications, because they believe that the pancreas can still release insulin with the help of an oral medication when food is eaten. With this method, the insulin at bedtime helps control glucose production by the liver during the night, thus controlling glucose levels in the morning. The oral medications then work to maintain reasonable blood glucose levels throughout the day. Both methods can work.

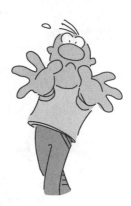

I am now taking the highest doses of Glucovance (metformin plus glyburide). My blood glucose level continues to rise, and my doctor has told me I will most likely need to begin insulin injections. Are there any other medications I can take to avoid this?

▼

TIP:

Maybe. You can try to delay insulin therapy through more rigorous attention to diet and exercise, or perhaps by adding yet another oral medication. However, currently up to 58% of people with type 2 diabetes must take insulin. Insulin is needed to achieve and maintain blood glucose levels that prevent or slow progression of kidney, eye, and nerve problems. If your pancreas is no longer able to make enough insulin (see page 411), you'll need to supplement this lost insulin with injections. Unfortunately, patients and health care providers alike may have an unreasonable fear of insulin injections. You'll be relieved to hear that insulin injections are virtually painless. This is because needles are now much sharper, thinner, and shorter than before. People who begin insulin therapy commonly report feeling much healthier and more energetic, so it's worth overcoming your fears to try this therapy.

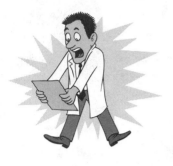

I have been injecting 40 units of NPH insulin each evening and taking metformin twice daily. I have very high blood glucose levels before dinner, and now my doctor has asked me to inject insulin twice daily, in the morning and before supper. Why do I need to do this?

▼
TIP:

The high dinner blood glucose values indicate that the effect of a single dose of NPH insulin is not lasting for 24 hours. NPH and lente insulins are both intermediate-acting insulins. They look milky because the insulin is contained in a small particle that takes some time to dissolve and reach the bloodstream once it is injected under the skin. Although these insulins are said to last for 12 to 24 hours, their duration of action will depend on the site of injection and dose. The larger the dose, the longer the duration. However, if a single dose of insulin is increased so that it will last for 24 hours, there is a greater danger of hypoglycemia, especially if you skip a meal during the day. By splitting the injections, very high and very low insulin levels are avoided and it becomes easier to maintain desirable blood glucose levels. See page 474 for an additional insulin therapy tip with insulin glargine (Lantus).

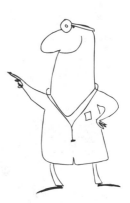

I have been taking two injections of NPH insulin each day. Now my doctor has asked me to begin "mixing" two different kinds of insulin. Why is this necessary?

▼
TIP:

Your doctor is trying to improve your blood glucose control. Although NPH insulin lasts for 12 to 24 hours, it may take 2 to 4 hours to begin working because the insulin particles dissolve so slowly. Because of this, NPH does not work very well to control the blood glucose that rises after you have eaten a meal. For this, you will need an insulin that gets into the body more quickly and has a shorter duration of action. Three types of insulins are available and used for this purpose: regular insulin, insulin lispro (Humalog), and insulin aspart (Novolog). (Insulin glulisine [Apidra] is a rapid-acting insulin that received FDA approval in April 2004. It is also used for mealtime blood sugar control.) If you look at these insulins, they are clear, like water, because the insulin crystals are dissolved. Thus, they reach the bloodstream much more quickly and are used to control the blood glucose at meals.

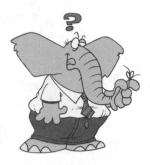

I'm supposed to inject regular insulin 30 minutes before I eat, but it seems I can never predict exactly when that will be. What happens if I take my insulin right when I start eating?

TIP:

You are not alone. Many people find it hard to time their insulin injections in relation to meals. In the ideal world, it is best to have high levels of insulin in the bloodstream at the same time glucose arrives there from a meal you have just eaten. Since it can take 30 to 60 minutes for regular insulin to reach your bloodstream after it is injected, if you wait until mealtime to inject it, you run the risk of hyperglycemia—too much glucose in the bloodstream and not enough insulin to handle it. Conversely, you may experience hypoglycemia 3 to 4 hours after a meal because regular insulin remains active for up to 6 hours. There are two rapid-acting insulins—insulin lispro (Humalog) and insulin aspart (Novolog)—that might be a good option for you (see page 417) since they can be injected right before a meal (within 15 minutes).

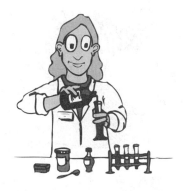

*I read about some "insulin analogs"
called insulin lispro (Humalog) and
insulin aspart (Novolog). What are these?*

▼
TIP:

These are rapid-acting insulins that can be taken immediately before a meal (within 5–15 minutes). This feature makes these insulins more convenient than regular insulin for people with very busy or unpredictable meal schedules. However, because lispro and aspart are very rapid-acting, you must eat within 15 minutes of taking them to avoid a possible low blood glucose reaction. A potential disadvantage of these insulins is that blood glucose can rise again before the next meal because they are so short-acting. To counteract this, many patients must take a long-acting insulin as well, such as NPH or insulin glargine (Lantus). Like regular insulin, lispro and aspart can be mixed with longer-acting insulins, but the mixture should be injected soon after the insulins are mixed to make certain the rapid-acting features of these insulins are retained. Insulin lispro and insulin aspart are available by prescription only.

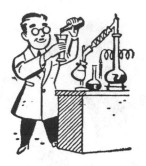

I currently have to mix two different types of insulin. I understand there is a type of insulin that comes already mixed. Can I be switched to this product?

▼

TIP:

Perhaps. It depends on the types of insulins you are mixing and the doses of each. You may have heard of 70/30 and 50/50 products, which are mixtures of intermediate-acting NPH and short-acting regular insulin. The first number refers to the percentage of NPH present and the second number refers to the percentage of regular present in the injected dose. For example, if you inject 10 units of 70/30 insulin, you are taking 7 units of NPH and 3 units of regular insulin. If you currently take NPH and regular insulin in this ratio, it is likely that you could use the premixed product instead with equal results. Premixed insulins can greatly simplify insulin therapy, but they offer very little flexibility in meal planning. This is because the dose of the short-acting insulin, in particular, is strongly determined by the amount of carbohydrate in each meal. Humalog Mix 75/25 and Novolog Mix 70/30 are premixed products containing an intermediate-acting insulin in combination with the rapid-acting insulin lispro (Humalog) or insulin aspart (Novolog), respectively. Premixed insulins are usually taken twice daily, before breakfast and before dinner.

I now have to inject insulin three and sometimes four times daily. Does this mean I have a more severe form of diabetes?

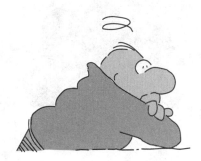

▼
TIP:

No. This means that your health care provider is trying to deliver insulin into your bloodstream in a way that mimics the normal release of insulin from the pancreas. In someone without diabetes, the pancreas constantly releases just the right amount of insulin to keep the blood glucose concentration between 70 and 120 mg/dl at all times. This means that rapid bursts of insulin are released every time food is eaten in amounts that exactly match the carbohydrate content of the meal or snack. In between meals, the pancreas releases very low levels of insulin that prevent the liver from producing and releasing too much glucose into the bloodstream. So you use shorter-acting insulins to provide bursts of insulin before meals and longer-acting insulins to provide low levels of insulin between meals. Often, it is possible to achieve better glucose control over 24 hours with lower total daily doses of insulin by using smaller doses of insulin injected more frequently. Insulin pumps deliver insulin by a similar mechanism.

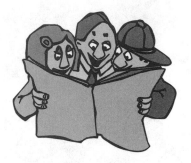

Everyone I know who is taking insulin seems to be on a different dose. What is a "normal dose" of insulin?

▼
TIP:

U nfortunately, there is no "normal dose" of insulin. Because some people are very resistant to the action of insulin, they require higher doses. Your own insulin requirement may vary, going up when you are ill, or coming down if you exercise or eat less. There is a way to evaluate your insulin dose, however. Someone without diabetes makes about 40 units of insulin a day. You can estimate the amount of insulin you would need if you didn't have diabetes by dividing your body weight in pounds by 4. For example, if you weigh 200 pounds, your estimated daily need would be about 50 units. Now, add together all your insulin doses to compute your total daily dose. A dose that is much higher than 50 units suggests that your body is resistant to insulin action and therefore requires more than the usual amounts of insulin. A dose that is far lower than 50 units suggests that your body is more sensitive to insulin and that your own pancreas is still making and releasing insulin.

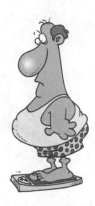

I am taking almost 100 units of insulin a day, yet my diabetes is still not controlled, and I keep gaining weight. Should my insulin dose be increased?

▼

TIP:

Maybe. This is a complicated issue. Obesity and high glucose concentrations decrease the body's ability to release and respond to insulin, so you need to take a higher dose. However, high insulin doses can lead to weight gain (see page 433) and cause hypoglycemia. Your body reacts by releasing hormones that increase blood glucose, and you get rebound hyperglycemia. To avoid this cycle, it is important to step up your efforts to incorporate meal planning and exercise into your daily plan. You should also begin self-monitoring your blood glucose levels four or more times daily to see if the type of insulin you inject and numbers of injections are ideal. It may also be possible to add an oral medication such as metformin (Glucophage), rosiglitazone (Avandia), or pioglitazone (Actos) to your insulin to improve your blood glucose control and decrease your insulin requirements (see page 422).

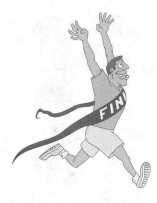

A friend of mine started taking rosiglitazone (Avandia) and is now using less insulin. If I took rosiglitazone, could I stop using insulin?

▼
TIP:

If you take high doses of insulin daily and your diabetes is still not controlled, you may be able to take less insulin and be under better glucose control with rosiglitazone (Avandia) or pioglitazone (Actos). Generally, low doses of these medications are added to your current dose of insulin while you keep careful track of your blood glucose levels. It is important to remember that rosiglitazone and pioglitazone take several weeks to begin working, and up to several months to reach their maximum effect in lowering blood glucose. When your morning (fasting) glucose values are consistently below 120 mg/dl, your total daily insulin dose will need to be decreased to avoid hypoglycemia. Keep in mind that the primary goal is to improve your blood glucose control, not to lower your insulin dose. In some studies insulin requirements declined by over one-half. Occasionally, patients are able to discontinue insulin altogether if they have been treated with relatively low doses of insulin initially. You may not be able to stop using insulin if you add rosiglitazone (Avandia) to your therapy, but it may decrease the amount of insulin you are using or the number of times you have to inject yourself each day.

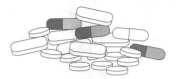

I have had type 2 diabetes for 10 years and was started on insulin before many new oral medications were available. Is it possible that I could once again be controlled on an oral medication or a combination of medications?

▼
TIP:

Yes. Some diabetes specialists have had success converting people with type 2 diabetes who have only been treated with insulin to a combination of oral medications. Generally, these people were switched from medications to insulin during a time when the only oral medications available to treat diabetes were sulfonylureas. Even though there were several different medications within this group, they all had a similar chemical structure and acted in the same way. When people failed to respond to these medications over time, the only other option was insulin. Now there are several new medications that lower blood glucose in different ways. In general, you have the best chance of responding to a combination of oral medications if your total daily insulin requirement is less than 40 units daily, your current plasma glucose values are within the target range recommended by the American Diabetes Association (between 90 and 130 mg/dl), and you have had diabetes for less than 15 years.

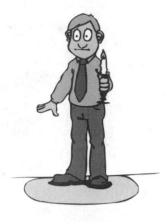

*H*ow do I know when my insulin is going *bad?*

▼
TIP:

It is not always easy to tell if your insulin has lost its potency, but you should make a habit of closely inspecting your insulin vial, pen, or delivery device every time you use it. First inspect the insulin for any changes in appearance. Is it discolored? Are there any large particles present in the liquid? Are there salt- or sugar-like crystals on the shoulder of the vial? Has your regular, insulin aspart, or insulin lispro that is supposed to be clear become cloudy? If any of these visible changes occur, the insulin should be discarded. However, keep in mind that other changes may not be observable with the naked eye, so always be alert for any indication that your insulin may not be working as well (such as high blood glucose levels), especially when there are no other explanations. To minimize this possibility, date your vial when you begin using it, store it properly (see page 431), and discard it after 1 month, or as recommended by the manufacturer. Some insulin pens or other delivery devices should be discarded sooner, some as early as 7 to 14 days.

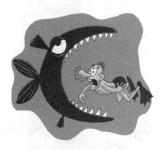

My health insurance company changed the brand of insulin it covers. Is it safe to switch brands?

▼
TIP:

Yes, with a few exceptions. Regular, NPH, and lente and ultralente human insulins made by different manufacturers have the same potency, onset, and duration of action. However, some products are unique to specific manufacturers and brands. Specific examples include insulin lispro (Humalog) made by Lilly, Humulin 50/50 made by Lilly, insulin aspart (Novolog) and Velosulin made by Novo Nordisk, and insulin glargine (Lantus) made by Aventis. If you are using insulin lispro (Humalog) as your rapid, short-acting insulin, it should be mixed only with Lilly brands of NPH, lente, or ultralente human insulins. It is not known whether lispro will retain its rapid-acting characteristics if it is mixed with other brands of intermediate- or long-acting insulins.

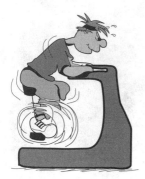

*H*ow does exercise affect my insulin *therapy?*

▼
TIP:

Exercise may lower your insulin requirements, and this effect can last for several hours if the exercise is strenuous. Since your muscles use glucose more efficiently during exercise, your usual dose of insulin can have a greater effect in lowering your blood glucose. Also, if you inject your insulin in an area near a major muscle group such as your thigh, the onset of effect from your insulin may be quicker. Therefore, if you anticipate that your activity level will be substantially increased, you should be alert for signs and symptoms of hypoglycemia, and you should take care not to delay or skip a meal. If you are planning to begin a more vigorous exercise plan, work with your health care provider to adjust your insulin doses before beginning your program.

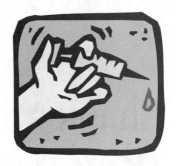

*W*ill I always have to take insulin by
injection?

▼
TIP:

Perhaps not. Several groups are studying ways to give insulin as a
nasal spray, an inhaler, or as a patch, but there are many
challenges that must be overcome to get enough insulin into the
bloodstream using these methods. Unfortunately, insulin cannot be
taken in pill form, because it is a fragile protein that is destroyed
and digested by the stomach and intestines before it reaches the
blood circulation. Therefore, to get an active form of insulin into the
blood, these organs must be bypassed. Injection is the most direct
way to get precise amounts of insulin into the body. When given as
a nasal spray or inhaler much of the dose is wasted, so up to 3 times
the dose of insulin is needed to produce an effect similar to an
injection. Not enough research has been done on insulin patches.
Currently, inhaled insulin (delivery into the lung) is in phase 3
clinical trials (the final phase before submission to the FDA for
approval) and will likely be the first non-injectable form of insulin
available. The long-term safety of these forms of insulin delivery
have yet to be established.

Chapter 5
HOW TO GET THE MOST OUT OF YOUR INSULIN THERAPY

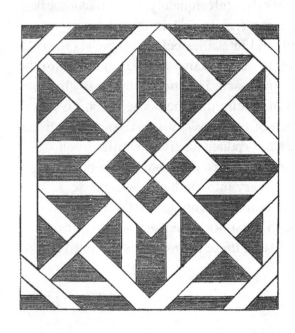

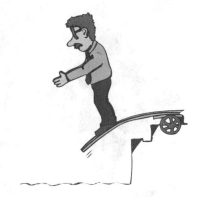

Where is the best place to inject my insulin?

▼

TIP:

There is no "best place" to inject insulin. The abdomen, arms, thighs, and hips may be used. However, many health care providers recommend the abdomen as the primary site because it is a large area that is easily reached and insulin gets into the bloodstream quickly. It is also the site least affected by exercise (see page 426). To avoid the development of lumps, you should rotate your insulin injections throughout the abdomen (move each injection 1 inch from the previous site and don't reuse the site for 2 weeks) and avoid the area around your belly button (see page 435). If you use various body sites, you should keep the site consistent based on the time of injection. For example, always use the outer thigh for morning injections, the upper arm for noontime injections, and the abdomen for evening injections. When using these other sites, remember to rotate your insulin injections throughout the area.

My mother has type 2 diabetes that is treated with regular and lente insulin. Because she has poor eyesight and arthritis, I prepare several syringes for her twice weekly and store them in the refrigerator. Is this safe?

TIP:

Yes, if you use good, clean technique and label the containers in which they are stored with the date of preparation. However, it probably is prudent to premix no more than a week's supply at a time and to discard any unused syringes. You should be aware that when regular insulin is mixed with lente insulin, the action of regular insulin may be slowed and prolonged if the mixture is not used within 15 minutes. If your mother is meeting her glucose control goals, this may not be an issue, but ask her to tell her health care provider that you are preparing her insulin injections in advance. Another alternative is to work with your mother's provider to change from lente to NPH insulin, which is more compatible with regular insulin and does not change its action when mixed together and stored for short periods.

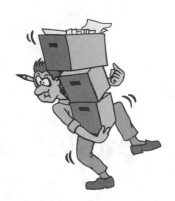

I don't like injecting cold insulin because it stings. Can I store my insulin at room temperature?

▼
TIP:

Yes. Insulin may be stored at room temperature for one month, but it should be kept in a place where the vial will not be exposed to temperature extremes (above 86° or below 36° Fahrenheit). During winter and summer months, this can be accomplished by keeping insulin in an insulated container. Insulin is a delicate protein molecule that can be changed or destroyed by heat, freezing, or too much agitation. Extra insulin that is not in use should be kept in the refrigerator. When you open a new vial, write on the label the date that it is opened or the date that it should be discarded (e.g., 28 days later). Instead of writing the date on the vial, some patients obtain a new insulin supply on the first day of the month (for insulins that are good for 1 month at room temperature). The expiration date printed on the label by the manufacturer signifies the date after which insulin should not be used under ideal, unopened, refrigerated storage conditions. The manufacturers of insulin pens and other delivery devices recommend devices in use **not** be refrigerated, as this can lead to clogging in the device.

Chapter 6
COMMON SIDE EFFECTS
OF INSULIN

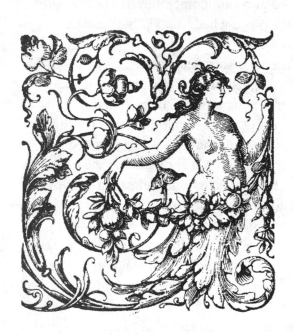

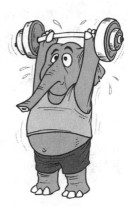

Since I started using insulin 6 months ago, I have gained 10 pounds. I feel frustrated because I have stuck to my meal plan. Is this weight gain caused by my insulin?

▼
TIP:

Probably. Most people who use insulin gain weight—sometimes up to 15 to 20 pounds. Although the added pounds can be discouraging, they may actually signal better diabetes control. People with poorly controlled diabetes lose tremendous amounts of glucose (and therefore calories) in their urine. However, when blood glucose concentrations fall to less than 180 mg/dl, little or no glucose is spilled into the urine. Also, remember that insulin is a "storage" hormone. It helps the body's cells pick up glucose and other fuels from food and store them for future use. Because producing fat is one of the most efficient ways to store fuel, people taking insulin will tend to gain weight. Weight gain can be minimized by properly adjusting your insulin dose to just the right amount you need to keep your blood glucose levels within the target range without causing too many lows. Low blood glucose levels cause hunger and overeating, and this also may contribute to weight gain.

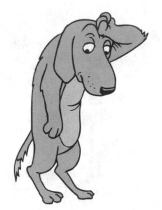

I have night sweats and often wake up in the morning with headaches. Is this related to my insulin?

TIP:

It could be. The symptoms you describe can be caused by hypoglycemia while you are sleeping. You may be injecting too much insulin in relation to your evening food. Or, you may be injecting too much of the wrong type of insulin. People who inject an intermediate-acting insulin such as NPH or lente in the early evening before dinner sometimes experience similar symptoms. These insulins have their most potent action 6 to 10 hours later, which corresponds to the early morning hours when glucose concentrations are normally at their lowest level. Discuss these symptoms with your health care provider. In the meantime, set your alarm for 2:00 A.M. and test your glucose level at that time and again first thing in the morning for several days in a row. You may want to delay the injection of NPH or lente from before your evening meal to bedtime. This shifts the peak action of these insulins to the early morning hours when you will be rising and ready to eat breakfast. Another option is to use a long-acting insulin that has a constant, smooth action without "peaks," such as insulin glargine (Lantus). Insulin glargine (Lantus) is often taken at bedtime, but it can be taken at any time of the day. However, it should be administered at the same time every day (see page 474).

I have developed lumps on my stomach where I inject my insulin. Is there anything I can do about this?

▼
TIP:

Give the lumps on your stomach a rest from insulin injections. Fat pads and lumps occur when insulin is repeatedly injected into the same place. By carefully rotating your injection sites, you should not have to use the same site more often than every 2 weeks or so. If the lump is in one area of your abdomen, rotate the injections around unaffected areas. If the lumps are all over the abdomen, you should probably begin injecting insulin in your thighs, buttocks, and arms. The lumps you describe are not dangerous or harmful, but some people are troubled by their appearance. When insulin is injected into these sites, it cannot get into the bloodstream as quickly and this can delay and prolong its action. If you give your abdomen a rest, the lumps may slowly go away after several weeks or months, depending on their size. But if they are large and bothersome, surgical removal may be the only solution.

Chapter 7
MEDICATIONS USED TO TREAT COMPLICATIONS OF DIABETES

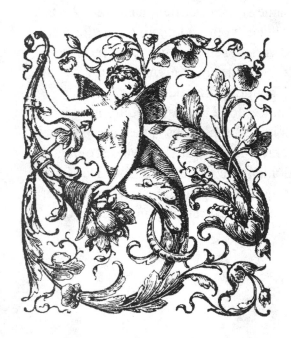

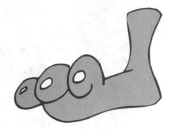

I have developed tingling and burning in both of my feet that seems to get worse at night. Are there medications I can take to treat this problem?

▼
TIP:

You are experiencing symptoms of diabetic neuropathy, a nerve disease caused by chronically high blood glucose levels. Medications used to treat this pain are not always effective. It will help you the most if you normalize your blood glucose levels and quit smoking (if you are a smoker). You can try nonprescription analgesics such as acetaminophen (Tylenol) and ibuprofen (Advil), but you may need prescription medications. Tricyclic antidepressants such as amitriptyline (Elavil) and nortriptyline (Pamelor) are the most commonly used. Although these medications are traditionally used to treat depression, they can be very effective for pain due to nerve damage. Other antidepressants used are fluoxetine (Prozac) and paroxetine (Paxil). Anti-seizure medications such as gabapentin (Neurontin), lamotrigine (Lamictal), and topiramate (Topamax) are also used to treat neuropathy. Narcotic analgesics such as codeine plus acetaminophen (Tylenol #3) or Vicodin are effective, but unfortunately lose their effectiveness over time. Because they can be addictive, narcotics are usually tried after all of the above medications have failed. Another analgesic, tramadol (Ultram), has been studied and shown to be effective in relieving pain caused by diabetic neuropathy.

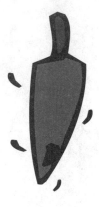

I have heard there is a "red pepper" cream that will improve the pain in my feet. Can I use it safely?

▼
TIP:

Yes. A "red pepper" cream is available to treat the pain in your feet caused by nerve disease. The active ingredient is capsaicin, a chemical found in hot chili peppers. When you apply it topically to your feet, it causes a depletion of a body chemical called substance P, which causes the pain. Initially, capsaicin causes substance P to be released from cells, which in turn causes a burning or stinging sensation (similar to how your mouth feels when you eat hot peppers). When capsaicin is applied regularly (3 to 4 times daily for several weeks), substance P is eventually depleted from cells and you'll feel relief from pain. Capsaicin cream can be used safely, but you must be careful to use gloves or to wash your hands thoroughly after application to avoid getting this medication into your eyes. Capsaicin does not work for everybody, but it may be an option for you. It is available without a prescription as a 0.025%, 0.05%, or 0.075% cream or ointment (Zostrix). A prescription strength (0.25%) product is also available (Dolorac).

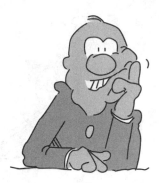

My doctor told me I have small amounts of protein in my urine and prescribed an ACE inhibitor for me. I thought this was a medication for high blood pressure. Why do I need to take this?

▼

TIP:

The ACE (angiotensin-converting enzyme) inhibitors are used to treat many conditions, including high blood pressure, heart failure, and diabetic kidney disease. Your doctor may have prescribed an ACE inhibitor so that you may benefit from its protective effect on your kidneys. Another group of medications, called angiotensin II receptor blockers (e.g., valsartan [Diovan], losartan [Cozaar], irbesartan [Avapro], and candesartan [Atacand]), can also be used to protect kidneys. Albumin is a protein that is normally found in the bloodstream but not in the urine. The small amount of albumin in your urine (called "microalbuminuria") is an early signal of kidney damage. Without treatment, microalbuminuria can worsen to a more severe form of kidney disease in 20 to 40% of people with type 2 diabetes. Many ACE inhibitors are available: captopril (Capoten), enalapril (Vasotec), benazepril (Lotensin), lisinopril (Prinivil), and ramipril (Altace). It is important to monitor your blood glucose levels when you start these medications because they sometimes lower them. Other measures that will protect your kidneys include very good control of your blood pressure (aim for less than 130/80 mmHg) and blood glucose levels.

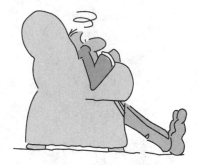

I get full easily and often feel sick and nauseated after I eat. Are there any medications that can help relieve this?

▼
TIP:

The nerve disease seen in people with diabetes can sometimes affect the nerves of stomach. This is called gastroparesis (or paralysis of the stomach). The stomach doesn't empty food as rapidly, causing an early feeling of fullness or nausea during a meal. Achieving good glucose control is important to help alleviate the symptoms. There are a couple of prescription medications used to help relieve gastroparesis: metoclopramide (Reglan) and erythromycin. Cisapride (Propulsid) was also used in the past, but it was removed from the market due to toxicity reasons. These medications all increase the stomach's ability to contract and aids in digestion. It is best to try these medications one at a time to see if one of them will work for you.

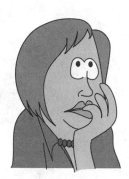

I *am often constipated. Are there any*
medications that I can take to help with this
problem?

▼

TIP:

The nerve disease seen in people with diabetes can also affect the
nerves in the bowel, leading to constipation. Try to exercise and
increase the amount of fluids and fiber in your diet. However, you
should avoid large amounts of juices and drink more water instead
in order to prevent fluctuations in your blood glucose levels. You can
try laxatives such as psyllium (Metamucil) and methylcellulose
(Citrucel). These are bulk forming laxatives that cause an increase in
pressure, leading to contraction of the bowel muscles and
defecation. Psyllium tends to cause more gas and cramping than
methylcellulose. Stimulant laxatives, such as Ex-lax and senna, are
effective as well. However, the bowel can become dependent on
them, which means you cannot have a bowel movement without
them. Since many medications can cause constipation, you should
ask your pharmacist or doctor to review your list of medications. It
may be possible to use an alternative medication or modify the dose
to avoid constipation.

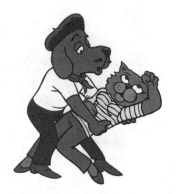

I have increasing difficulty maintaining an erection during intercourse. Are there any medications that can help improve this problem?

▼
TIP:

Yes, depending on the cause of impotence. Men with diabetes can develop impotence, which is defined as the consistent inability to achieve or maintain an erection sufficient for satisfactory performance during intercourse. About 50% of men with diabetes become impotent during their lifetime. The main causes of impotence are decreased blood flow to the penis from plaque deposits in the circulatory system or diabetic nerve disease. Many non-medication approaches are used, including psychotherapy, penile implants or prostheses, and vacuum constriction devices. The FDA-approved medication therapies include alprostadil (Muse), vardenafil (Levitra), and tadalafil (Cialis), and sildenafil (Viagra). Muse must be injected into the penis or inserted as a pellet into the urethra; Viagra, Levitra, and Cialis are tablets that are taken 30 minutes to 4 hours before intercourse. These medications inhibit the breakdown of one of the chemical components involved in an erection and improves intercourse success rates in about 50% of men with diabetes. Side effects are mild and can include facial flushing, headache, and indigestion. These medications cannot be used by men who take nitrates (such as Nitrostat, Isordil, or Imdur) in any form or alpha blockers (medications used to treat high blood pressure) because a dangerous drop in blood pressure can result.

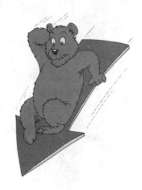

I have high blood pressure. What medication should I take?

▼
TIP:

High blood pressure contributes to the development and worsening of complications, such as stroke, eye problems, and kidney damage, due to diabetes. The target blood pressure in people with diabetes is less than 130/80 mmHg, which is lower than the recommended blood pressure for the general population. There are many groups of medications that are effective in lowering blood pressure in people with diabetes. To achieve this goal, two or three medications may be necessary. However, because the ACE inhibitors also help protect the kidneys, they are preferred (see page 439). Angiotensin receptor II are used for similar reasons (see page 444). Beta-blockers, often used in patients for angina pectoris (chest pain) or after a heart attack, have also been used as initial therapy to treat high blood pressure in people with diabetes. A group of water pills called thiazide diuretics is very effective in lowering blood pressure when used in combination with ACE inhibitors. A group of calcium channel blockers called nondihydropyridines are considered "second-line" agents, to be used after the medications discussed above. Another group, the dihydropyridines, are used in addition to, but not instead of, ACE inhibitors or beta-blockers.

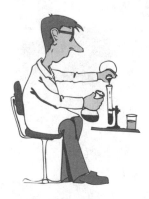

My doctor started me on the ACE inhibitor Altace (ramipril) for my kidney disease and I have developed a dry cough that won't seem to go away. Are there other medications that can be used for my kidneys instead?

▼
TIP:

Yes. Another group of medications called angiotensin receptor II blockers work similarly to the ACE inhibitors, but do not cause a cough. Examples include losartan (Cozaar), valsartan (Diovan), and irbesartan (Avapro). Studies have shown that they too will prevent the worsening of diabetic kidney disease in patients with type 2 diabetes. Some practitioners will try another ACE inhibitor, but typically, once you have developed a cough from one ACE inhibitor, it is unlikely that you will be able to tolerate others. Therefore, switching to an angiotensin receptor II blocker is probably your best option.

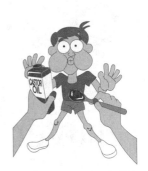

I feel like I am taking so many medications for my heart, cholesterol, high blood pressure, and diabetes. Do I really need to take them all?

▼

TIP:

Yes. It is quite common for people with type 2 diabetes to be taking many medications at the same time. This is because people with diabetes often have other conditions, such as high blood pressure, heart disease, high cholesterol or triglycerides, obesity, and insulin resistance. This collection of conditions has been termed "Syndrome X," "Metabolic Syndrome," and "Insulin Resistance Syndrome." It is well known that people with type 2 diabetes don't usually die from the diabetes itself. The major cause of death in people with this type of diabetes is heart disease. Thus, it is very important to treat the conditions that will increase your risk of heart disease, such as high blood pressure, high blood cholesterol levels, diabetes, obesity, and smoking.

Chapter 8
EFFECT OF MEDICATIONS ON DIABETES

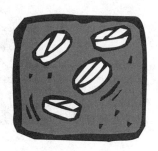

*W*hat are the most common medications
     that can increase my blood glucose
levels?

▼

TIP:

Agroup of steroids called glucocorticoids can significantly raise
your blood glucose by causing insulin resistance. This group
includes medications such as prednisone, hydrocortisone, dexamethasone, and cortisol. Glucocorticoids are used to treat a variety
of conditions, such as rheumatoid arthritis, asthma, cystic fibrosis,
and severe allergic reactions. Your blood glucose levels are likely to
rise if you take large doses of these medications as pills or by
injection. When you inhale them or rub them on your skin as an
ointment or cream, they have low potential to increase blood
glucose, because very little of the steroid is absorbed into your
bloodstream. Fortunately, the effect of steroids on blood glucose is
usually reversible. Niacin (nicotinic acid) can also increase blood
glucose (see page 453), as can protease inhibitors (medications used
to treat people with HIV/AIDS) and certain antipsychotics
(medications used to treat schizophrenia and bipolar disease). When
treating medical conditions with drugs, you and your doctor must
weigh the benefits against the risks of therapy. Sometimes the
benefit gained from treating your condition will outweigh the risk of
increasing your blood glucose. In that case, the effect on blood
glucose can be managed by adjusting your diabetes treatment plan.

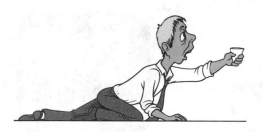

Is it OK for me to drink alcohol? How much can I drink?

▼
TIP:

The effect of alcohol on blood glucose depends on how much you drink in what period of time. Large amounts of alcohol over a short time can cause hypoglycemia by preventing the liver from making glucose. You can get severe hypoglycemia if you drink alcohol and take medications that also can cause hypoglycemia, such as insulin, sulfonylureas, repaglinide, and nateglinide. Unfortunately, the signs and symptoms of hypoglycemia may not be recognized, because they can be confused with drunkenness. You are most vulnerable to this effect if you drink heavily, drink large amounts on an empty stomach, or do not eat while you are drinking. You should know that heavy drinking (defined as more than 2 drinks daily, every day) can worsen your blood glucose control (one drink is 12 ounces of beer, 5 ounces of wine, or 1 1/2 ounces of distilled spirits). If you take chlorpropamide (Diabinese), you may experience flushing of your face and body while drinking. It is best to discuss alcohol intake with your physician or dietitian. Keep in mind that alcohol is a source of calories and needs to be included in your meal plan.

*I*s it safe for me to take birth control pills, or
will they make my diabetes worse?

▼
TIP:

E strogens and progestins, the two active ingredients found in
most birth control pills, will not generally make your diabetes
worse. Birth control pills can increase your risk for blood clots if
you have peripheral vascular disease (blood circulation problems).
However, the doses of estrogen used in most birth control pills now
are much lower than doses used in the past, so this problem is not
quite as frequent as it used to be. Women who smoke or have
diabetes are at an increased risk of cardiovascular events, such as
stroke and clots in peripheral blood vessels. To minimize this risk,
use a low-dose estrogen product, keep your blood glucose levels
under control, and do not smoke. Women over 35 who are heavy
smokers (more than 15 cigarettes a day) should not take birth
control pills due to a substantially increased risk for stroke, heart
attack, and blood clots. All women should quit smoking, preferably
with the help of a counseling program. At the very minimum, an
alternate type of birth control is recommended.

I know most people with type 2 diabetes die of heart disease. I am postmenopausal; should I take hormone replacement therapy (HRT)?

▼
TIP:

Women are thought to be protected against heart disease before menopause by their natural estrogen hormones. Unfortunately, if you have diabetes, you are already at a greater risk for heart disease. While estrogen replacement therapy has been shown to increase the good cholesterol (HDL) as well as decrease the bad cholesterol (LDL), it is no longer recommended for this purpose. Cholesterol-lowering agents, such as the statins (like simvastatin or atorvastatin) are the preferred treatment. Furthermore, studies have called into question the cardioprotective effects of hormone replacement therapy. Another concern with the use of estrogen therapy is the small but increased risk for breast or endometrial cancer. Also, you should not be on estrogen if you have a family history of endometrial or breast cancer, clotting disorders, or liver disease. Some women will be prescribed estrogen to treat symptoms of deficiency, such as hot flashes or flushing. Because so many factors must be taken into account, the decision to use HRT requires extensive discussion with your health care provider.

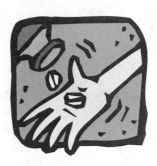

After I had a heart attack, my doctor put me on a beta-blocker. I've heard this kind of medication is bad for someone with diabetes. Should I take it?

▼
TIP:

Yes. Medications called beta-blockers are commonly prescribed after a heart attack because people who take them are more likely to survive one year after their first heart attack. The beta-blockers metoprolol (Lopressor) or atenolol (Tenormin) may be prescribed for this use. Previously, doctors were warned to use beta-blockers cautiously in people with diabetes because they might block or "mask" warning symptoms of hypoglycemia, such as heart palpitations and shakiness. Beta-blockers can also slow the body's recovery if hypoglycemia occurs. However, the benefits of preventing future heart attacks far exceed these risks. If you are taking medications for diabetes that could cause hypoglycemia and are started on a beta-blocker following a heart attack, you should test your blood glucose level more frequently and be aware that your normal warning symptoms of hypoglycemia may be blunted. Sweating, a common symptom of hypoglycemia, is not affected by beta-blockers.

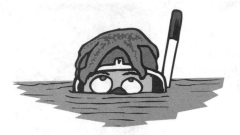

I take a water pill called hydrochlorothiazide for high blood pressure. Doesn't this increase blood glucose levels? Is it okay to take?

▼
TIP:

Hydrochlorothiazide, a thiazide diuretic that is often referred to as a "water pill," can increase your blood glucose by causing insulin resistance. However, the effect on your blood glucose depends on the dose you take. In the past, doses of 50 mg or higher daily were commonly used to treat high blood pressure. But these days it's more common to take doses as low as 12.5 mg, which are as effective for blood pressure control and have minimal effects on the blood glucose level. The thiazide diuretics have also been shown to elevate blood lipid levels (e.g., triglycerides), but this is much less of a concern if doses are 25 mg per day or lower.

*M*y daily multivitamin contains niacin. I've
heard this can cause my blood glucose to
rise. Should I stop taking it?

▼
TIP:

No. Niacin, or nicotinic acid, can increase your blood glucose,
but generally at much higher doses than those contained in a
multivitamin tablet. Niacin is a form of vitamin B3, as is
niacinamide (also called nicotinamide). The amount usually
contained in these products is 50 to 100 micrograms. People who
take niacin to lower their cholesterol levels take 20 to 60 times this
amount or 2 to 6 grams daily. These higher amounts usually do
increase blood glucose levels.

Chapter 9
NON-PRESCRIPTION
MEDICATIONS

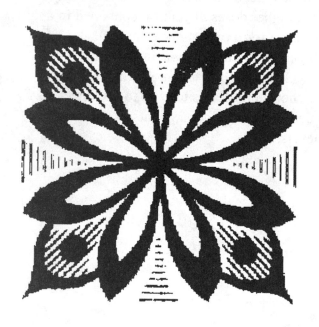

*M*any medications you can buy without a prescription say "consult with your physician before using if you have diabetes." Should I heed these warnings? Are there any general rules to use when buying medications without a prescription?

▼
TIP:

Yes. Always read the labels carefully. It is important to see if a product contains sugar or alcohol. Look in the "active" and the "inactive" ingredients sections. Use tablets or capsules when possible, since they generally contain less sugar and alcohol compared to liquid products. Avoid combination products, which tend to have hidden ingredients that could potentially be harmful. Some over-the-counter products may have side effects that can be harmful if you have diabetes. Some can increase or decrease your blood glucose. Others may worsen diabetic complications such as nerve or kidney disease. Some have a negative effect on other conditions such as high blood pressure or high blood lipids. Therefore, it is very important to read the labels of these products to see if there are any warnings regarding diabetes, high blood pressure, or heart disease. If such warnings are present, ask your physician or pharmacist if the product is safe for you to take.

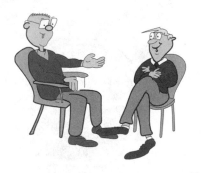

Should I tell my physician if I am taking any medications I purchased without a prescription?

▼
TIP:

Yes. Always tell your physician, pharmacist, and other health care providers about any over-the-counter products you take. Like all medications, these products can cause harmful side effects, even though you don't need a prescription for them. Your physician and pharmacist can check the product to see if it interacts with any medications you are currently taking or if it could make any of your current medical conditions worse. When telling your physician or pharmacist which over-the-counter medications you are taking, be sure to include dietary supplements, such as vitamins and minerals, and herbal products, including herbal teas.

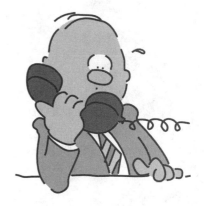

I read a newspaper article indicating that I should take one aspirin every day since I have diabetes. How much aspirin is recommended?

▼
TIP:

The American Diabetes Association (ADA) recommends that people with diabetes who have had a heart attack, undergone heart bypass surgery, suffered a stroke, have angina, or have poor circulation in the legs take an aspirin daily. People who are over the age of forty or who have a family history of heart disease, high blood pressure, kidney disease, high blood cholesterol, or who smoke should also take a daily aspirin. People with diabetes who are under the age of 40 and do not have heart disease risk factors or those who have an aspirin allergy, bleed easily, are taking a blood thinner such as warfarin (Coumadin), or have serious liver disease are not advised to take aspirin. The ADA recommends anywhere from 75 mg (equivalent to a "baby" aspirin) up to 162 mg of enteric-coated aspirin daily. The warning labels advising against aspirin use often placed on vials of diabetes medications applies only to large doses of aspirin (for example, 12 tablets daily for arthritis). Always ask your pharmacist to clarify what the warning label on a prescription means.

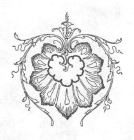

If I take aspirin, should I take a buffered or coated aspirin pill to protect my stomach?

▼
TIP:

The American Diabetes Association recommends use of an enteric-coated aspirin tablet. The risk of stomach bleeding depends on the amount and for how long you have taken aspirin. Enteric coating allows the aspirin tablet to bypass the stomach so that it dissolves in and is absorbed from the upper intestines. This decreases the chance of indigestion due to direct irritation of the stomach lining. However, because coated aspirin is absorbed into your bloodstream, it can still get back to your stomach lining where it can cause bleeding through another mechanism. Buffered aspirin tablets contain a "buffer" or antacid, which allows the aspirin to dissolve much more quickly. Unfortunately, the amount of antacid contained in each tablet is not likely to protect the stomach lining. Symptoms of a bleeding stomach include a substance that looks like coffee grounds in your vomit, black tarry stools, and a weak or dizzy feeling. Alert your physician if you have any of these symptoms. Many manufacturers use different terms to indicate enteric coating of their aspirin products, such as "safety-coated." Make sure to read the label carefully.

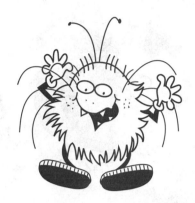

I have a cold and am terribly congested. Most cough and cold products warn against use if you have diabetes or blood pressure. I have both. What general advice can you give me in selecting a product?

▼
TIP:

G enerally, you should avoid any product that claims to be a "nasal decongestant." These work by constricting the blood vessels in your nose to relieve congestion, but if taken by mouth, they also can constrict the blood vessels throughout your body, thereby raising your blood pressure. If your blood pressure is well controlled, your physician may decide a low dose of decongestant is safe for you to use. Examples of decongestants are phenylephrine (Actifed) and pseudoephedrine (Sudafed). These medications can also cause your blood glucose to rise. Unlike tablet or liquid decongestants, nasal sprays will not affect your blood glucose because they act locally and little of the medication reaches the bloodstream. Examples include Afrin and Dristan nasal spray. These topical sprays are very effective, but should be used only occasionally and for no longer than 3–5 days at a time to avoid "addicting" your nasal passages. If your congestion is due to allergies, you can probably take antihistamines.

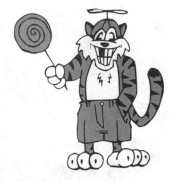

*H*ow important is the sugar content of medication I can buy without a prescription?

▼
TIP:

Not too important. Liquid formulations of nonprescription medications commonly contain sugar in order to make them taste better. Often the amount of sugar is minimal and will not greatly affect your blood glucose levels. Of course, it depends on the amount of nonprescription medication you take and how long you use it. If you notice your blood glucose is greatly affected when taking a product, ask your pharmacist whether a sugar-free formulation is available. If you require an over-the-counter product on a regular basis, consider taking a pill or capsule form if it is available, since the sugar content in these products is minimal.

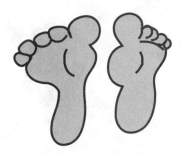

I have developed a corn on my little toe as well as some athlete's foot. Can I use medications that do not require a prescription to self-treat my feet?

▼
TIP:

It is best not to self-medicate corns, calluses, or blisters on your feet. The salicylic acid used in most products can irritate and damage your skin. You may not detect skin damage early because of decreased sensation in your feet. Furthermore, if an ulcer or infection occurs, healing may be difficult and prolonged because blood flow to your feet may be diminished. Ask your physician or podiatrist to treat and monitor any corns, calluses, or blisters. It is probably safe to treat your athlete's foot, but do let your physician or podiatrist know that you have this condition. You should inspect your feet daily using a hand mirror to look for sore, red spots that can turn into blisters and skin cracks that can become infected. If your feet don't improve, inform your physician or podiatrist, since you may need a prescription-strength medication. Be sure to wear well-fitting cotton socks that absorb excess moisture and shoes that support and fit your feet; change your socks daily to avoid reinfecting your feet; and dry your feet well after bathing or showering.

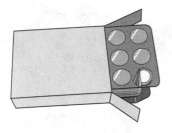

*W*hat are the safest medications I can use to treat a headache or fever?

▼
TIP:

Aspirin, nonsteroidal anti-inflammatory agents (NSAIDs), and acetaminophen (Tylenol) can be used to treat a fever and headaches and are all equally effective. Examples of NSAIDs available without prescription include ibuprofen (Advil and Motrin IB), ketoprofen (Orudis KT and Actron), and naproxen (Aleve). Aspirin and NSAIDs often are considered less preferable because of their potential for stomach irritation and kidney toxicity. However, when used for a few days, they generally are safe. In contrast, chronic use of NSAIDs and large doses of aspirin are of particular concern for people with kidney disease, and acetaminophen can be toxic to the liver if taken in high doses. Even with a healthy liver, you should not use more than 4 grams (eight 500 mg tablets or capsules) daily of acetaminophen. If you currently have or have had any problems with your kidney or liver or if your fever persists for longer than 72 hours, contact your health care provider. Check the ingredient labels to make sure the product is safe for people with diabetes. Ask your pharmacist if you have any concerns or, better yet, use a simple analgesic product that contains a single ingredient.

*I've had a vaginal yeast infection in the past
and I know the symptoms. Can I buy
something at the drugstore to treat this
problem myself?*

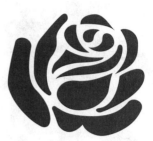

▼
TIP:

Vaginal yeast infections may be a sign of poorly controlled
diabetes, because organisms thrive when blood glucose levels
are high. High blood glucose levels also impair the body's ability to
fight infection, and the infection itself is a stress factor that makes
blood glucose control more difficult. For these reasons, this problem
should be brought to your physician's attention. Women with poorly
controlled diabetes may not respond to nonprescription products for
vaginal yeast infections and may require a prescription antibiotic.
Improving your blood glucose control also is important to prevent
repeat vaginal yeast infections.

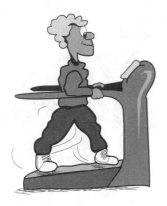

*M*y doctor told me my diabetes would improve if I lost weight. Should I try something like Dexatrim?

▼

TIP:

Several nonprescription products are available for weight loss. While products that provide "bulk" and a feeling of fullness are generally safe to use, many nonprescription products that suppress the appetite contain ephedrine or ephedrine-like compounds. Ephedrine, which acts like adrenaline, is a stimulant that can increase your blood glucose level and blood pressure, both of which are undesirable effects. Ephedra-containing compounds, such as ephderine, have also been associated with heart attacks and strokes. In April 2004, the FDA issued a regulation prohibiting the sale of supplements containing ephedra because of their unreasonable risk of illness or injury. Some herbal weight loss products, although called "natural," also contain similar stimulant-like drugs. For example, the herb ma huang is just ephedra, the botanical source of ephedrine. These weight loss products can also contain other stimulants, such as caffeine and botanical sources of caffeine (such as kola nut and guarana). As you probably know, exercising regularly and eating less are key components to successful and permanent weight loss. If these lifestyle changes are ineffective, you can discuss other options with your physician or dietitian. Although some prescription medications are available, people often gain weight back after they stop taking them. You'll have more luck with a comprehensive, behavioral approach to weight loss.

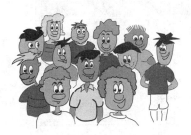

I read about some special vitamin and mineral supplements for people with diabetes. Do people with diabetes have special needs for vitamins? If so, which ones should I take?

TIP:

Yes. People with diabetes do have special needs for vitamins and minerals. When your blood glucose levels are high, glucose spills into your urine, leading to an increase in urination. This may lead to excessive losses of magnesium, zinc, and water-soluble vitamins such as vitamin C. Also, many people with diabetes are on weight-reduction diets and may not be eating a well-balanced diet. Nonprescription multivitamin and mineral products can be used to replace these possible deficits, but be sure to discuss any additional supplementation with your physician. Try to eat a well-balanced, healthy diet and take an inexpensive, all-purpose multivitamin and mineral product daily (see page 466).

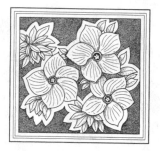

I have been reading a lot about
antioxidants such as vitamins A, C, and E,
as well as alpha-lipoic acid. Should I be
taking these vitamins?

TIP:

This depends. Vitamins A, C, and E and alpha-lipoic acid are
antioxidants that neutralize substances called free radicals that
can cause damage to cells throughout the body. Evidence is quite
convincing that taking the antioxidant vitamins E and C can protect
your heart against heart disease. The recommended dose of vitamin
E for heart protection is usually 400 to 800 IU (international units)
and the dose of vitamin C is generally 500 to 1,000 mg daily. Since
vitamin E may decrease the ability of your blood to clot, you should
not take it if you are also taking a blood thinner such as warfarin
(Coumadin). There is less evidence that vitamin A works as well as
an antioxidant, and high intakes can build up in the liver and cause
toxicity, especially if the dose exceeds 25,000 IU daily. Smokers or
former smokers should not take more than the recommended adult
daily requirement of vitamin A (5,000 IU) or excessive beta-
carotene (a form of vitamin A), since this could increase the
incidence of lung cancer. Alpha-lipoic acid has also been studied for
the treatment of neuropathy. If you have this condition, alpha-lipoic
acid may be beneficial.

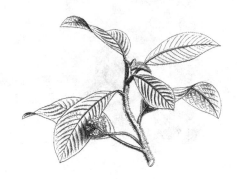

A re "natural" vitamins more
effective than synthetic ones?

▼

TIP:

Not necessarily, but they can be more costly. Synthetic vitamins, or those made by a chemical process, are the same molecules as those found in "natural" sources. Your body cannot distinguish between a vitamin derived from a natural or synthetic source. "Natural" or "colloidal" vitamins may be more readily absorbed by your intestines, but vitamin products are standardized to ensure an equivalent amount is absorbed by your gastrointestinal tract. For example, "natural" and "synthetic" vitamin E both contain alpha-tocopherol. The natural product also contains gamma-tocopherol, but it is not clear whether or not this provides a benefit. The active compound is measured by international units (IU). Selecting a product based on IU content guarantees that the amount of active ingredient absorbed will be the same, regardless of the vitamin source.

I've seen chromium advertised a lot by health food stores. Will it help lower my blood glucose?

TIP:

Most likely not. Chromium is a trace mineral that is used by the body in tiny quantities to regulate glucose metabolism. Most people have plenty of chromium in their daily meal plans. Some ads say chromium can lower blood glucose, reduce "sugar cravings," reduce weight, and improve insulin sensitivity, but there are few scientific studies to back up these claims. A chromium deficiency could lead to elevated blood glucose, but this is extremely rare. Because chromium deficiency is highly unlikely in most people with diabetes, routine supplementation is not necessary. If you are concerned about chromium deficiency, take a multivitamin and mineral product that contains the recommended daily allowance. If you choose to take a chromium supplement, make sure your supplement only contains chromium, since some supplements also contain ingredients that should be avoided by people with diabetes, including ma huang (ephedra) and kola nut (caffeine). Your daily dose of chromium should not exceed 50 to 200 micrograms.

Chapter 10
COMMON DRUG INTERACTIONS THAT OCCUR WITH MEDICATIONS FOR DIABETES

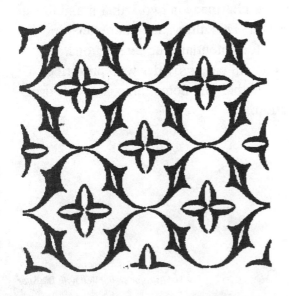

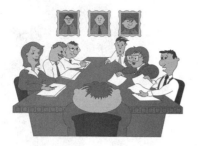

Lately, I have been seen by many physician specialists and each of them has been prescribing medications for me. How will I know if these medications will affect my diabetes or interact with other medications I am taking?

▼
TIP:

This is a difficult problem for many people with diabetes. When reviewing medication profiles, pharmacists commonly identify medications prescribed by various physicians that potentially interact with one another. They also recognize medications that may not be ideal if another medical problem exists. There are several ways for you to help minimize this problem. First, keep your own medication record and show it to every health care provider (physician, pharmacist, and nurse) you see whenever you are starting a new medication. Second, try to get all of your medications filled at one pharmacy or in one pharmacy network that maintains a single medication record for you. This allows the pharmacist to screen all of your medications for potential drug interactions. Finally, every time you see a health care provider who prescribes a new medication for you, ask whether any potential exists for a drug-drug or drug-disease interaction.

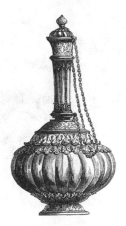

*A*re there any medications I shouldn't use if I
take pioglitazone (Actos)?

▼
TIP:

Yes. Pioglitazone decreases blood levels of oral contraceptives
and perhaps estrogen. This could lead to a contraceptive failure
resulting in pregnancy or a return of signs of estrogen deficiency,
such as hot flashes. If you are taking oral contraceptives, you should
stop and use alternative forms of contraception. If this is undesirable, ask your doctor if you should take a different diabetes
medication or if you should take an oral contraceptive with a higher
dose of estrogen. Ketoconazole (Nizoral), a medication used to treat
fungal infections, can increase blood concentrations of pioglitazone.
Therefore, blood sugar levels should be checked more frequently in
patients taking these agents in combination. Pioglitazone (Actos) is
a relatively new medication and, because of this, other drug
interactions may be discovered as more and more people use it.
Therefore, if you are taking pioglitazone, ask your pharmacist and
physician about potential drug interactions each time a new
medication is prescribed for you.

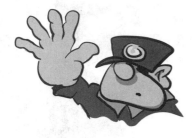

I am on a "statin" called atorvastain
*(Lipitor) to lower my cholesterol. Are
there any medications that I should avoid?*

▼
TIP:

Yes. There are several prescription medications that can interact
with atorvastatin (Lipitor) and other medications that belong to
this group. The other available statins include fluvastatin (Lescol),
rosuvastatin (Crestor), pravastatin (Pravachol), simvastatin (Zocor),
and lovastatin (Mevacor). Your physician and pharmacist will check
the particular statin you are taking for any drug interactions. Gem-
fibrozil (Lopid), a medication that lowers triglyceride levels,
interacts with all of the statins and can lead to a muscle or kidney
disorder on rare occasions. For this reason, many physicians will not
use these two medications together. However, some people with
high levels of cholesterol and triglycerides may take these drugs
together with careful monitoring of their kidney and muscle function. A group of antibiotics that treat fungal infections (fluconazole,
ketoconazole, and itraconazole) also can cause a muscle or kidney
disorder and should not be given with the statins. The same is true
for another antibiotic, erythromycin, the antidepressant nefazodone,
and cyclosporine. The effects of the blood thinner warfarin
(Coumadin) can be enhanced by the statins, but this can generally be
monitored with careful blood testing.

Chapter 11
MISCELLANEOUS
INFORMATION

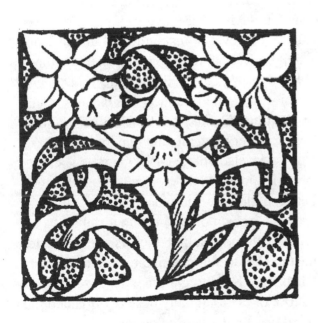

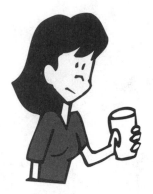

My doctor has suggested that I switch from using two daily injections of NPH to a single bedtime injection of insulin glargine. How is this insulin different from NPH?

▼
TIP:

Insulin glargine (Lantus) is different from NPH in several ways. Once injected, insulin glargine is released very slowly into your bloodstream and provides a low level of insulin for 24 hours. This translates into a single daily injection, usually administered at bedtime. In contrast, NPH has a "peak," or maximum effect, between 4 and 12 hours following injection and often lasts less than 24 hours. Thus, two injections of NPH per day may be needed. The timing of the NPH peak is different for every patient, and may result in overnight low blood glucose levels. Unlike NPH, glargine is clear and does not need to be rolled in the vial before injection. Another important difference between glargine and other longer-acting insulins (NPH and Ultralente, among others) is that it cannot be mixed in the syringe with mealtime insulins, such as regular, lispro, and aspart. The manufacturer of insulin glargine recommends that when a patient is switched from NPH to glargine, the dose of insulin glargine be reduced by 20% of the total daily dose of NPH and then adjusted as required based on blood glucose readings.

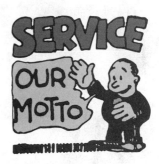

I receive a bigger discount from my insurance company if I have my prescriptions filled by mail. What services can I expect?

▼

TIP:

Many mail-order pharmacies offer good, efficient service when it comes to filling your regular medications. However, most cannot quickly fill prescriptions for medications you need right away, nor are they able to give personalized advice about over-the-counter products. Some have toll-free hotlines to answer your questions about prescriptions they have filled for you or educational programs about diabetes. Ideally, one pharmacy or pharmacy network should have a record of all of the prescription medications you are taking, a history of any bad effects from medications that you have experienced (especially allergies), and your most basic medical history. This allows the pharmacist to screen every new medication that is added to your regimen. Because records of mail-order pharmacies are not always linked to your local pharmacy, potential problems could be missed. You should keep your own detailed medication record (include medication name, strength, dose, and dates of use) and share it with all of your health care providers. Be sure to include nonprescription medications, herbal remedies, vitamins, and minerals in your records.

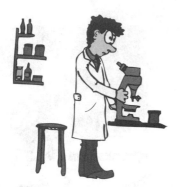

What qualities should I look for in a pharmacist who oversees my medications?

TIP:

A good pharmacist can be a valuable resource for people with type 2 diabetes because they take more medications than most other people. Therefore, it is important to find a pharmacist who is willing to take the time to review any changes in your medication history each time you get a new prescription and to carefully review the new medication's proper use with you. Your pharmacist should also quickly assess whether you are responding to your medications and whether you have developed any common side effects. The pharmacist should advise you about over-the-counter medications in order to avoid side effects or drug-drug interactions. Although many pharmacists are busier than ever, there are still highly qualified pharmacists who are willing to meet with you by appointment to review your medication use and to contact physicians or other health care providers on your behalf. These pharmacists can provide many other services, such as teaching you how to use glucose meters, giving you immunizations, taking your blood pressure, and providing smoking cessation counseling.

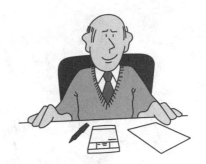

*W*hat questions should I ask my
pharmacist each time I begin
taking a new medication?

▼
TIP:

To protect yourself and to increase the chances that you will get
the best effect from your medications, ask the pharmacist these
questions:

- What is the name of this medication and why am I taking it?
- How should I take it to get the best effect? (For example, with or
  without meals? What time of the day?)
- What good effects can I expect and when?
- How will I know if the medication is working?
- How long should I take it?
- What are the common side effects and how will I know if I have
  them?
- Are there any ways to avoid or diminish these side effects?
- Are there any side effects serious enough to discontinue the
  medication?
- Should I avoid certain foods, activities, and alcohol?
- Will my medical conditions make me more susceptible to any of
  this medication's side effects?
- Will this medication interact with any other medications I am
  taking? What is the effect of the interaction?
- Can I take my medications if I become pregnant or breast-feed?
- How should I store my medication?

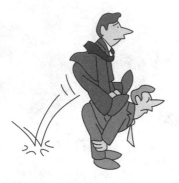

I have been taking Micronase (glyburide) for many years. When I last refilled my prescription, I noticed that the pill was a different color. The pharmacist told me she had filled my prescription with a generic brand because this was covered by my insurance. Is this medication likely to have the same effect as Micronase?

▼ TIP:

Yes. A generic brand of a medication has the same chemical structure as the brand name medication and is provided in the same strength and dosage form (for example, tablet, syrup, or ointment). The Food and Drug Administration has strict standards for manufacturers of generic medications to ensure that they will have the same effects as the brand-name medication. Once a brand medication has lost its patent status, other manufacturers may produce a generic product. In some cases, the primary source of the generic products is the original manufacturer. Because generic medications generally are less expensive than their brand-name equivalents, insurance companies give patients, doctors, and pharmacies incentives to prescribe and dispense generic drugs.

I have been taking lovastatin (Mevacor), but when I refilled my prescription, the pharmacist told me this medication was no longer included in the "formulary" used by my insurance company. I received simvastatin (Zocor), which the pharmacist said worked in the same way. Will this medication have the same effect?

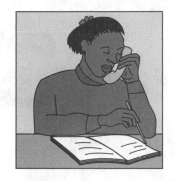

▼
TIP:

You have experienced what the industry calls a "therapeutic interchange." Often several manufacturers make medications that belong to the same class of agents, have a similar chemical structure, work by the same mechanism, and generally have the same effects. A group of health professional experts pronounces the medications in this group "therapeutically equivalent." The insurance company or health maintenance organization (HMO) then decides which medication to include in the formulary (medications approved for use within a health care insurance plan) based on price. Other factors, such as ease of use (a single daily dose versus a twice-daily dose), may also be considered. However, each medication is likely to have a unique dose and dose regimen, and side effects may differ slightly. You should carefully review how to take the medication with your pharmacist and check with your doctor to make sure you are still getting good effects from the new drug.

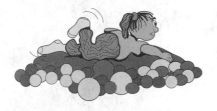

I have several young grandchildren who visit me on occasion. I have asked my pharmacist not to use childproof caps because I have such a hard time opening them. Is there any danger to the children if they accidentally take the medications I use to treat my type 2 diabetes?

▼

TIP:

Yes, depending on the type of medication you are taking. The sulfonylurea medications, repaglinide (Prandin), and nateglinide (Starlix) are most likely to cause acute problems if a child ingests a large amount. These drugs are likely to cause severe hypoglycemia that could last up to 24 hours, depending on the specific medicine ingested. High doses of metformin could cause lactic acidosis. Pioglitazone (Actos) or rosiglitazone (Avandia) are not likely to cause any acute effects. Acarbose (Precose) may cause temporary abdominal pain, gas, and diarrhea. Nevertheless, whenever an ingestion of any sort is suspected, you should call the local poison control center or the emergency number (911) for advice. Since it is difficult to predict the toxic potential of medications, especially if several medications are taken at once, prevention is key. Take time to store all medications and toxic cleaners out of the reach of children, preferably in a locked cabinet, when you are expecting a visit.

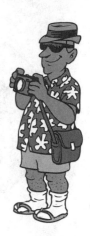

I *will be traveling abroad for 4 weeks. What*
precautions should I take in case I misplace my
medications?

▼

TIP:

First, be aware that the medication you are taking may or may not
be available in the country to which you are traveling. There is a
good chance that even if the medication is available, it will have a
different name or will be available in different strengths. Before you
leave, you should ask your doctor to provide a letter that briefly
describes your medical conditions and their current treatments.
Bring extra prescriptions for the medications you are taking so
pharmacists or physicians in other countries can provide them for
you in an emergency. Write down a detailed list of all the medications you are taking and ask your pharmacist to provide extra
supplies of them that you can store in separate bags. Always keep a
2-week supply of medications with you at all times in case your
luggage is lost. Make an effort to store all medications in an air-
tight, insulated case to minimize exposure to temperature and
humidity extremes. Finally, wear a bracelet and carry an ID in your
wallet that identifies you as someone with diabetes.

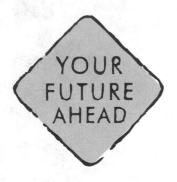

Many members of my family have diabetes, and now I am worried about my children. Are there any medications they can take to prevent or delay the onset of type 2 diabetes?

▼
TIP:

Perhaps. The National Institutes of Health sponsored a study called the Diabetes Prevention Program to answer this question. People in the study were at high risk for developing diabetes. These individuals had "impaired glucose tolerance" (IGT). That is, they had blood glucose levels higher than normal, but not high enough to be diagnosed with diabetes. People in the study were assigned to one of three groups for 3 years. One group received a placebo (inactive pill), another group participated in an intensive diet and exercise program, and the last group received metformin (Glucophage). The purpose of the study was to determine if people taking metformin or those assigned to a diet and exercise group were less likely to develop type 2 diabetes over time compared to the group taking a placebo. Compared to the placebo group, people in the intensive diet and exercise program reduced their risk of getting diabetes by 58%. Individuals in the metformin group reduced their risk by 31%. Participants in the study will be followed to determine how long such interventions are effective in preventing diabetes. In the meantime, patients with IGT should be counseled on weight loss and exercise. Further research is needed to determine the role of drug therapy in the prevention of type 2 diabetes.

101 NUTRITION TIPS

FOR PEOPLE WITH DIABETES

▲

A project of the
American Diabetes Association

▼

Written by

Patti B. Geil, MS, RD, FADA, CDE
Lea Ann Holzmeister, RD, CDE

101 NUTRITION TIPS FOR PEOPLE WITH DIABETES

▼

TABLE OF CONTENTS

Chapter 1
NUTRITION:
THE BIG PICTURE

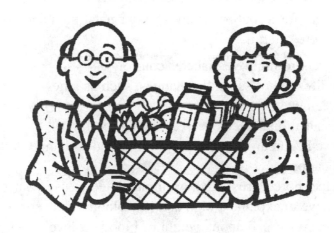

How do I know when I should see a registered dietitian?

▼
TIP:

See a registered dietitian (RD) when your diabetes is first diagnosed, when a new doctor changes your treatment plan, or twice a year for a routine review of your meal plan and goals. See the RD more often if

- You want to improve diabetes control
- Your lifestyle or schedule changes, such as a new job, marriage, or pregnancy
- Your nutritional needs keep changing (children)
- You've begun an exercise program or had a change in diabetes medication
- You feel bored, frustrated, or unmotivated to use your meal plan
- You have unexplained high and low blood glucose levels
- You're concerned about weight or blood fat levels
- You develop nutrition-related complications, such as high blood pressure or kidney disease

You may have an RD on your diabetes team. Ask your doctor or hospital for a referral. You can call the American Diabetes Association (800-342-2383), The American Dietetic Association (800-877-1600), or the American Association of Diabetes Educators (800-338-3633) for referrals. Many RDs are certified diabetes educators (CDEs) and have additional training in diabetes care.

What should I eat until I can meet with the registered dietitian?

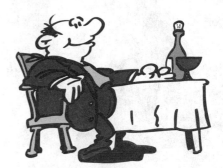

▼
TIP:

E at the foods that are healthy for everyone—grains, beans, vegetables, fruits, low-fat milk, and meat. Cut down on foods and drinks with a lot of added sugar (soda, desserts, candy) and fat (fried foods, lunch meats, gravy, salad dressings). You do not need special or diet foods.

It is important to eat about the same amount of food at the same time each day. Don't eat one or two large meals. Try to eat at least three small meals each day, especially if you are taking diabetes medication. You may need a snack between meals and before you go to bed. Avoid drinking alcohol until you learn how it fits into your diabetes treatment plan. Remember, you can make a big difference in your diabetes control through what you choose to eat. Before you see the RD, keep a record of everything you eat and drink for 3–5 days and bring this record to your appointment. This will help the RD personalize the meal plan to you.

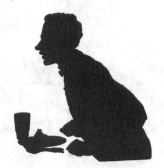

*H*ow often do I need to eat for good
diabetes control?

▼
TIP:

This depends on the type of diabetes you have, your medications,
your physical activity, and where your blood glucose level is at
the moment. An RD can help you decide.

For type 1 or type 2 using insulin: Have food in your system
when your insulin is peaking. You may need three meals and an
evening snack. If you take two injections of short- and intermediate-
acting insulin, you may need three meals and three snacks. If you
use rapid-acting insulin, eat within 15 minutes of taking your
insulin. You may need a snack for physical activity (see page 547).
A common mistake is not waiting 1/2 hour to eat after taking
regular insulin. If you start eating before insulin activity is peaking,
you have higher blood glucose levels after meals.

For type 2: Eat a small meal every 2–3 hours. When you eat
smaller amounts of food, your blood glucose levels are lower after
eating. Mini-meals spread over the day may help control your
hunger and calorie intake, leading to better blood glucose control
and weight loss. Your blood cholesterol levels will also be lower.

*W*hat can I eat for snacks?

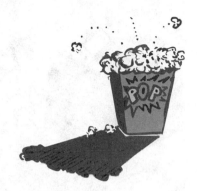

TIP:

hoose from the same healthy foods that you eat at meals. Often, snacks are based on foods with 15 grams of carbohydrate per serving. Good snack choices begin at the bottom of the food pyramid. Choose foods from the grain group, such as air-popped popcorn, baked tortilla chips and salsa, graham crackers, pretzels, bagels, or cereal. Fresh fruits and vegetables make excellent snacks, and they're also portable! To make a snack more substantial, add a source of low-fat protein, such as low-fat milk, reduced-fat peanut butter on a slice of bread or a bagel, low-fat cheese on crackers, or a slice of turkey breast on whole-wheat bread.

Be prepared! Always carry a snack with you in case of a delayed meal or unexpected change in your schedule. Snacks can be stashed in your desk, briefcase, backpack, or glove compartment. Having good food on hand will save you from hypoglycemia and from having to settle for less nutritious fast foods.

*How can keeping a food diary help my
diabetes?*

TIP:

The food you eat raises your blood glucose. Until you write it
down, you probably are not aware of how much or what you
are eating. A food diary helps you make important decisions about
your medication, meal plan, and exercise plan.

■ Record information you need. If you want to lose weight,
measure your serving sizes and write down how many calories or
fat grams you're getting for several days. Looking up the nutrient
values of foods helps you learn what nutrients each food gives
you.

■ Keep records that are easy to use—a notebook, calendar, or form
created on your computer. Write it down when you eat it; don't
wait until later.

■ Use the information. Bring your record to the next appointment
with your RD. Look for patterns in your eating behaviors and
blood glucose levels. For example, your records may show that
high-fat snacks in late afternoon result in high blood glucose at
dinner. You also notice that your lunch is much smaller than
other meals and causes you to be too hungry before dinner. You
may want to adjust the size of lunch and decrease your afternoon
eating.

Why are serving sizes important? Is there an easy way to remember them?

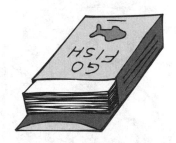

▼
TIP:

No matter what meal plan you follow—carbohydrate counting, exchanges, or the food guide pyramid—serving size is the key. An extra ounce of meat or tablespoon of margarine doesn't sound like much, but it can quickly add up to higher blood glucose levels and weight gain.

Begin by using standard kitchen measuring cups, spoons, and food scales until you train your eyes to see correct serving sizes. Once you've weighed, measured, and looked at 1/2 cup of green beans or 5 oz of chicken, you'll have a mental picture no matter where you dine. Every few months, measure some servings again to keep your eyes sharp and your servings the right size.

Mental pictures can help you eat correct serving sizes.

Food	Looks like
1 cup pasta or rice	a clenched fist
1/2 cup vegetables	half a tennis ball
1 cup broccoli	a light bulb
3 oz meat, chicken, or fish	a deck of cards or palm of a woman's hand
1 oz cheese	two saltine crackers or a 1-inch square cube

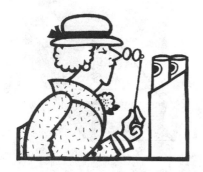

Nutrition Facts	
Serving Size 1 cup (228g)	
Servings Per Container 2	

Amount Per Serving	
Calories 260 Calories from Fat 120	

	% Daily Value*
Total Fat 13g	**20%**
Saturated Fat 5g	**25%**
Cholesterol 30mg	**10%**
Sodium 660mg	**28%**
Total Carbohydrate 31g	**10%**
Dietary Fiber 0g	**0%**
Sugars 5g	
Protein 5g	

Vitamin A 4%	•	Vitamin C 2%
Calcium 15%	•	Iron 4%

* Percent Daily Values are based on a 2,000 calorie diet. Your daily values may be higher or lower depending on your calorie needs:

	Calories:	2,000	2,500
Total Fat	Less than	65g	80g
Sat Fat	Less than	20g	25g
Cholesterol	Less than	300mg	300mg
Sodium	Less than	2,400mg	2,400mg
Total Carbohydrate		300g	375g
Dietary Fiber		25g	30g

Calories per gram:
Fat 9 • Carbohydrate 4 • Protein 4

*W*hat should I be looking for on food labels— carbohydrate or fat?

TIP:

Most people with diabetes should be looking at both carbohydrate and fat on the Nutrition Facts panel on food labels. Carbohydrate is what raises your blood glucose the most, so it's important to you. Fat carries the most calories per gram, so it affects your weight. Also, diabetes puts you more at risk for developing heart disease. Eating foods lower in fat (especially saturated fat) may help you lose weight and lower your risk for heart disease.

The total amount of carbohydrate you eat affects your blood glucose. The carbohydrate listed in the Nutrition Facts can be from beans, vegetables, pasta, grains, and sugars (added or naturally present in foods such as milk and fruit). Keeping track of the total grams of carbohydrate you eat and drink is more important than where it came from. The food label will tell you exactly how many grams of carbohydrate and fat are in a serving of food.

*H*ow do I deal with comments such as, *"Are you allowed to eat that?"*

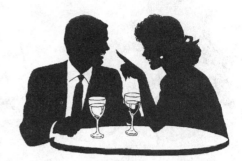

▼

TIP:

Y our family and friends mean well. When this happens,

- **Recognize your own feelings.** Part of adjusting to diabetes is recognizing the difficult emotions that come with it. How do you feel about the lifestyle changes and pressures of self-care?

- **Recognize the feelings of family and friends.** Your family and friends are also adjusting to your diabetes and the ways it affects them. They may feel anxious, intimidated, guilty, or overwhelmed.

- **Use positive reframing.** Change the way you see the situation. If you feel angry at someone's comment, take a moment to acknowledge your own feeling and then the other person's feeling. Then look at the situation in a positive way. For example, you may say, "Thanks for reminding me. I know you want to help. I've already planned to adjust my insulin (or exercise) to handle the additional calories and carbohydrate in this food."

- **Develop an interaction plan.** Changing years of old thinking and communication patterns takes time. In a calm moment, discuss a new way to talk about food and diabetes issues.

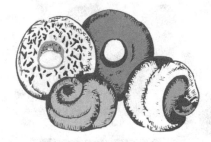

*N*ow that sugar is no longer
forbidden for people with
diabetes, can I eat all the sweets I
want?

▼
TIP:

It's true that the carbohydrate in table sugar has the same effect on
your blood glucose as any other carbohydrate, such as that in
bread, potatoes, or fruit. Different carbohydrates do raise blood
glucose in different ways; however, for blood glucose control, it's
more important to focus on the total amount of carbohydrate you
eat, rather than where it comes from. You substitute sweets into your
meal plan for other carbohydrates—don't add them on top.

No, don't have sweets at every meal. Sugary foods don't have the
nutrients, vitamins, and minerals that your body needs to be healthy.
That's why we call these calories "empty" and list these foods in the
top of the food pyramid. If you include sweets in a meal, eat a small
serving, and check your blood glucose before and 1–2 hours after
you eat to see how it affects you. Keep an eye on your weight and
blood glucose levels over time. Hold back on the sweets if you see
your numbers creeping up.

I went to lunch with three friends who also have diabetes. We all follow different types of meal plans. What happened to the "diabetic" diet?

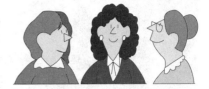

▼
TIP:

Just as there is no one medication that works for all people with diabetes, there is no single meal-planning approach. The standard 1,800-calorie preprinted diet sheet is gone. Individualization is the key to good diabetes control.

The best meal plans are designed by you and an RD and are based on your health, other medications, activity level, and treatment goals. Your friend with type 1 diabetes may be taking multiple insulin injections and using the carbohydrate counting approach with frequent blood glucose monitoring. Her food choices would be quite different from your friend with type 2 diabetes and high blood fat levels who needs to lose weight. She may be trying to lower her carbohydrate intake and increase the monounsaturated fats in her diet by eating more nuts, olives, or canola oil. And the friend who works swing shift is probably using an entirely different approach to the timing and food choices in her meals and snacks. The important thing is to use a meal plan that works for you.

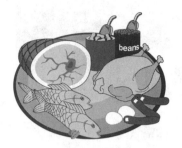

I've heard that a low-carbohydrate, high-protein, high-fat diet will help me lose weight without cutting calories. Should I change from the high-carbohydrate, low-fat diet I've always followed?

▼

TIP:

Probably not. A low-carbohydrate diet is very difficult to follow for a long period of time. On this diet, you eat meat, eggs, and cheese but very few carbohydrate foods, such as pasta, breads, fruits, and vegetables. You eat too few fruits and vegetables to get all the vitamins and minerals you need.

The rapid weight loss on a low-carbohydrate diet comes from an unhealthy loss of water and muscle tissue. Side effects include dehydration, low blood pressure, and increased work for the kidneys. The high fat certainly isn't good for heart health. Other side effects include constipation, fatigue, and nausea. And as with all very restricted diets, once you go back to a normal way of eating, your weight is going to come back.

Until there's more evidence, it's probably best to continue with a balanced carbohydrate meal plan. If you have insulin resistance, you may do better substituting some monounsaturated fats for carbohydrates (see page 532). Get your health care team's help to decide on a nutrition approach for you.

*W*ill fiber help my diabetes control?

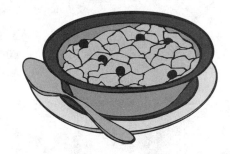

▼

TIP:

Fiber can keep your blood glucose from going high after a meal because it slows down the speed at which the food is digested. A high-fiber, low-fat way of eating can also reduce your risk for cancer, cardiovascular disease, high blood pressure, and obesity. Fiber has a favorable effect on cholesterol, too.

Fiber in a food is made up of two types: insoluble fiber, such as that in vegetables and whole-grain products, and soluble fiber, found in fruits, oats, barley, and beans. Insoluble fiber improves gastrointestinal function, while soluble fiber can affect blood glucose and cholesterol. Unfortunately, most Americans eat only 8–10 grams of fiber daily, not the recommended 20–35 grams a day from a variety of foods. You can increase fiber by eating foods such as the ones in this chart.

Food	Serving Size	Total Fiber (g)	Soluble Fiber (g)
Beans	1/2 cup cooked	6.9	2.8
Oat bran	1/3 cup dry	4.0	2.0
Barley	1/4 cup dry	3.0	0.9
Orange, fresh	1 small	2.9	1.8
Oatmeal	1/3 cup dry	2.7	1.4

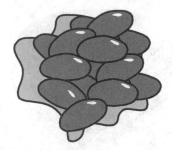

*I*s it true that beans can improve *diabetes control?*

▼
TIP:

Y es. Beans are very high in carbohydrates and need to be eaten in the proper portions, but beans digest slowly, resulting in only a small rise in blood glucose and insulin levels. Several research studies have shown that eating 1 1/2–2 1/2 cups of cooked beans daily leads to beneficial effects on the control of diabetes. Beans also reduce the risk of cardiovascular disease, a common complication for people with diabetes. Eating 1–3 cups of cooked beans a day will lower total cholesterol in the range of 5–19%. Beans are also an excellent source of folate, which may reduce the risk of cardiovascular disease.

Packed with protein, fiber, vitamins, and minerals, beans are also low in fat, cholesterol, and sodium. They can be included in all types of diabetes meal plans. Beans can be used in salads, soups, or entrees. Canned beans require less preparation time and have the same beneficial effects as dried beans.

Soak dried beans overnight and rinse well before cooking. Introduce beans gradually into your diet, chew thoroughly, and drink plenty of liquids to aid digestion. Enzyme products such as "Beano" can also help you avoid gastrointestinal distress.

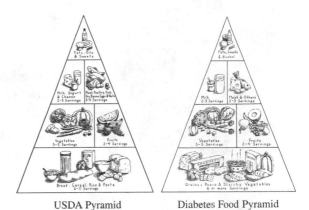

USDA Pyramid   Diabetes Food Pyramid

*W*hat is the
difference
between the Diabetes
Food Pyramid and the
USDA Food Pyramid?

▼
TIP:

T he Diabetes Food Pyramid in *The First Step in Diabetes Meal
Planning* is based on the USDA Food Guide Pyramid. There are
only a few differences between the two pyramids. Each has six food
groups, but the names are a little different. In the USDA Food
Pyramid, cheese is in the Milk, Yogurt, and Cheese group, but in the
Diabetes Food Pyramid, cheese is in the Meat and Others group.
Cheese is mostly protein and fat, like foods found in the meat group.
In the USDA Pyramid, beans are in the Meat group, but in the
Diabetes Pyramid, beans are in Grains, Beans, and Starchy
Vegetables because beans are a good source of carbohydrate and
fiber. The food group at the tip of the Diabetes Pyramid includes
alcohol with fats and sweets. This suggests limiting all three.

Both pyramids were designed to encourage you to include more
foods in your diet from the largest groups—grains, beans and
starchy vegetables, vegetables, and fruits—and fewer foods from the
small groups at the top. As of this publication, the USDA Food
Guide Pyramid is in the process of being revised. Look for changes
in the USDA Pyramid, as well as the Diabetes Pyramid, in the years
to come.

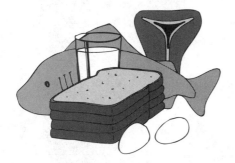

I keep hearing about carbohydrate counting. Is it still okay to use exchanges?

▼

TIP:

Yes. The exchange system is a valuable way for people with diabetes to plan meals. It can also help if you want to count carbohydrates. The *Exchange Lists for Meal Planning* group foods with similar carbohydrate content, so the "carb" counting is already done for you. For example, all the foods on the starch list (1 slice of bread, 3/4 cup cold cereal, etc.) contain 15 grams of carbohydrate.

To use exchanges, you need an individualized meal plan that tells you how many exchanges from each list to eat daily for meals and snacks. You can choose a variety of foods from the exchange lists to fit into your meal plan. An RD can help you design a meal plan and teach you how to use this system. In 2003, the *Exchange Lists* were updated. The food groupings were changed and more foods were included. A pocket-sized guide is now available.

Many people prefer to use exchanges because it helps keep their food choices balanced and healthy. If this system works for you, there is no reason to switch to another.

What is carbohydrate counting?

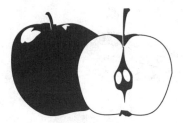

▼

TIP:

It is a precise method of meal planning for people with diabetes. Foods containing carbohydrate (grains, vegetables, fruit, milk, and sugar) have the largest effect on blood glucose level. A small amount of carbohydrate (1 apple) raises blood glucose some; a larger amount of carbohydrate (3 apples) raises blood glucose more. You track how the carbohydrate affects you by monitoring your blood glucose.

You have to invest some time in monitoring blood glucose, record keeping, measuring food servings, and learning about nutrients in foods.

Carbohydrate counting has two levels: basic and advanced. Basic carbohydrate counting is generally used by people with type 2 diabetes and consists mostly of counting and eating consistent amounts of carbohydrate. Advanced is often used by people taking insulin and is made up of recognizing and managing patterns in blood glucose, food, medication, and exercise for intensive management of blood glucose. You may only need to learn about basic carbohydrate counting. The amount of work may seem overwhelming at first, but most people find the improvements in blood glucose control are worth it! An RD can help you learn carbohydrate counting.

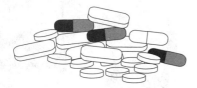

*D*o I need special vitamins
and minerals because I
have diabetes?

▼
TIP:

Y ou don't need special vitamins because of diabetes. You do
need vitamins and minerals for a well-functioning body,
whether you have diabetes or not. If you are eating a variety of
foods, you don't need a special vitamin or mineral supplement.
There is currently no scientific evidence to show that certain
vitamins or minerals can improve your blood glucose control, except
in rare cases of deficiencies of the minerals chromium, copper,
magnesium, manganese, selenium, or zinc. (See pages 565–567)

Discuss your diet with your physician or RD. You may need a
vitamin and mineral supplement if you are

On a diet of fewer than 1,200 calories a day

Following a strict vegetarian diet

At risk for bone disease

Over age 65

Pregnant or breastfeeding

Taking diuretics

I really don't feel like eating in the morning. Do I have to eat breakfast?

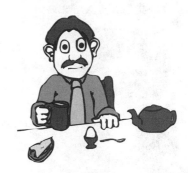

▼
TIP:

Yes. Breakfast is crucial for people with diabetes. Your body has been without food for 8–12 hours. If you have type 1 diabetes, you need food to balance your injected insulin. If you have type 2 diabetes, you may skip breakfast to cut calories and lose weight, but it can lead to overeating later. In fact, research shows that breakfast skippers have higher blood cholesterol levels and extra pounds!

The best breakfast has carbohydrate, protein, and fiber. Save high-fat foods like bacon, sausage, and eggs for special occasions. You can choose cereal or an English muffin, low-fat milk or yogurt, and fruit, but there's no rule that says breakfast can't be pasta tossed with low-fat ricotta cheese or a leftover chicken breast with a piece of fruit.

Once you experience the dividends that breakfast pays in mood, performance, and diabetes control, you'll never skip your morning meal again!

Hint: People who eat a smaller evening meal (spread the calories out over the day) are more likely to wake up hungry for breakfast.

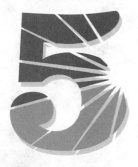

I've heard I'm supposed to eat five fruits and vegetables a day. Why?

▼
TIP:

Increasing the fruit and vegetables in your diet gives you better health, particularly in the prevention of cancer and heart disease. Fruits and vegetables are low in fat and are rich sources of vitamin A, vitamin C, and fiber. The average American eats only one serving of fruit and two servings of vegetables a day. You can find ways to put five or more servings in your salads, soups, sandwiches, main dishes, and snacks.

Fruits and vegetables affect diabetes in different ways. Fruit has 15 grams of carbohydrate per serving and affects your blood glucose within 2 hours. The amount blood glucose rises depends on whether you eat the fruit on an empty stomach, the form of the fruit (cooked or raw, whole or juice), and your blood glucose level when you eat. Check your blood glucose level after eating fruit to see what it does to you. Nonstarchy vegetables contain only 5 grams of carbohydrate per serving, few calories, and lots of vitamins and minerals. Moderate portions of vegetables have little effect on blood glucose but major effects on your health. Eat up!

Why does it seem that I need less food—and enjoy it less—now that I'm older?

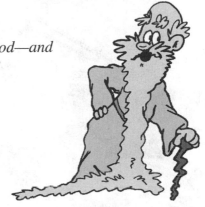

▼
TIP:

If you are not as active as you were when you were younger, you probably don't need to eat as many calories. However, it may be that your appetite and enjoyment are being affected by one of the following changes in

- Taste buds—affecting taste and interest in food
- Smell—affecting interest in food and the amount you eat
- Vision—making it difficult to read labels or recipes
- Hearing—affecting your ability to enjoy the social events around eating
- Touch—making it difficult to prepare food
- Teeth or poorly fitting dentures—making it painful to eat anything but soft, easy-to-chew foods

For reasons such as these, you may skip meals or eat fewer calories than you need, which affects your diabetes control. Limitations on movement can keep you from exercising, leading to loss of energy and appetite. Poor nutrition itself can bring on fatigue and a general sense of not feeling well. Work with your RD to overcome any challenges to following your meal plan.

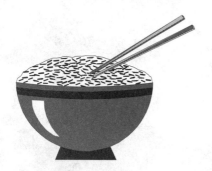

*A re plant sources of protein better
for me than animal protein?*

▼
TIP:

M aybe. Plant proteins have benefits for people with diabetes.
Plant foods are low in fat, especially saturated fat, and high in
fiber. Animal protein adds cholesterol and saturated fat to our diets.
People with diabetes have a greater risk of heart disease earlier in
life. It is important to decrease saturated fat and cholesterol. For
people with diabetic kidney disease, changing the source of protein
in the diet as a treatment is being studied. Whether plant protein
(beans, nuts, vegetables, tofu) is preferred over animal protein
(meat, poultry, fish, milk, eggs) has not been decided. Discuss the
latest research with your diabetes professionals. We do know that
people in other countries who eat less meat and more soy protein
and rice have fewer cancers and heart disease than Americans who
eat lots of animal protein.

Animal protein contains all eight essential amino acids that you
need to build cells in the body. Because your body can't make them,
your food choices must supply them. However, eating a variety of
plant proteins each day can also provide all the amino acids that you
need (see page 510).

*I*s there a benefit to
including more soy
foods in my diet?

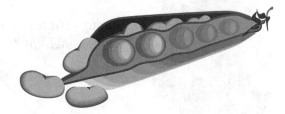

▼
TIP:

Yes. Soy foods are low in saturated fat, have no cholesterol, and contain high-quality protein. Scientists are learning about compounds in soybeans that may reduce your risk of certain chronic diseases, such as heart disease, osteoporosis, and cancer. Eating soy foods may reduce blood cholesterol levels and decrease your risk for heart disease. In soy protein is a group of phytochemicals called isoflavones that may directly lower blood cholesterol levels. In certain stages of kidney disease, vegetable protein may be easier on the kidneys than animal protein.

Soybeans are made into a variety of foods, from ice cream to burgers, and they can be eaten whole or used in your recipes.

Soy Food (serving size)	Calories	Carbo-hydrate (g)	Protein (g)	Isoflavones (mg)
Soybeans (1/2 cup, cooked)	149	9	14	35
Tempeh (1/2 cup)	165	14	16	40
Tofu (1/2 cup)	94	2	10	40
Soy nuts (1 oz)	128	9	11	40
Soy milk (1/2 cup)	40	2	3	40
Miso (2 Tbsp)	72	10	4	10

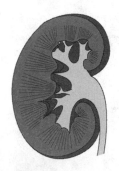

Should I eat less protein to keep my kidneys healthy?

▼ TIP:

Not necessarily. The American Diabetes Association recommends you eat the same amount of protein as the general public. The RDA guidelines suggest eating 15–20% of calories as protein or 0.8 grams per kilogram for healthy adults. For a 132-pound person, this would be about 50 grams of protein per day. Some plant and animal protein choices are listed below. Some with poor blood glucose control may benefit from more protein than the RDA recommended amount. However, most Americans eat more than enough protein. If you already have kidney disease, you may want to eat less protein. Your doctor will consider the stage of kidney disease and your overall nutrition before prescribing a low-protein diet.

Animal Proteins	Protein (g)
1 oz lean meat, poultry, or fish	7
1 cup milk or yogurt	8
1 egg	7

Plant Proteins	Protein (g)
1/2 cup cooked lentils, peas, or beans	7
2 Tbsp peanut butter	8
1/3 cup nuts	7
4 oz tofu	7
1 slice bread, 1/2 cup rice	2–3

Chapter 2
MANAGING
MEDICATION

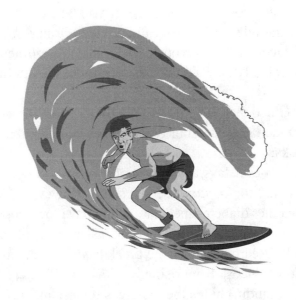

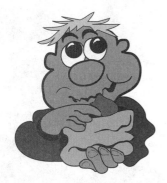

*D*o I need to eat snacks now that I'm taking diabetes pills?

TIP:

The way your pills work tells you whether you need snacks. Diabetes pills called sulfonylureas help the pancreas secrete insulin and can cause low blood glucose. If you take chlorpropamide (Diabinese), tolazamide (Tolinase), tolbutamide (Orinase), glipizide (Glucotrol or Glucotrol XL), glyburide (Glynase), or glimepiride (Amaryl), you probably need snacks, especially in the afternoon and evening.

Metformin (Glucophage) helps your body use insulin and decreases how much glucose your body makes and absorbs, so you don't need snacks.

Acarbose (Precose) delays absorption of glucose and does not cause hypoglycemia, so you don't need a snack. However, if you take acarbose with another diabetes medication and have low blood glucose, treat it with glucose tablets or milk instead of fruit (or sugar-sweetened) drinks. Acarbose slows the breakdown of sugar and may prevent your blood glucose from rising.

Rapaglinide (Prandin) helps the pancreas release insulin and is taken with meals or large (more than 250-calorie) snacks. Other snacks are not necessary.

If you take insulin injections and pills, you will probably need to eat healthy snacks.

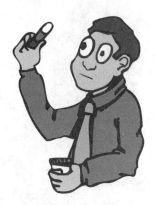

*C*an I adjust my diet to avoid the side effects of acarbose (Precose)?

▼
TIP:

A carbose is a pill for type 2 diabetes that slows down the digestion of carbohydrates. This helps lower your blood glucose level after a meal. It is often used along with another kind of diabetes pill and is taken three times a day with meals.

Acarbose may cause gas, diarrhea, and abdominal pain. This is because the carbohydrate you eat is not completely digested. It may help to increase the amount of medication slowly over a period of months. Eating a low-fiber diet may help. Avoid seeds, nuts, or beans. Select low-fiber cereals, breads, pasta, and rice. Peel and seed fruits and vegetables. It may also help to avoid gas-forming foods, such as beans and vegetables in the cabbage family. Other foods that may cause gas are milk, wheat germ, onions, carrots, celery, bananas, raisins, dried apricots, prune juice, and sorbitol. Sorbitol is a sugar alcohol used in dietetic or diabetic foods, such as sugar-free chewing gum, ice cream, candy, or cookies.

When you add fiber back to your diet, do it slowly and be sure to drink plenty of water.

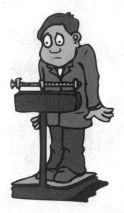

*M*y doctor wants me to start insulin, but I'm afraid I'll gain weight. How can I prevent weight gain while I'm taking insulin?

▼

TIP:

When your blood glucose is high, you lose calories as sugar in your urine. Taking insulin will give you better blood glucose control, which makes you feel better every day and lowers your chances of developing complications. This is important! However, when you stop losing calories in your urine, you can gain weight.

Review your eating habits, total calories, types of food, and how much fat and carbohydrate you eat with your RD. You may not need to eat as many calories, or you may need more exercise. This will help you take advantage of the more efficient job your body is doing at capturing and storing glucose.

There is another way that insulin can cause weight gain. If you take more insulin than you need, then you have to eat to "feed" the insulin and avoid low blood glucose. If you find yourself eating more than you want just to avoid hypoglycemia, your insulin dose may need adjusting. Discuss your medications, weight goal, and meal plan with your health care providers if you are concerned about gaining weight.

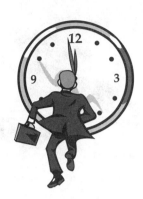

*M*y doctor just switched my insulin to
Humalog. How will this affect my blood
glucose and meal plan?

▼
TIP:

You may have better blood glucose control and more flexible
mealtimes. Humalog is a rapid-acting insulin that starts working within 10 minutes and peaks in 30–90 minutes, the way a normal pancreas responds to food. You may not need snacks between
meals as you did with regular insulin, because rapid-acting insulin
does not stay in your body as long. You may need less Humalog
than your regular insulin dose but more intermediate- or long-acting
insulin.

When you take a rapid-acting insulin and your blood glucose is
in target range, you must eat within 15 minutes. This is quite
different from waiting 30–45 minutes with regular insulin. If your
blood glucose level is low before your meal, you might take
Humalog after your meal.

It is easier to fine-tune your insulin dose to a meal with rapid-
acting insulin because it works only on the food eaten right then.
Monitor your blood glucose levels when you begin using Humalog
to learn how the medication works for you.

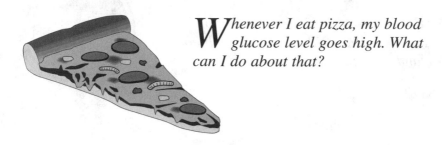

Whenever I eat pizza, my blood glucose level goes high. What can I do about that?

▼
TIP:

You might try eating a smaller serving. The type of crust, sauce, toppings, and size of slice varies a lot, so it is easy to overeat pizza. When you order pizza, ask for nutrition information. If you purchase it in the grocery store, check the Nutrition Facts panel. Exercising after you eat pizza can help bring down your blood glucose level.

For some people, high blood glucose occurs several hours after eating, perhaps because pizza is digested at different rates. Each person has a unique response to each food. Monitor your blood glucose up to 9 hours after eating pizza to find your response. If you take insulin, increasing premeal rapid-acting insulin may not be enough. Your intermediate- or long-acting insulin may need an adjustment also. Talk with your health care providers.

If you take diabetes pills, count the carbohydrates in your pizza serving. Is this more than you usually eat? Monitor blood glucose before and after eating to find your response.

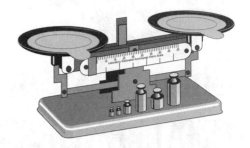

What is a carbohydrate-to-insulin ratio? Can I use this to eat what I want?

TIP:

A carbohydrate-to-insulin ratio is used by people who manage diabetes with multiple daily injections or an insulin pump. The relationship between the food you eat and the insulin you take can be shown as a ratio—a carbohydrate-to-insulin ratio. This ratio tells you how much rapid-acting insulin to use, which is very useful when you eat more (or less) carbohydrate than usual. So, yes, you can eat unusual meals and determine the correct insulin dose. You have more flexibility in food choices and timing of meals. Take care, however, to choose foods that give you the nutrients you need and don't overindulge. To figure the insulin dose, you also take into account any exercise that you do.

Your carbohydrate-to-insulin ratio varies according to the meal or time of day. Many people have a lower carbohydrate-to-insulin ratio at breakfast than at dinner. The amount of fat, protein, and fiber in the meal will also affect the insulin's action. Blood glucose monitoring helps you adjust the ratio for different kinds of meals and mealtimes. Diabetes professionals can help you determine whether this approach will work for you.

Chapter 3
CHALLENGES OF CHILDREN

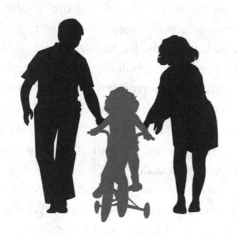

How often should my child have sweets?

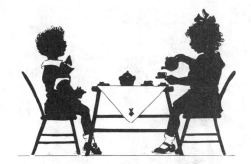

TIP:

O ccasionally. Sweets are in the tiny top portion of the Diabetes Food Pyramid, telling you to enjoy them when your nutrient needs from the other five groups have been met. If your child eats ice cream, cookies, and candy often or in large amounts, he or she won't have room for the foods he or she really needed. Some experts recommend offering sweets as part of a meal. This avoids making children think that sweets are special. Having sweets in appropriate amounts as part of the meal plan prevents the guilt feelings children may have about eating them. This approach also teaches that high-sugar foods are part of the carbohydrates in the meal plan, instead of an addition.

Many kid-friendly foods may seem healthy, but the nutrient value is similar to candy or desserts. A fruit snack pouch is handy but may contain 100% sugar with only fruit flavoring. Look closely at labels to see how much of the carbohydrate content is sugar. A juicy piece of fresh fruit is also handy and supplies essential vitamins, minerals, and dietary fiber.

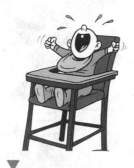

*W*hat do I do if my toddler refuses to eat his or her meal?

▼
TIP:

If you gave insulin before the meal, give your child a peanut butter and jelly sandwich or milk or a bigger portion of a food you know she or he will eat to cover the insulin given and prevent low blood glucose.

It is not uncommon for a toddler to refuse to eat. This can make parents anxious, especially if rapid- or short-acting insulin has already been given. Keep in mind that during the toddler stage, growth and appetite are slowing down, and your child is becoming an independent self-feeder. Your toddler may be eating adult table foods but is not ready for adult-size servings. Are you serving appropriate types and amounts of foods? Is your child joining the family in a regular schedule of meals and snacks? Be sure your child has enough time between meals and snacks so he or she will have an appetite. In some cases, you can give rapid-acting insulin after the meal and adjust the dose to the amount of food the child has eaten.

*What if my child is napping
and it's time for a snack?*

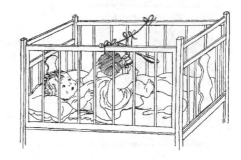

▼
TIP:

If your child's nap will pass snack time, you might test his or her
blood glucose if your child is not startled and awakened by the
finger stick. Some children sleep through a stick. However, waking
your child this way may be too traumatic. It may be better to simply
wake your child and feed him or her.

For very young children, preventing low blood glucose is your
goal. Low blood glucose levels are dangerous because they can
affect the developing brain. Know your child's insulin types and
doses and understand when they peak and how long they keep
acting. You have to learn to balance the amount and type of insulin
with food and eating times.

Discuss the following approaches to naptime snacks with your
diabetes professionals:

- If your child's nap is 30 minutes to 1 hour after a meal, you don't
  need to test blood glucose or feed him or her before the nap.

- If your child's snack is scheduled for 3:00 P.M. and nap starts at
  2:00 P.M., offer part of the snack before the nap and the rest after
  the nap.

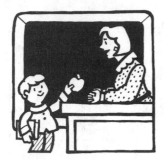

*I*s it okay for my child to eat school lunches?

▼
TIP:

Probably. School lunches can fit into your child's meal plan, but you'll have to do some homework. Review menus with your child and select those that your child likes. Evaluate foods and serving sizes with your child's food and insulin plan in mind. Often, the cafeteria staff or your child must adjust the serving size. Food items may need to be added by the cafeteria or brought from home by your child, and some food items (sweetened fruit, fruit punch, or desserts) may need to be left off the tray.

Your child's comfort level with making changes in the menu, which may single him or her out as different, could cause a problem. Also, how willing are school personnel to work with you? A change in the menu may complicate things. Help your child learn how to choose basic foods. In junior high and high school, menu choices are more varied but may not be as healthy. Review nutrition information from fast food restaurants with your child to help him or her select foods that fit the meal plan. Carrying a lunch from home part of the time can help balance meals.

*H*ow do I handle trick-or-treating or other
holiday activities for my child with
diabetes?

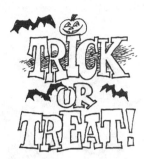

TIP:

*P*art of growing up with diabetes is learning to make decisions
about eating in special situations. Deciding *with your child*
when, what kind, and how much candy he or she will eat can help
form positive attitudes and feelings. If you talk with your child, you
may find that food or treats are not what is most important to him or
her about holiday activities.

Read the Nutrition Facts label on candy with your child and
discuss the nutritional value of candy. Help your child make adjustments to the meal plan to include favorite treats from time to time.
Some Halloween candy can be put in the freezer for later, if your
child is not tempted by having it in the house. Discuss monitoring
blood glucose carefully. Ask your diabetes team to explain the
option of adjusting insulin upward to cover extra treats. Other family members can help by offering to trade some of the child's candy
for money, movie passes, sleepovers, staying up late, or use of a big
brother or sister's stereo. Plan ahead to prevent frustration and
disappointment.

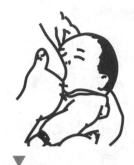

I have type 1 diabetes. Will I be able to breastfeed?

▼
TIP:

Yes, you and your baby can enjoy all the benefits of breast-feeding. Enroll in a prenatal program for women with diabetes. Develop a breastfeeding meal plan and blood glucose goals with an RD. Breastfeeding lowers blood glucose and requires an extra 500 calories a day, but your insulin needs will drop to about half of what you used during pregnancy. You must monitor blood glucose carefully to adjust your insulin to your new eating and sleeping patterns and your infant's demands for milk. Checking blood glucose right before breastfeeding is wise. To avoid low blood glucose, eat a snack such as a glass of milk, piece of fruit, or a few crackers before or during breastfeeding and before taking a nap. A meal 1–2 hours before nursing works as well. Discuss all this with your diabetes team.

High blood glucose levels may lead to breast infections (masti-tis). To prevent infection, alternate breasts when feeding; clean the breasts with water after feedings and let them air dry; learn proper infant latching-on techniques; drink plenty of water; and avoid wearing tight bras.

Chapter 4
THE SKINNY ON FAT

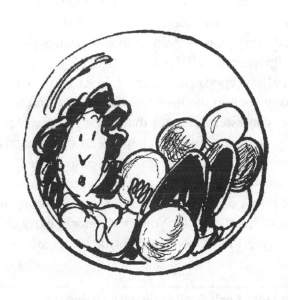

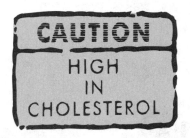

What should my cholesterol level be? What is the difference between "good" and "bad" cholesterol?

▼

TIP:

The target for total cholesterol in adults is less than 200 mg/dl. For children and adolescents, it is less than 170 mg/dl.

The ADA recommends that people with diabetes have blood lipids checked every year. A lipid profile measures the levels of high-density lipoprotein (HDL), low-density lipoprotein (LDL), and triglycerides. HDL (good) cholesterol carries cholesterol from every part of the body back to the liver for disposal. If you have high levels of HDL cholesterol (higher than 40 mg/dl for men, 50 mg/dl for women), you are less likely to have heart disease. LDL (bad) cholesterol carries cholesterol from the liver to other tissues. Along the way, it forms deposits on the walls of arteries and other blood vessels. High levels of LDL cholesterol (above 130 mg/dl) show an increased risk of heart disease. Your body stores extra fat and calories as triglycerides. Good triglyceride levels are less than 200 mg/dl.

Blood Lipid Goals for People with Diabetes*	
Total Cholesterol	<200 mg/dl
LDL (bad) Cholesterol	<100 mg/dl
HDL (good) Cholesterol	>40 mg/dl
Triglycerides	<150 mg/dl

*2004 American Diabetes Association Clinical Practice Recommendations

*H*ow *much can changes in
diet lower my blood
cholesterol level?*

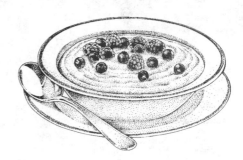

▼

TIP:

Diet changes may decrease your LDL (bad) cholesterol by
15–25 mg/dl. For every 1% decrease in your total cholesterol,
you decrease your risk for heart disease by 2%. Wouldn't you rather
improve your risk factors for heart disease without medications,
using diet changes only?

A heart-healthy eating plan is low in saturated fat and dietary
cholesterol with total fat around 30% of total calories. This helps
reduce blood cholesterol. Eating foods containing more fiber, such
as beans, can also help reduce blood levels of cholesterol (see page
500). An RD can help you find the best amount of fat, carbohydrate,
and protein in your food choices to lower your cholesterol, maintain
healthy weight, and have good blood glucose control.

The following suggestions can help you eat low-fat meals:

■ Select lean meats and cook with little or no fat.

■ Choose low-fat or fat-free milk products.

■ Eat less meat, cheese, and bacon.

■ Eat low-fat breads and starchy foods, such as potatoes, rice, and
beans.

■ Remember that sweets, such as pastries and chocolate, are often
also high in fat.

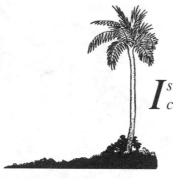

Is it more important to decrease the cholesterol or the saturated fat in my diet?

▼
TIP:

Focus on the saturated fat. Decreasing saturated fat in your diet has a more significant effect on your blood cholesterol level. Saturated fats come mainly from animal foods, such as meat, poultry, butter, and whole milk, and from coconut, palm, and palm kernel oils. Foods high in saturated fats are firm at room temperature.

To eat less saturated fat, use liquid vegetable oils instead of shortening, margarine, or butter whenever you can. Cut back on total fat and you'll likely reduce saturated fats, too. Check for saturated fat on Nutrition Facts panels on food labels. Check the ingredient list also. A food labeled "low in saturated fat" must contain one gram or less saturated fat per serving and no more than 15% of calories from saturated fat.

Your liver makes most of the cholesterol in your body, but every cell can also make cholesterol. When the body makes too much, the risk for heart disease goes up. Cholesterol also comes from animal foods. Cholesterol is found in milk, meat, poultry, eggs, fish, and dairy foods. However, dietary cholesterol doesn't automatically become blood cholesterol.

*H*ow can I boost good (HDL) cholesterol and
lower bad (LDL) cholesterol?

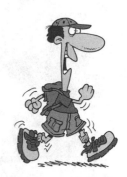

▼
TIP:

To increase HDL cholesterol and lower LDL cholesterol

- Stay physically active. It keeps HDL levels normal, reduces blood pressure, helps control stress, helps control body weight, gives your heart muscle a good workout, and improves blood glucose control.
- Lose weight.
- Reduce the fat in your diet to no more than 30% of calories from fat and 10% from saturated fat. Replace some saturated fat in your diet with monounsaturated fats.
- Stop smoking. Smoking may lower HDL cholesterol levels and is a key factor in sudden death from cardiovascular disease. Smoking seems to raise blood pressure and heart rate and may increase the tendency of blood to clot and lead to a heart attack.

Other ways to decrease your LDL cholesterol are to

- Improve blood glucose control. It may decrease LDL cholesterol by up to 10–15%.
- Eat high-fiber foods, such as beans, oatmeal, oat bran, wheat bran, barley, and some fruits and vegetables. They contain soluble fiber, which seems to lower LDL cholesterol levels.

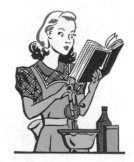

*H*ow do I know if I'm eating the right
amount of fat?

▼
TIP:

Talk to an RD about the right amount of fat for you, based on
your weight and blood glucose and lipid goals. Most people eat
too much fat. Fats contain 9 calories per gram, which means they
contain a lot of calories in a small amount of food.

Write down what you eat for a few days, including the fat grams
in your foods. The Nutrition Facts panel on food labels gives this
information. For most people, fat should contribute about 30% of
total calories for the day. Here is how to figure the number of grams
of fat to eat if 30% of your 1,800 calories come from fat:

To find 30% of 1,800 calories,
    1,800 × 0.30 = 540 calories from fat
To find the number of fat grams in 540 calories
    (9 calories per 1 gram of fat)
    540 ÷ 9 = 60 grams of fat per day

Total Calories	Fat (g) for 30% of Calories
1200	40
1500	50
1800	60
2100	70
2400	80
2600	87

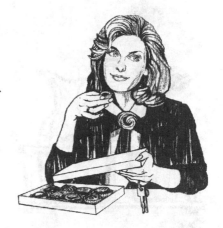

*C*an I have an unlimited amount of
fat-free foods?

▼
TIP:

No. Fat free does not mean the food is calorie free or carbohydrate free. Nor does it mean that it is a "free food." A free
food is a term used by people with diabetes for foods that have less
than 20 calories or less than 5 grams of carbohydrate per serving.

Fat-free foods have fat taken out and sometimes replaced by fat
replacers. Some fat replacers, such as those used in fat-free salad
dressings, contain carbohydrate and can affect your blood glucose
level. Also, many fat-free foods have more sugar added to them for
taste, and this will affect your blood glucose level.

If your weight and blood lipids are in a healthy range, you don't
need fat-free foods. If your goal is to lower blood lipids and lose
weight, moderate portions of some fat-free foods may help you.
Read the Nutrition Facts on food labels to get the serving size,
calories, and carbohydrate content to help you decide how fat-free
foods fit into your meal plan.

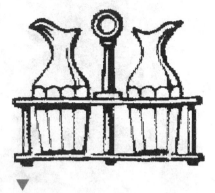

How can I eat more monounsaturated fats?

▼
TIP:

Use olive oil, canola oil, or nuts in your meals. The ADA recommends that you replace part of your dietary fat, especially saturated fat, with monounsaturated fats. Keep in mind, these healthier fats must *replace* saturated or polyunsaturated fat in the diet rather than be added to it. In other words, don't increase the total fat content of your meal plan.

Nuts can substitute for animal protein in recipes or be eaten in small servings as snacks. Garnish vegetables with slivered almonds, hazelnuts, or pine nuts instead of butter. Use nut butters (such as peanut, cashew, or almond butter) without partially hydrogenated oils. Avocados can be sliced and added to a sandwich of tomato, sprouts, or other vegetables.

Prepare salad dressings or pastas with olive oil. Cook (sauté, stir-fry, or broil) with small amounts of olive or canola oil. Canola oil is a monounsaturated fat that is less expensive than olive oil and lighter in taste. When you substitute a liquid oil for a solid shortening in a recipe, use 1/4 less oil.

*W*hat are trans fatty acids and how do
they affect my diabetes?

▼
TIP:

Trans fatty acids are formed in processed foods during hydrogenation. Hydrogenation makes a fat solid when it is at room temperature. For example, liquid vegetable oil is partially hydrogenated to make stick margarine. Partially hydrogenated vegetable oil is used in fried foods, baked products, and snack foods.

Trans fatty acids don't affect blood glucose levels but do increase blood cholesterol levels, which increases your risk for heart disease. If less than 30% of your calories come from fat and 10% from saturated fat, you're probably okay. If you eat a moderately high-fat diet, your trans fatty acid intake may be too high. Don't eat many processed foods. Choose soft table spreads instead of stick margarine. Read food labels and select margarine that contains no more than 2 grams of saturated fat per tablespoon and liquid oil as the first ingredient. Look for baked products, convenience dinners, and snack foods with less than 2 grams of saturated fat per serving. Use vegetable oil instead of solid shortening in cooking. By January 2006, food manufacturers will be required to list trans fats on the Nutrition Facts label of food products. Check with your RD if you have questions about trans fatty acids.

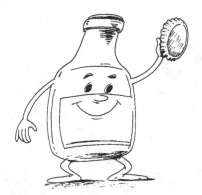

*D*oes it matter what kind of
margarine and vegetable oil I use?

▼
TIP:

It depends on the fatty acids they contain—saturated, polyunsaturated, and monounsaturated. Saturated fats (butter and lard)
are the least healthy. Polyunsaturated fats (corn or soybean oil) are
healthier. Monounsaturated fats (canola or olive oil) are the best. All
fats are actually mixtures of these three fatty acids.

All margarines are made of vegetable oil. However, the fat is
hydrogenated (saturated), so it is less healthy than oil. Tub and
squeeze margarines also contain water and air to lower fat and
calories. Read the food label to find margarine with only 2 grams of
saturated fat per serving and liquid oil as the first ingredient.

Canola and olive oil are the best vegetable oils because they are
low in saturated fat and have the largest amount of monounsaturated
fats. Safflower, sunflower, corn, and soybean oil are also low in
saturated fat.

Hint: If you want the taste of butter but not all the saturated fat,
whip 1 cup of canola oil into 1 cup of butter!

*W*hat are fat replacers and how do they affect my diabetes?

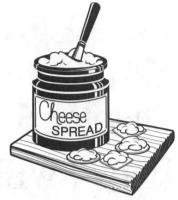

▼
TIP:

Fat replacers are used to give reduced-calorie foods the texture, appearance, and taste of full-fat products. Most fat replacers are made from carbohydrates and can raise your blood glucose level. The ones made of protein or fat are not so likely to affect blood glucose. Remember that food with a fat replacer can still have lots of calories.

Fat replacers made from carbohydrates include polydextrose, cellulose gum, corn syrup solids, dextrin, maltodextrin, hydrogenated starch hydrolysate, carrageenan and modified food starch. They combine with water to provide thicker texture, as in fat-free salad dressings. Fat replacers made from protein include Simplesse and whey protein concentrate. They are used in cheese, sour cream, salad dressings, baked goods, butter, and mayonnaise spreads.

Olestra is a fat replacer found in salty snacks. Made from sugar and fat, it does not act like fat. It is not digested, so it contributes no calories. It may cause cramping, diarrhea, and inhibit the absorption of some fat-soluble vitamins.

Check the Nutrition Facts panel for calories and the amount of carbohydrate, fat, and protein in foods with fat replacers. Ask your RD to help you work these foods into your meal plan.

Chapter 5
HOW SWEET IT IS

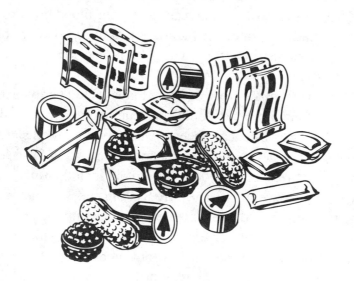

*D*oes eating sugar cause
diabetes?

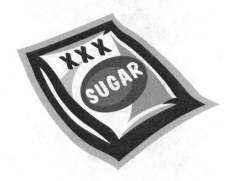

▼
TIP:

No. Although diabetes has been called "sugar diabetes" for many years, eating sugar does not cause it. Type 1 diabetes happens when your body's immune system destroys the insulin-producing beta-cells in the pancreas. Factors that may cause the immune system to do this are autoantibodies, cow's milk (see page 593), genes, and oxygen-free radicals (see page 566). Type 1 diabetes is probably triggered by one of these environmental factors in people who have the genes for developing the disease.

Type 2 diabetes is different from type 1. The bodies of most people with type 2 make insulin but can't use it well. Genetics play a strong role in type 2 diabetes, as does age, obesity, and lifestyle. Obese individuals who eat a high-calorie diet and don't participate in physical activity are more likely to develop type 2 diabetes. In this case, too much sugar may provide excess calories, in the same way excess fat does. The resulting weight gain and obesity, which interfere with the action of insulin, can lead to the development of type 2 diabetes.

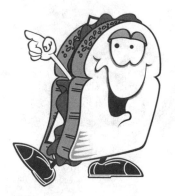

I'm confused about sugars and starches. Will a brownie or a piece of bread raise my blood glucose the most?

TIP:

Sugars and starches are carbohydrates and, eaten in equal amounts, they raise blood glucose about the same. A small brownie (15 grams of carbohydrate) raises blood glucose the same as one slice of bread (15 grams of carbohydrate).

For years, we thought that the body absorbed sugar more quickly than starch, and people were told to avoid sweets. Research has shown that sugar is okay for people with diabetes if it is part of a meal plan. It is substituted for other carbohydrate foods. Certain carbohydrates are absorbed at different rates, but when combined with other foods in a meal, this effect can be hard to predict. Focus on the total amount of carbohydrate that you eat rather than on whether it comes from starch or sugar.

Certain factors affect the way your blood glucose responds to sugars and starches. When you eat sweets, observe whether other foods are eaten at the same time, how quickly you eat, how the food was prepared, and the amount of protein and fat in the food. Measure your blood glucose 1–2 hours after eating and note the effect sugar has on it. Use this information to make decisions about including sweets in your meal plan.

*H*ow *many grams of sugar am I allowed to eat in a day?*

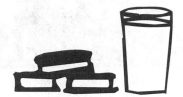

▼

TIP:

There is no magic number of grams for each day, but eat sugar sparingly. Sugar has calories but few vitamins or minerals. Foods high in sugar are usually high in fat, which can lead to poor diabetes control and weight gain.

The Nutrition Facts label gives the number of grams of sugar in the food. This number includes both natural and added sugars. Natural sugars are found naturally in foods, such as fructose in raisins or lactose in milk. These sugars provide some vitamins and minerals. Added sugars are put into foods to make them sweet, such as sugar in cookies or high fructose corn syrup in soft drinks. These sugars provide calories but no other nutrients.

When you read the food label, check the type of sugar the food contains, but focus on the grams of total carbohydrate rather than the grams of sugar. Sugar and sweets are fine occasionally, in small portions, if you substitute them for other carbohydrate foods in your meal plan and check your blood glucose to see how the food affects you.

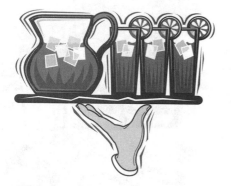

A re there sweeteners that are free foods? How can I tell which to use?

▼
TIP:

Y es. "Nonnutritive" sweeteners are free foods because they have no calories or carbohydrate. They don't raise blood glucose levels. None of them are perfect for all uses. Some are great in cold beverages but won't work in baked goods. While the sweeteners themselves are calorie free, don't forget to count the calories, fat, and carbohydrate in the foods they are sweetening.

Sweetener	Calories (per gram)	Other Names	Description
Saccharin	0	Sweet 'n Low	200–700 times sweeter than sucrose; suitable for cooking and baking
Aspartame	0	Nutrasweet, Equal	160–220 times sweeter than sucrose; may change flavor if heated
Acesulfame-K	0	Sunette, Sweet One	200 times sweeter than sucrose; suitable for cooking and baking
Sucralose	0	Splenda	600 times sweeter than sucrose; suitable for cooking and baking

*W*hat calorie-containing sweeteners can I use instead of sugar?

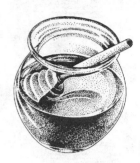

▼

TIP:

Sugar and all the other calorie-containing sweeteners provide about the same amount of calories and raise your blood glucose in the same way. Fructose, honey, and other "natural" sweeteners have no advantages over the other sweeteners that contain calories. You can substitute the nutritive sweeteners listed below for other carbohydrates in your meal plan. Remember to count the calories and carbohydrate they contain.

Sweetener	Calories (per gram)	Other Names	Description
Sucrose	4	granulated sugar, table sugar, powdered sugar, brown sugar, molasses	sweetens; enhances flavor, texture, and appearance of baked goods
Fructose	4	fruit sugar, high fructose corn syrup	sweetens; functions like sucrose in baking; may produce a lower rise in blood glucose than sucrose; in large amounts raises LDL (bad) cholesterol
Sugar alcohols	2–3	sorbitol, mannitol, xylitol, isomalt, lactitol, malitol, hydrogenated starch hydrolysate	25–90% as sweet as sucrose; may produce laxative effect in large doses

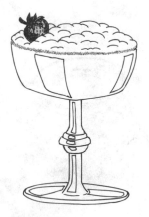

*C*an I eat all I want of food that is labeled *"sugar free"?*

TIP:

No. A food labeled sugar free must contain less than 0.5 grams of sugar per serving, but it may have calories and carbo-hydrate. For example, sugar-free pudding has 0 grams of sugar, but it also has 70 calories and 6 grams of carbohydrate in a 1/2-cup serving. If you were to eat unlimited amounts, you could easily add enough calories and carbohydrate to sabotage your diabetes and weight-control efforts over time.

Although the sweetener used in a sugar-free product may be calorie free (such as acesulfame potassium, aspartame, saccharin, or sucralose), the other ingredients in the food usually contain fat, carbohydrate, protein, and calories. Nonnutritive sweeteners may be used along with other sweeteners that contain calories, so don't rely on the "sugar-free" symbol on the front of the package alone. Read the ingredient list and food label carefully so you can make the best choices for healthy eating (see page 494).

*W*hat are sugar alcohols? Will
foods with sugar alcohols cause
my blood glucose to rise?

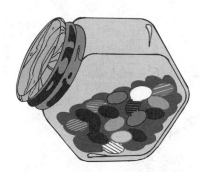

▼
TIP:

S ugar alcohols (also known as polyols) are used to sweeten a
variety of foods, such as candy, chewing gum, baked goods, ice
cream, and fruit spreads. They are also found in toothpaste, mouth-
wash, and medications, including cough syrups and throat lozenges.
Sugar alcohols have 2–3 calories per gram, compared to 4 calories
per gram in other sugars. Sugar alcohols are absorbed more slowly
than other sugars and cause a smaller rise in blood glucose levels
after they are eaten.

Because sugar alcohols are not completely digested in the stomach, you may experience side effects such as diarrhea, intestinal
cramping, or gas if you eat too much of them. One recommendation
is to eat no more than 20–50 grams of sugar alcohol in a day, which
is the amount found in 12–33 pieces of sugar alcohol–sweetened
hard candy.

The sugar alcohols you'll see on food labels include:

Hydrogenated starch hydrolysate	Mannitol
Isomalt	Malitol
Lactitol	Sorbitol
	Xylitol

What is stevia?

▼
TIP:

Stevia is a sweetener 30–300 times sweeter than sugar, but it has no calories. It is made from an herb and comes in three forms. The greenish-black liquid is 70 times sweeter than sugar and is used to sweeten cereal, tea, coffee, and hot chocolate. It's also used in baking but may change the color of foods. The crushed leaf form is 30 times as sweet as sugar. It comes in small tea-bag packets and is sprinkled on cereal and other foods. The leaf particles do not dissolve. The third form of stevia is a white, heat-stable powder that is 300 times sweeter than sugar. The liquid and leaf forms have a slight taste of anise (licorice).

Although it is used in Brazil and Japan, stevia has not been approved as a food additive by the Food and Drug Administration (FDA) here. However, health food stores sell it for personal use. There is no research available describing the effects of stevia when used by a person with diabetes. Side effects are also unknown, so discuss the product with your health care team and use caution until more information is available.

Chapter 6
FOOD AND FITNESS

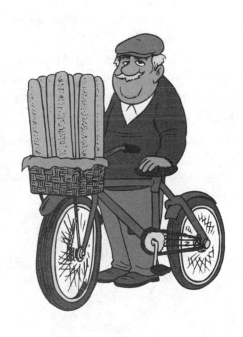

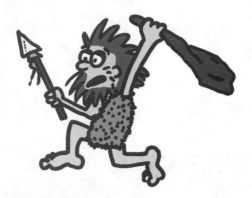

*W*hat kind of exercise burns off enough calories to lose weight?

▼
TIP:

To lose a pound of body weight you need to burn 3,500 calories—not all at once, but over several days. Most people lose weight by getting more exercise each day and cutting back their food by about 500 calories a day.

The more frequently and more intensely you exercise, the more calories you burn. And exercise includes everyday activities such as vacuuming and gardening. If you are moderately active every day, you will burn about 150 calories, or about 1,000 calories a week. With exercise alone and no diet changes, you would lose 1 pound in 3–4 weeks. A combination of exercise and chores gives you variety.

Activity (30 minutes)	Body Weight	
	120 lbs	**170 lbs**
Aerobic dance	165 calories	230 calories
Bicycling	110	155
Bowling	85	115
Gardening	140	195
Golf (walking)	125	175
Hiking	165	230
Housework	70	95
Mowing lawn	150	215
Swimming, leisurely	165	230
Tennis	195	270
Walking, brisk	110	155

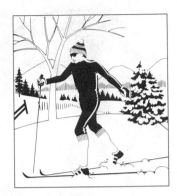

*D*o I need a snack when I exercise?

▼
TIP:

If you take insulin or oral diabetes medication, it will depend on your blood glucose level. Check before and after exercise and during long, hard exercise. (If blood glucose is more than 250 mg/dl, do not exercise until it is under control.)

- **30 minutes of low-intensity exercise** (walking): If blood glucose is less than 100 mg/dl before exercise, eat a snack with 15 grams of carbohydrate.

- **30–60 minutes of moderate-intensity exercise** (tennis, swimming, jogging): If blood glucose is less than 100 mg/dl before exercise, have a snack with 25–50 grams of carbohydrate. If blood glucose is 100–180 mg/dl, eat 10–15 grams of carbohydrate.

- **1–2 hours of strenuous-intensity exercise** (basketball, skiing, shoveling snow): If blood glucose is less than 100 mg/dl before exercise, add a snack with about 50 grams of carbohydrate. If blood glucose is 100–180 mg/dl, add a snack with 25–50 grams of carbohydrate. If blood glucose is 180–250 mg/dl, have a snack with 10–15 grams of carbohydrate. At this intense level of exercise, always monitor blood glucose carefully.

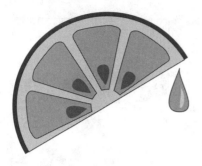

What are some foods or beverages to use with exercise?

▼
TIP:

If you take insulin or oral diabetes medicine, you may need a snack before, during, or after you exercise. Muscles keep burning glucose even after you stop exercising. It may take the body up to 24 hours to replace glucose stores used during exercise. After strenuous exercise, you may need to monitor your blood glucose every 1–2 hours (see page 547).

When you are exercising, don't wait to be thirsty to drink plenty of fluid. Dehydration can hinder your strength and endurance. Cool water is absorbed faster than warm water. Diluted fruit juice or sports drinks provide carbohydrate and fluids for exercise that lasts more than 1 hour.

Food for Exercise
(15 g carbohydrate)

- 1 small piece fresh fruit
- 2 Tbsp raisins
- 3 graham crackers
- 1/2 English muffin or bagel
- 1 small muffin
- 6–8 oz sports drink

- 1 cup yogurt
- 4–5 snack crackers
- 1/4 cup dried fruit
- 1/2 cup fruit juice
  (can be diluted)

*C*an I use sports drinks when I exercise?

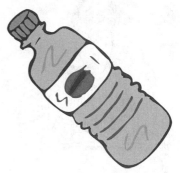

▼
TIP:

W ater is the best drink when you're exercising less than 1 hour. Every human needs carbohydrate during exercise that lasts more than 1 hour and is moderate to high intensity (swimming, jogging, soccer, shoveling heavy snow). When muscle stores of fuel are used up, blood glucose supplies the fuel for prolonged exercise. Sports drinks provide fluids, are easy to take, and are easier to digest than food during prolonged exercise. Certain sports drinks are better than others. Drinks with a concentration of carbohydrate or sugars greater than 10% (such as fruit juice and regular soda) may not be absorbed well and cause cramps, nausea, diarrhea, or bloating. Diluted fruit juice (1/2 water, 1/2 juice) works better.

	Portion Size	Calories (g)	Carbo-hydrate	Carbohydrate Concen-tration (%)
All Sport Body Quencher	8 oz	70	20	8
Exceed Energy Drink Powder	2 Tbsp + 8 oz water	70	17	7
Gatorade Thirst Quencher	8 oz	50	14	6
Power Ade Thirst Quencher	8 oz	70	19	8

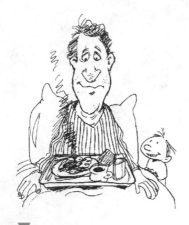

When should I eat breakfast and take my insulin if I work out early in the morning?

▼
TIP:

To exercise before breakfast: First check your blood glucose. If it is 100 mg/dl or higher, eat or drink 10–15 grams of carbo-hydrate, then exercise. If it is lower than 100 mg/dl, add another 10–15 grams of carbohydrate (total of 20–30 grams) and wait 10–15 minutes. Test again and if it is above 100 mg/dl, go exercise. You may need more carbohydrate during exercise, depending on the type of exercise. After exercise, check your blood glucose again, take your insulin, and eat breakfast. You may need to decrease your usual morning dose of insulin, depending on the time and intensity of exercise.

To exercise after breakfast: If you work out 1–2 hours after breakfast, eat your usual breakfast. You may need more carbo-hydrate at breakfast or to adjust your insulin, but you need to keep a record of your blood glucose levels before, during, and after exercise to learn your response to exercise at particular times of the day. This helps you decide whether food and insulin adjustments are needed.

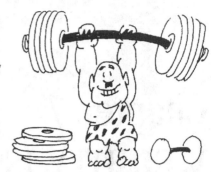

I'm 65. Can I start a weight-training program now? Do I need an amino acid (protein supplement)?

▼
TIP:

Weight (or resistance) training can give you more strength and endurance for your daily activities and help prevent osteoporosis. Building muscle mass is not just for young people. As you get older, your body loses muscle mass and tone unless you do something about it. You want muscle mass because muscles burn calories even when you are doing absolutely nothing. So the benefits of weight training go way beyond those you see in the mirror.

If you get serious about weight training, your protein needs are only slightly higher (about 2–4 oz more meat, chicken, or fish a day). Excess protein can actually be harmful by causing dehydration and strain on the kidneys. You can get enough amino acids—and all the other essential nutrients that supplements don't supply—from the food you eat. Food also costs less than protein in powder or pill form.

Chapter 7
WEIGHTY ISSUES

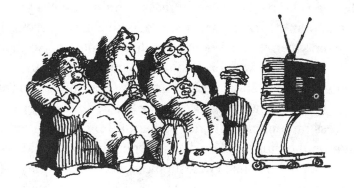

What is BMI and why is it important?

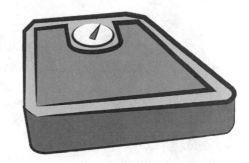

▼

TIP:

Body mass index, or BMI, combines your weight and height into one number. BMI applies to both men and women and is related to total body fat. The risk for type 2 diabetes, high blood pressure, lipid disorders, cardiovascular disease, gallbladder disease, osteo-arthritis, sleep apnea, respiratory problems, and cancer rises in people whose BMI is over 25.

To find your BMI
1. Multiply your weight in pounds by 705
2. Divide your answer by your height in inches
3. Divide this answer by your height again

For example, a 5'6", 185-pound individual has a BMI of about 30. Recent guidelines define overweight as a BMI of 25–29.9 and obesity as a BMI of 30 and above. Keep in mind that the BMI is only a guideline. A very muscular, active person could have a high BMI without health risks. On the other hand, a couch potato may have a lower BMI, yet have too much body fat.

If you are overweight or obese, the good news is that losing just 10% of your body weight will bring significant improvements in your health and diabetes control!

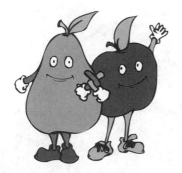

*H*ow can I determine my ideal body weight?

▼
TIP:

There is actually a range of body weights associated with good health. For example, a 5'5" man or woman should weigh between 114 and 150 pounds. You must consider your age, gender, body shape, and location of body fat. Talk to your health care providers about the best weight for you.

People with fat around the upper body, waist, and abdomen ("apple" shape) tend to have more health problems than those who put on fat on the lower body, hips, and thighs ("pear" shape). Health problems associated with apple shapes include insulin resistance, higher blood cholesterol, tendency toward heart and blood vessel disease, and high blood pressure.

To determine your body shape (waist-to-hip ratio):
1. Measure around waist or 1 inch above navel
2. Measure hips at biggest point
3. Divide waist measurement by hip measurement

For a woman, a ratio of greater than 0.8 means an apple shape; a ratio of less than 0.8 means a pear. For a man, a ratio greater than 1.0 means an apple, and a ratio of less than 1.0 means a pear.

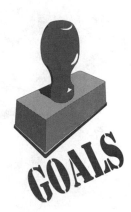

I need to lose weight to improve my blood glucose levels, but I can't get started. How can I set a reasonable weight loss goal and achieve it?

TIP:

Setting realistic goals is the key. If you start with a modest weight loss goal of 10–15 pounds, you are more likely to achieve and maintain it. (A weight loss of as little as 10–15% of your weight can lower your health risks.) Once you've reached your first goal, you can assess your progress and set your sights on the next target.

When you have chosen a weight loss goal, these tips can help you get started.

■ Write down your goal and keep it where you can be reminded of it each day.

■ Share your goal with someone who will see your progress, such as your health care team or a caring friend.

■ Take one immediate action to get started. For example, schedule an appointment with an RD or join an exercise class. Taking action improves your chances for success!

■ Commit to small daily actions, such as packing a healthy lunch rather than going out for fast food.

■ Find new ways to deal with stress, such as taking a walk or doing yoga.

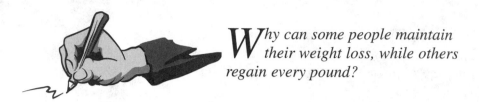

Why can some people maintain their weight loss, while others regain every pound?

▼
TIP:

Researchers have found that people who maintain their weight loss have done certain things to succeed. You can try the following:

Get help in developing a personalized meal plan that works for you, rather than following a preprinted diet from a magazine or book.

Exercise. Increased physical activity is one of the best ways to keep lost weight from returning.

Keep records of blood glucose levels, physical activity, and the food you eat.

Surround yourself with friends or relatives who support your efforts. They help you keep going!

Stay away from a quick-fix approach and commit to long-term weight control.

Don't deny yourself. Occasionally eat small portions of your favorite foods.

Find other ways to cope with everyday problems instead of smoking, sleeping, drinking, or eating too much.

Do your best, but don't make excuses, pity yourself, or put yourself down if you aren't perfect in your efforts.

Be upbeat. Believe that you will succeed and attempt to make your life happier and more fulfilling.

*H*elp! *My diet isn't working any more. What am I doing wrong?*

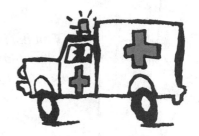

▼

TIP:

It may not be your diet. Diabetes and its treatments can affect how you lose weight. People who achieve tight glucose control may gain weight because they start absorbing all the energy from their food, rather than losing calories through urine (see page 514). Improvement in your diabetes control is the best measure of health success, rather than the numbers on your scale. Ask yourself:

■ Do I have the wrong goal? Your goal is not a certain weight but improved diabetes control. Don't step on the scale too often.

■ Can I increase my physical activity? Look for ways to add activity every day—walking more, using stairs instead of elevators.

■ Am I snacking on too many fat-free foods? Fat free doesn't mean calorie free. Fruit, cut-up vegetables, and whole grains are better snacks.

■ Am I eating a variety of foods? A rigid weight loss plan may keep you from learning how to add variety to your meals. Diet boredom can lead to overeating.

■ How are my serving sizes? Too much of a good thing can make a difference in weight and diabetes management (see page 493).

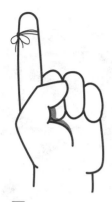

I'm having a hard time sticking with my weight-loss plan. Are there any quick tips to keep me on the right track?

TIP:

Here are some tried and true tips:

☐ Keep weight loss goals reasonable. You can't lose 25 pounds, stop smoking, *and* begin walking 3 miles a day all in one week!

☐ Set small weight loss targets. Aim for 5-pound goals.

☐ Record your weight and blood glucose levels. It's encouraging to see improvements in blood glucose, even if your weight doesn't change.

☐ Periodically, write down what you eat for one day. Measure your serving sizes.

☐ Drink a large glass of water before every meal.

☐ Use a smaller plate.

☐ Eat slowly and stop when you just begin to feel full.

☐ Put your fork down between mouthfuls and chew thoroughly.

☐ Keep low-calorie snacks on hand—sugar-free gelatin, cut-up fresh vegetables, and fresh fruit.

☐ Don't deprive yourself of your favorite food. Cut back on how often you eat it or on your serving size.

☐ Expect setbacks and don't give up. Begin again tomorrow.

*W*on't skipping meals help me cut back on calories and lose weight?

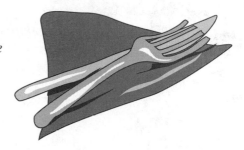

▼
TIP:

No. Eating all your calories in one or two big meals can send your blood glucose levels sky-high. Eating smaller meals more often keeps the amount of carbohydrate entering your system small and consistent, so your glucose level stays within your target range. This can keep your weight under control. And you'll need less insulin.

When to eat depends on many factors, particularly the type of diabetes medication you use. If you take insulin, skipping meals can result in dangerous hypoglycemia. Skipping meals can make you hungrier, moody, and unable to focus. This may lead to overeating later in the day. Breakfast-skippers are particularly at risk for grabbing sugary, high-fat foods later in the day (see page 505). Always eat within a few hours of getting up.

Your metabolism slows down when you do not eat. Eating regularly keeps your energy level high and helps your body burn calories. Eating more often doesn't mean that you eat more calories. See an RD to learn to spread your calories throughout the day. You may find that three meals and three snacks work better for you!

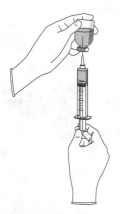

*W*on't skipping a few doses of insulin help me
lose weight?

TIP:

If you take too little insulin on purpose, your body will not use all the calories you eat, and this will result in weight loss. However, it is a very dangerous way to lose a few pounds. An inadequate dose of insulin means you will have higher blood glucose levels and poor diabetes control. This can affect growth and development in children and adolescents. In the short term, high blood glucose levels cause headache, blurred vision, and upset stomach and make you feel tired, hungry, and thirsty. Underdosing insulin puts you at greater risk for ketoacidosis and having to be hospitalized. It can be life-threatening.

Long-term diabetic complications such as nerve damage, kidney damage, and diabetic eye disease are more likely to develop if you deliberately underdose insulin to control your weight. Some researchers have found that people who misuse insulin have a high rate of psychological problems and may have more difficulty dealing with the diagnosis of diabetes.

Don't skip your insulin shot. Stick to a sensible, health-promoting plan of eating and physical activity to lose weight!

*W*ill *a very-low-calorie diet work for me?*

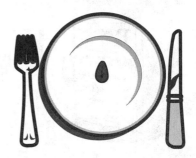

▼ TIP:

Probably not. They are for people with type 2 diabetes who are extremely obese and at immediate risk for serious health problems. Weight loss on a very-low-calorie diet (VLCD) is rapid, and blood glucose levels fall within a few days of beginning this restrictive way of eating. VLCDs are not for people with type 1 diabetes, because of the risk of hypoglycemia. A person with diabetes and kidney disease should not try VLCDs because of the high-protein content of the diet.

Most VLCDs are based on drinking a beverage or eating very lean meat. These diets are high in protein to prevent muscle tissue from wasting away and supplemented with vitamins and minerals because so little food is eaten. Because of the side effects, VLCDs should only be used under the supervision of a physician who specializes in the care of people with diabetes and obesity.

Unfortunately, a VLCD can be costly, and most people regain all the weight they lost within five years. It might jump-start a weight loss effort, but for truly permanent weight loss, you must make lasting changes in your lifestyle.

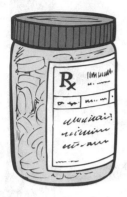

Why can't I just take diet pills to help me lose weight faster?

▼
TIP:

There is no "magic bullet." To lose weight, you eat less or exercise more—or both. Diet pills are meant to be used along with meal planning and exercise, not in place of them. These pills have side effects and should not be taken without your health care provider's advice. Weight loss medications are not for everyone and cannot be used long term.

Weight loss drugs work by controlling your appetite, increasing your sense of fullness, or changing the absorption of the fat you eat. Pills that control appetite and feelings of fullness act on brain chemicals. They cause you to feel less hungry, making it easier to stick with a low-calorie diet. Side effects include dry mouth, insomnia, jitteriness, and increased heart rate and blood pressure.

Drugs that change fat absorption don't reduce appetite but prevent the absorption of about 30% of the calories from the fat you eat. The fat is lost in the stools, leading to side effects of oily or loose stools and intestinal gas.

*W*hat is leptin? When will it be available for people with type 2 diabetes?

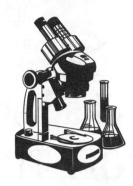

▼
TIP:

L eptin is a hormone made in fat cells that may regulate food intake and body weight by telling the brain when the body contains enough fat. A study of 123 humans reported that daily injections of leptin, in combination with a reduced-calorie diet, led to significant weight loss (average of 16 pounds over 6 months for those on the highest doses). The most common side effects were redness and itching or swelling at the injection site—common when human proteins are injected.

None of the participants in the study had diabetes, but the data suggest that leptin had a beneficial effect on blood glucose levels. It is not clear whether the effect was due to the leptin or the weight loss, but both weight loss and improved blood glucose levels are beneficial for people with type 2 diabetes. The journey from research laboratory to drugstore shelf is often a long one (3–5 years). The next steps are more research studies and then approval from the FDA.

Chapter 8
OFF THE BEATEN TRACK

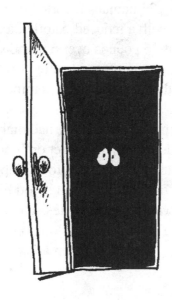

Should I take chromium supplements or can I get enough from foods?

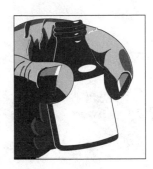

▼
TIP:

If you eat a healthy diet, you are getting enough chromium. Ads claim that chromium supplements will help overcome obesity, help the body use insulin better, prevent hypoglycemia, and take away sugar cravings. The body needs chromium to metabolize protein, carbohydrate, and fat and to produce the glucose tolerance factor, which is believed to help insulin work better. The estimated safe and adequate daily dietary intake of chromium is 50–200 mcg per day for healthy adults—a tiny amount. Chromium is found in Brewer's yeast, wheat germ, corn oil, whole-grain cereals, meats, cheese, bran, liver, kidney, oysters, potatoes with the skin left on, peanuts, and peanut butter.

People who do not eat healthy foods and suffer from malnutrition, especially the elderly, may be at risk for chromium deficiency. Supplements are recommended only for people with signs and symptoms of a deficiency, which is difficult to detect. Let the buyer beware. Most chromium supplements contain more than chromium, are poorly absorbed, and are not regulated by the FDA. Chromium supplements can be expensive, using up money that might be better spent on healthy foods.

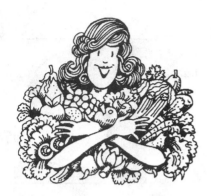

I've heard so much about
antioxidants. Will taking them help
my diabetes?

▼ TIP:

It may. Antioxidants include vitamins A, C, and E; beta-carotene;
and the mineral selenium. They protect the body from harmful
substances known as *free radicals*. Free radicals are by-products of
metabolism that disrupt our natural cancer-fighting defenses and
destroy important structures such as cell membranes and DNA. High
blood glucose helps free radicals form in the body, and free radicals
may be involved in diabetic complications.

Research shows that people who eat antioxidant-rich foods have
less cancer and heart disease. However, we don't know whether it is
because of the antioxidants or the food in which they're contained.
Your best bet is to eat a variety of foods rich in antioxidants. You
find

- Beta-carotene and vitamin A in green leafy vegetables (broccoli,
  collard greens, kale, spinach) and red, orange, and yellow fruits and
  vegetables (apricot, cantaloupe, carrots, mango, peach, pumpkin,
  sweet potato, tomato, watermelon, squash)

- Vitamin C in broccoli, cantaloupe, citrus fruit (orange, grapefruit,
  lemon), kiwi, potato, red pepper, strawberries, tomato

- Vitamin E in almonds, nuts, seeds, vegetable oil, wheat germ

- Selenium in cashews, halibut, meat, oysters, salmon, scallops,
  tuna

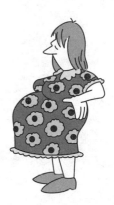

*W*ill a magnesium supplement improve my diabetes control?

TIP:

O nly if you are magnesium deficient. Magnesium deficiency may play a role in causing insulin resistance, carbohydrate intolerance, and hypertension. But only people at risk for a magnesium deficiency should have a blood test for magnesium levels. People at risk are those with congestive heart failure, with potassium or calcium deficiency, or who are pregnant. Others at risk have had heart attacks, ketoacidosis, long-term feeding through the veins, long-term alcohol abuse, or have taken drugs such as diuretics for long periods of time. Symptoms of magnesium deficiency might include irregular heartbeat, nausea, weakness, and mental derangement.

Magnesium is found in all kinds of foods. The best sources are legumes, nuts, whole grains, and green vegetables. The RDA for adult males is 350 mg a day; for females, it is 280 mg daily.

If a blood test shows that you are low in magnesium, your doctor will prescribe a supplement. People with kidney disease should only take a magnesium supplement under a doctor's care.

Food (serving)	Magnesium (mg)
spinach, boiled (1/2 cup)	80
peanut butter (2 Tbsp)	50
black-eyed peas (1/2 cup)	45
whole-wheat bread (1 slice)	25

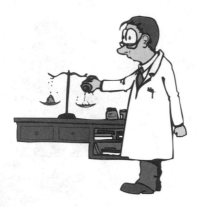

*C*an vanadium (vanadyl sulfate) supplements improve my blood glucose levels?

▼
TIP:

We don't know. At this time there is not enough information to say. This trace element is being studied for its effect on insulin sensitivity and glucose-lowering ability in people with diabetes.

Vanadyl sulfate is marketed in health food stores as a supplement that "mimics the effect of insulin in the body, thereby lowering blood glucose levels." Some ads say that it "enables some people to use less insulin, or stop taking insulin altogether." Because supplements are not regulated in the same way as drugs in the United States, this type of claim is legal. But little is known about this supplement, and the side effects are unclear. Before taking it or adjusting your diabetes medications, talk with your diabetes professionals.

Recommended levels of vanadium have not been determined. If research proves a connection to blood glucose control and insulin action, vanadium would likely be regulated as a drug rather than a supplement.

What is fenugreek? Can it lower blood glucose and cholesterol?

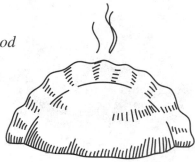

▼

TIP:

Fenugreek is a plant used since ancient times for managing diabetes and obesity. Its seed is a spice found in Indian, Middle Eastern, and Mediterranean dishes. Fenugreek contains concentrated amounts of soluble and insoluble fiber and can lower blood cholesterol and slow the rise in blood glucose after eating. It is on the *Generally Recognized as Safe Food and Spice List* from the FDA.

A form of fenugreek is marketed under the name Limitrol in capsule, wafer, or pudding form. The manufacturer's data from unpublished research show the product diminishes the rise in blood glucose levels after eating by about 40%. They also claim that when the product was taken daily before the two largest meals, it reduced the average total blood cholesterol by 20% and LDL cholesterol by 26% after six weeks. Side effects are common to dietary fiber—excess gas, diarrhea, and poor absorption of glucose and fats.

The jury is still out. The manufacturer's studies have not been published in a medical journal nor have the health claims been evaluated by the FDA. Speak with your health care providers about fenugreek as a suitable product for you.

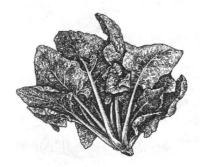

I've heard that folate will reduce my risk of heart attack. Do I need to take a folate supplement every day?

▼
TIP:

Because people with diabetes are at risk for heart and blood vessel disease, it may be wise for you to pay attention to the amount of folate in your diet. For several years, scientists have known that a daily 400-mcg supplement of the B-vitamin folate helps prevent certain birth defects when the mother takes it before conception. More recently, research has shown that 400 mcg of folate may reduce the risk of heart attacks by lowering elevated levels of homocysteine in the blood. Homocysteine is an amino acid that in excess amounts is toxic to blood vessels.

Ask your provider and RD whether they recommend a folate supplement for you. If you are interested in increasing the amount of folate you eat, the following list has some of the best food sources:

Food (serving)	Folate (mcg)
Spinach (1/2 cup)	130
Cooked navy beans (1/2 cup)	125
Wheat germ (1/4 cup)	80
Avocado (1/2)	55
Orange (1 medium)	45
Bread (1 slice, fortified)	40
Dried peanuts (1 ounce)	30

Chapter 9
FOOD FOR THOUGHT

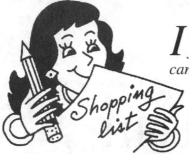

I don't have lots of time to spend shopping for food and making healthy meals. What can I do?

▼
TIP:

Here are some tips:

■ Plan your meals for the week, using your diabetes meal plan as a guide. Do all your grocery shopping at once.

■ Make a shopping list and move through the store quickly.

■ Grated, chopped, precooked, and presliced foods will save preparation time. For example, use prechopped broccoli florets from the salad bar.

■ "Cook once, serve two or three times." Plan to use leftovers. For example, if you are making pasta for a hot dish at supper, cook an extra handful to use in a cold pasta salad tomorrow. Make a pot roast with vegetables on Sunday and plan to use the leftover beef in beef stew, burritos, or vegetable beef soup later in the week.

■ Take a few minutes in the morning to assemble a slow-cooker recipe. Your reward: a ready-to-eat meal at the end of the day.

■ Take advantage of the time you have on weekends. Cook and bake in large quantities and freeze portions for future meals and snacks.

*H*ow *can I make my favorite*
recipes lower in fat?

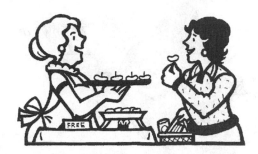

▼

TIP:

These tips may help:

■ Most recipes (except some baked goods) will taste fine if you cut 1/3–1/2 of the butter or oil.

■ When baking, substitute 2 egg whites for a whole egg; use fat-free instead of whole milk. Reduced-calorie butter or margarine has too much water to be used for baking. Because fat gives texture to baked goods, decreasing it can be tricky. Try replacing oil, margarine, or butter with applesauce. Use an equal amount of fruit for fat to retain moisture and flavor. Puréed prunes taste great in chocolate desserts.

■ Marinades need acid, such as lemon juice, vinegar, or wine, more than oil for tenderizing.

■ Use lower-fat substitutes. Low-fat yogurt replaces sour cream in dips and dressings. Use evaporated fat-free milk instead of heavy cream. Replace half the ground meat in casseroles with mashed beans or cooked brown rice.

■ Use butter-flavored spray on cooked vegetables, baked potatoes, or popcorn.

■ Cocoa powder gives chocolate flavor without the fat. Use 3 Tbsp unsweetened cocoa powder and 1 Tbsp vegetable oil to replace 1 oz unsweetened chocolate.

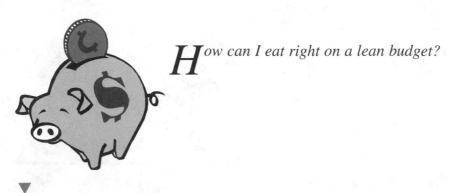

*H*ow can I eat right on a lean budget?

▼
TIP:

Y ou don't need expensive diabetic or sugar-free foods. The
foundation foods of your meal plan are inexpensive—beans,
rice, and whole-grain breads. For snacks, try popcorn, pretzels, and
cereal.

Fresh vegetables in season are a great buy. Otherwise, canned,
fresh, and frozen vegetables are all quite similar nutritionally. Or,
you can grow or pick your own!

Buy fruits in season for best taste and bargain prices. Try the local
farmer's market. Think about the cost per serving—if apples and
melon are the same price per pound, buy the apples. You throw away
the rind of the melon, getting less fruit for the price.

Use fat-free dry milk for cooking and baking. It's inexpensive and
stays fresh for a long time if the box is refrigerated. Preshredded
cheese saves time but costs more. Buy cheese in blocks and grate it
yourself. Buy or make plain yogurt and add your own fresh fruit.

Make meat a side dish, rather than the whole meal. Enjoy
meatless meals several times a week. Use leftovers wisely.

Choosing fats, sweets, and alcohol less often will be good for
your diabetes and your budget.

*W*hich frozen dessert is best for me?

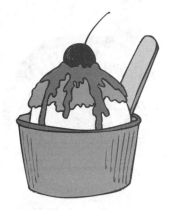

▼
TIP:

Y ou can eat frozen desserts occasionally if you substitute them
for other carbohydrates in your meal plan. The following
information can help you choose:

■ Watch the serving size (1/2 cup). If you eat more, double or triple
the nutrient information to keep your count accurate.
■ Watch the fat content, particularly the saturated fat. Light ice
cream or yogurt contains about half the fat of the regular kind.
Fat-free ice cream still has sugar, carbohydrate, and calories.
■ A no-sugar-added frozen dessert may still contain carbohydrate,
fat, and calories. Sweeteners commonly used in frozen desserts
include aspartame and sugar alcohols such as sorbitol (see p. 543).
■ Check your blood glucose after eating a frozen dessert to see
how it affects you.

Frozen Dessert (1/2 cup)	Calories	Carbohydrate (g)	Fat (g)	Saturated Fat (g)
Regular ice cream	145	17	8	5
Light ice cream	120	20	3	2
Fat-free ice cream	90	20	0	0
No-sugar-added ice cream	100	12	4	2
Sherbet	107	23	2	1
Sorbet	100	24	0	0

A re frozen dinners a good choice for quick meals?

▼

TIP:

Frozen dinners have come a long way, but keep the following tips in mind:

■ Check the Nutrition Facts panel for the amount of fat and sodium. You want no more than 30% of calories from fat, 10% of calories from saturated fat, and 200 mg of sodium for every 100 calories.

■ Most "healthy" frozen dinners are based on small servings. If your meal plan calls for 1,500 calories a day, don't skimp by eating a meal with less than 400 or 500 calories. You'll find yourself hungry later and may overeat on snacks.

■ Be aware that although most healthy frozen dinners contain fruits and vegetables, the serving size of these foods is as small as 1 tablespoon in some cases.

You can improve a frozen dinner by adding a salad, some steamed vegetables, and a piece of fruit. It may be better to make your own frozen dinners by putting the extras from home-cooked meals onto microwave-safe dishes in your serving sizes.

*A*re eggs off-limits now that I have diabetes?

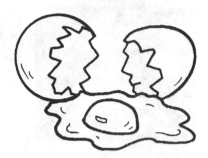

▼

TIP:

No. Contrary to the widely held belief that cholesterol-rich eggs are bad for heart health, several research studies have found that for most people, dietary cholesterol has little effect on the cholesterol level in blood. Saturated fat has a more significant effect on your blood cholesterol level (see page 528). A person's response to dietary cholesterol is highly individual and genetically determined. About 20% of us have little or no response to dietary cholesterol, 50% show a small response, and the remaining 30% are responders, particularly sensitive to high-cholesterol foods. There is no easy test to determine who is cholesterol sensitive, so just be cautious when using eggs and other cholesterol-rich foods.

An egg is an economical source of protein, providing 70 calories, less than 1 gram of carbohydrate, 4.5 grams of fat, and 1 gram of saturated fat. One egg contains vitamins, minerals, and about 215 mg of cholesterol.

Don't eliminate eggs from your diet. Use them wisely or follow the American Heart Association guideline—no more than four a week.

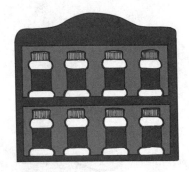

How can I use herbs and spices?

▼
TIP:

Herbs and spices taste good, smell good, and best of all, have no effect on diabetes control. They are free foods on every meal plan. Herbs and spices come fresh or dried. Dried herbs have more intense flavor. (When substituting fresh for dried herbs, double or triple the amount.) The amount of herb or spice that you use in a recipe depends on individual taste.

Here is a list of traditional spice partners:

Beef: bay leaf, chives, garlic, marjoram, savory
Lamb: garlic, marjoram, mint, oregano, rosemary, sage, savory
Pork: cilantro, cumin, ginger, sage, thyme
Poultry: garlic, oregano, rosemary, sage, thyme
Seafood: chervil, dill weed, fennel, tarragon, parsley
Pasta: basil, oregano, fennel, garlic, paprika, parsley, sage
Rice: marjoram, parsley, tarragon, thyme, turmeric
Potatoes: chives, garlic, paprika, parsley, rosemary
Fruits: cinnamon, cloves, ginger, mint
Salads: basil, chervil, chives, dill weed, marjoram, mint, oregano, parsley, tarragon, thyme

Be aware that some herb blends contain sodium or are salts, such as garlic salt or lemon pepper.

Chapter 10
SPECIAL SITUATIONS

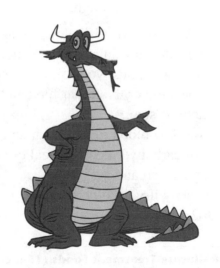

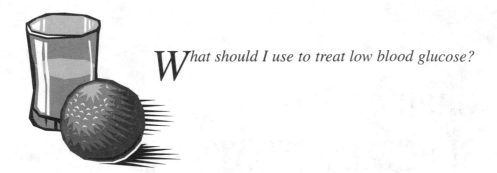

*W*hat should I use to treat low blood glucose?

▼
TIP:

Always carry something with you to treat low blood glucose. Do not use chocolate or candy bars because they may not bring your blood glucose up quickly enough.

1. Check your blood glucose. If it is below 70 mg/dl or you have signs of hypoglycemia but cannot test, eat one of the foods below.
2. Rest for 15 minutes and retest your blood glucose.
3. If it is still low, eat another treatment food and retest. If it is normal, go to the next step.
4. After treating your low blood glucose, eat an extra snack with about 15 grams of carbohydrate. If a meal or snack is scheduled within an hour, go ahead and eat it now.
5. Get help immediately if your blood glucose is still low after 30 minutes and 2 treatments.

Low Blood Glucose Treatment Foods (15 g carbohydrate)

1/2 cup juice or regular soft drink	10 jelly beans
1 Tbsp honey	8 LifeSavers
4 tsp sugar	2 Tbsp raisins
3 pieces of hard candy	Glucose or dextrose tablets or gel

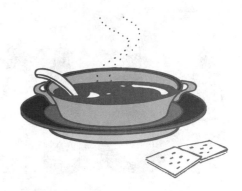

*W*hat foods can I eat when I
am sick?

TIP:

*W*hen you are sick, take your usual medication, check your
blood glucose, and test your urine for ketones. If you can't
eat regular food, have carbohydrates in liquids or soft foods. Drink
plenty of fluids—at least 4–6 oz every hour. If you can't eat at your
usual times, have 15 g carbohydrate every hour to keep blood
glucose from dropping. (See list below.)

These tips can help you handle sick days:

■ Sip clear liquids, such as apple juice, sports drinks, or regular
soda, if you can't keep anything else down.
■ Use broth, vegetable juices, and sports drinks to replace potassium and sodium lost from diarrhea and vomiting.
■ Ask your RD for sick-day meal plans.

Sick-Day Foods (15 g carbohydrate)	
1 cup broth soup	1/4 cup sherbet
1 cup cream soup	1/2 cup regular soda
1/2 cup fruit juice	1 small frozen juice bar
1 cup milk or yogurt	1 cup sports drink
1/3 cup plain pudding	1/2 cup unsweetened
1/2 cup ice milk or ice cream	applesauce
1/2 cup regular gelatin	6 saltines

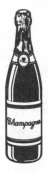 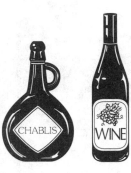

*C*an I safely drink alcohol?

TIP:

It depends. Alcohol can make blood glucose too high or too low. Eat a meal when you drink alcohol to prevent low blood glucose. Alcoholic beverages with mixers, wine, and beer have carbohydrates and can cause your blood glucose to go too high. Choose lower-calorie mixers such as mineral water, club soda, diet tonic water, diet soda, coffee, or tomato juice. Choose light beer or a glass of wine.

If your diabetes is in control, you may have a moderate amount of alcohol—one drink each day for women, two for men. One drink is a 12-oz beer, 5 oz of wine, or 1 1/2 oz of liquor. If you have type 1 diabetes and you are not overweight, this serving would be an addition to your meal plan. If you have type 2 diabetes or are overweight, any alcohol you drink should be substituted for another food in your meal plan. Ask your RD for help.

Avoid alcohol if your blood glucose is out of control, you have an empty stomach, you are pregnant, have neuropathy, have problems with alcohol abuse, take prescription or over-the-counter medications that react with alcohol, or have just had vigorous exercise.

*H*ow can I eat less fat when I eat out in restaurants?

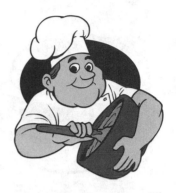

▼
TIP:

Identify your habits by answering these questions:

- How often do you eat out?
- What meals do you eat out most often?
- What type of restaurants do you choose most often?
- What foods do you order?

Select restaurants that have some lower-fat choices. Get copies of menus and decide what you will eat before you arrive. Plan ways to balance your restaurant meal with food choices the rest of the day. Save fat choices for your meal out.

Choose menu items or foods that are baked, braised, broiled, grilled, poached, roasted, steamed, or stir-fried instead of au gratin, fried, breaded, buttered, creamed, sautéed, scalloped, or with gravy or thick sauce. Look for menu items called *light* or *lean.* Ask about food preparation and ingredients. Ask that sauces and salad dressings be served on the side. Decline any extra bread or tortilla chips.

If a serving seems too big, order an appetizer instead, split a main dish with your dining companion, or take home leftovers. Set aside the portion you want to take home as soon as the food arrives.

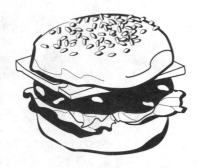

Which fast foods can I eat?

▼

TIP:

The following tips can help you decide:

Watch the serving size. Order a regular serving or split the super-size with someone.

Most restaurants have free nutrient information. Ask for it.

Go for grilled, broiled, baked, or rotisserie sandwiches. Skip meats with breading and cheese.

Remember your fruits and vegetables. Order juice or fruit, a salad or raw vegetables, tomato slices or vegetables for sandwiches, vegetable toppings for potatoes, or vegetables on pizza.

Bagels, muffins, French fries, baked potatoes, and sandwich buns can be extra large and give you too much carbohydrate. Cut them in half or split an order.

Low-fat frozen yogurt, low-fat milk shakes, and fresh fruit are good dessert choices. Order small sizes or share.

For breakfast, order cereal, English muffins, fruit, and milk.

Ask that ketchup, barbecue sauce, mayonnaise, salad dressing, tartar sauce, honey, cream cheese, and others be left off your sandwich or salad.

*H*ow can I avoid overeating at a
salad bar or buffet?

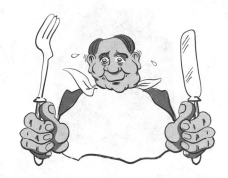

▼
TIP:

An average plate from the salad bar can give you more than
1,000 calories, depending on choices and portions. Consider
these tips:

- Don't go to restaurants that only offer buffet-style eating or
  salad bar.
- Take a stroll around the salad bar, breakfast bar, or buffet to size
  up your choices before you decide.
- If you are tempted to overdo, use a smaller plate. Single trips are
  usually less expensive.
- Enjoy plenty of vegetables, legumes (such as kidney and gar-
  banzo beans), and fresh fruit.
- Dark green leafy vegetables (such as spinach and romaine)
  supply more vitamins than iceberg lettuce. Choose fresh fruit
  instead of juice or sweet breads at breakfast bars.
- Become familiar with calories and fat in typical salad bar foods.
  A 2-Tbsp ladle of salad dressing adds 150 calories to a salad.
  Choose low-fat or fat-free salad dressing.
- Side dishes such as potato salad, pasta salad, and creamy soups
  add calories and fat quickly. Avoid these or take small servings of
  less than 1 Tbsp.

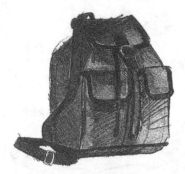

*W*hat do I do if my meal is delayed for an hour?

▼
TIP:

Don't let your blood glucose get too low. If your scheduled meal is delayed for an hour, take your diabetes medication at your usual time before the meal. Then eat 15 g of carbohydrate at your usual mealtime. Always keep quick and easy carbohydrate foods (see ideas below) with you in your purse, briefcase, locker, glove compartment, or backpack. Eat your dinner when it is ready.

For meals that are delayed for more than 1 1/2 hours, adjustments depend on when and what kind of diabetes medications you take. Many times you can switch a snack with a meal. Check with your diabetes professionals for a specific plan.

Emergency Foods (15 g carbohydrate)	
6 saltines	1/2 oz dried fruit
2 rice cakes	3 prunes
3/4 oz pretzels	Cereal bars (may be
3 graham crackers	more than 15 g)

*H*ow can I eat healthy when I travel on the
airlines?

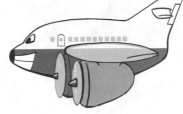

▼
TIP:

T he following tips should help:

■ If the airline meal won't fit your meal plan, bring your own.
Having food with you is essential for any kind of travel.

■ If a meal is to be served, call your agent or airline several days
before the flight and order a special meal. Major airlines offer free
diabetic, vegetarian, low-calorie, low-fat, and low-sodium meals.
When you board, tell the flight attendant that you ordered a special
meal and need it on time. After your meal arrives, take your
diabetes medication. If your special meal isn't available, eat the
regular meal and substitute other food that you have brought.
Foods such as bagels, cereal, fruit, crackers, cheese, raisins, and
bottled water travel easily.

■ Drink plenty of liquids before, during, and after the flight to
avoid dehydration and jet lag. Beverage choices include milk,
vegetable and fruit juice, and bottled water. Don't drink too many
caffeinated beverages.

■ Check your blood glucose. Your activity level during airline
travel is low, so you may need to adjust your meal plan or
medication. For help, contact your RD.

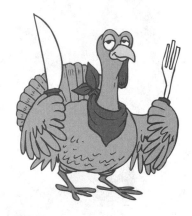

How can I keep my weight and blood glucose levels in control during the holiday season?

TIP:

You can keep your holiday spirit by using the following tips:

- **Holiday meals:** Thanksgiving dinner can add up to 4,500 calories if you include appetizers, eggnog, turkey, trimmings, and dessert. Redesign dinner with delicious lower-fat dishes. Serve grain, fruit, and vegetable dishes. Substitute white turkey meat for dark meat; make your own cranberry sauce; skim the fat off the gravy.
- **Holiday parties:** Have a small snack before you go. Don't socialize by the food table, but do socialize. For potlucks, bring a dish you know you can enjoy. Watch the alcohol; it can lower your resistance to tempting treats.
- **Holiday travel:** Pack healthy, portable snacks to see you through the trip. Good ones include fresh or dried fruit, pretzels, low-fat chips, ready-to-eat cereal, and low-fat cheese (see page 587).

Take advantage of opportunities for exercise. Walk the mall before you shop or take a stroll with your family after dinner to see neighborhood decorations. Keep things in perspective, and if you overindulge, make good choices the rest of the year.

*H*ow *do I adjust food and insulin for a swing-shift schedule?*

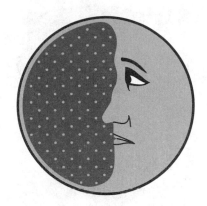

▼
TIP:

Y our RD and physician must help you plan insulin doses, mealtimes, and physical activities. Multiple daily injections are usually recommended. Learning to adjust rapid-acting insulin to your meal size and carbohydrate content (see pages 503 and 517) gives you flexibility for unpredictable meals. Frequent blood glucose monitoring on workdays and days off helps you make adjustments. Your activity varies from workdays to days off, so your food and/or insulin need adjustments then, too.

If you work the 11:00 P.M.–7:00 A.M. shift, try this:

1. Eat before you go to work and take rapid-acting insulin and intermediate- or long-acting insulin (usual before breakfast injections).
2. Eat your next meal around 3:00 A.M. and take rapid-acting insulin.
3. Eat a snack, if needed, between 3:00 –7:00 A.M.
4. Eat a meal at home 8:00–8:30 A.M. and take rapid-acting insulin and intermediate- or long-acting insulin (usual before dinner injections).
5. Sleep between 9:00 A.M.–4:00 P.M.
6. Eat a snack between 5:00–8:00 P.M.

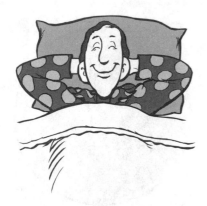

Should I use a slow-release carbohydrate snack bar to prevent hypoglycemia?

▼
TIP:

Products such as Extend Bar and Nite Bite are medical foods that reduce hypoglycemia for hours, particularly at night. These snack bars are based on a long-acting carbohydrate (such as cornstarch) and come in fruit flavors, chocolate crunch, and peanut butter.

These bars were developed when researchers found that in children with glycogen storage disease and hypoglycemia, blood glucose levels could be stabilized for nine hours by feeding uncooked cornstarch. This was also true in children with diabetes who followed an intensive insulin regimen. Snack bars were created as a tasty alternative to plain cornstarch.

The Diabetes Control and Complications Trial (DCCT) showed that hypoglycemia accompanies tight diabetes control. If you are taking multiple daily insulin injections, these bars may help you. They contain 22 grams of carbohydrate per bar (1 1/2 starch exchanges) and are added to an evening snack to reduce the risk of nighttime and early-morning hypoglycemia. Blood glucose monitoring will help you determine the effect these snack bars have on you. Consider the cost and taste, and discuss using them with your diabetes care providers.

*D*o I need to drink a nutritional
supplement now that I'm a senior?

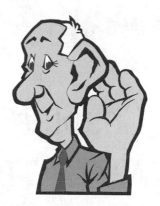

▼
TIP:

Maybe. For some people, keeping a balance of nutrients may be
more difficult because calorie needs decrease with aging,
food budgets get tight, appetite decreases, social contact is reduced,
or eating problems arise.

If you are in good health and have a varied diet, you probably
don't need these supplement drinks. However, there are drinks and
shakes designed specifically for people with diabetes, such as those
from Glucerna and Enterex, and many people use them simply for
convenience. Check the Nutrition Facts panel for calories, carbohydrate, protein, and fat content. Some are high in sugar. Ask your
RD whether these drinks fit your meal plan. Monitor your blood
glucose levels when you use these nutrition drinks to see how they
affect your diabetes. You may not be able to find these products in
stores near you, or they may be too expensive for your budget. Ask
your RD about supplemental drinks you can make at home. If you
are concerned about being underweight, ask for high-calorie meal
ideas, too. Try eating five or six small meals a day.

Chapter 11
NUTRITION POTPOURRI

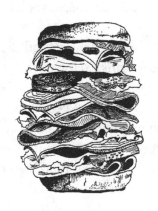

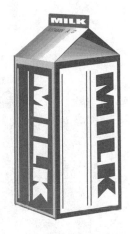

*D*oes cow's milk cause type 1 diabetes?

▼
TIP:

The answer remains a mystery. Researchers are studying early exposure to cow's milk (before age 3–4 months) as a cause of type 1 diabetes. Infant formulas are made from cow's milk. Children with type 1 diabetes have shown higher amounts of antibodies that recognize a specific protein in cow's milk. The immune response to the milk proteins might be related to the destruction of insulin-producing beta-cells in the pancreas and to type 1 diabetes. Other studies have not found this same link between cow's milk and type 1 diabetes.

Breast milk is the best source of nutrition during the first year of life for infants with or without diabetes. Breast milk offers physical, emotional, and practical benefits. The baby benefits even when breastfed for only a short time.

However, breastfeeding may not be right for every woman. Commercial infant formula is a healthful alternative or supplement to breastfeeding. The cow's milk used to make infant formula has been modified to meet an infant's special needs. The decision to breast-feed or use commercial infant formula is a personal one. Discuss questions or concerns with your diabetes professionals and your pediatrician.

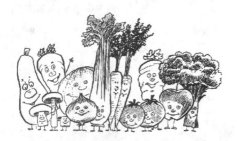

*W*ill becoming a vegetarian
help my diabetes control?

▼
TIP:

Yes, a vegetarian diet can be a healthy choice for people with diabetes. There are several types of vegetarian diets.

■ **Lacto-ovo-vegetarian:** no flesh foods, including meat, fish, seafood, poultry, and their by-products, but includes some dairy products and eggs

■ **Lacto-vegetarian:** no flesh foods, eggs, and their by-products, but includes some dairy products

■ **Vegan:** no foods of animal origin

Vegetarian diets are based on fruits, vegetables, grains, beans, lentils, soybeans, nuts, and seeds. As a result, they are low in fat, cholesterol, and calories. Decreasing your use of animal products offers you several diabetes health advantages. Vegetarians are less likely to be overweight, have high cholesterol levels, or have high blood pressure. They are also less likely to suffer from heart and blood vessel disease and certain cancers. If you have type 1 diabetes, becoming a vegetarian may enable you to use less insulin. If you have type 2 diabetes, the weight loss from a vegetarian diet may improve your blood glucose control. An RD can help you plan vegetarian meals and ensure that you get all the vitamins, minerals, and protein you need.

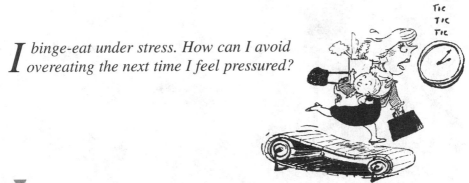

I binge-eat under stress. How can I avoid overeating the next time I feel pressured?

▼
TIP:

Learn the difference between hunger and appetite. Hunger is a physical sensation that tells you that your body needs food. Appetite comes from the mind and is triggered by sensation and emotion. The following are several ways to deal with the urge to "stuff your feelings" or binge:

■ Identify the situations that cause you to overeat. Keep a diary of how much you eat, when you eat, and what the triggers are.
■ Establish regular eating patterns. Skipping meals or not eating enough leads to overeating.
■ Limit foods that tempt you. If it's chocolate, don't bring full-sized candy bars into the house; a fun-sized bar may satisfy the craving.
■ Change the ways you cope with stress. Rather than eat,
   ■ Exercise. Being active (walking, biking) is good for your mind and your body.
   ■ Talk with a supportive friend or family member.
   ■ Enjoy a warm bath or long shower.
   ■ Take good care of yourself. Listen to music you enjoy, go to a movie, get a massage.

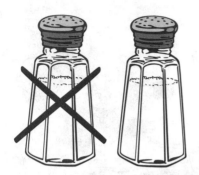

*S*hould I follow a low-sodium diet?

▼
TIP:

The recommended sodium intake for people with diabetes is less than 2,400 mg per day. People with high blood pressure and kidney disease should eat less than 2,000 mg per day.

While most people aren't affected by excess sodium, some are. If you are one of the 30% of Americans who have sodium-sensitive blood pressure, decreasing sodium intake will reduce your blood pressure.

To lower your sodium intake

■ Check Nutrition Facts for sodium.
■ Don't use processed foods. Buy fresh meats, fruits, and vege-tables instead of high-salt meat products (bacon, cold cuts, ham), canned soups, or frozen dinners.
■ Be cautious with condiments and sauces. Cut back on pickles, ketchup, soy sauce, salad dressing, steak sauce, and teriyaki sauce.
■ Cook with less salt. Try herbs, spices, lemon juice, pepper, or garlic (see page 578).
■ Remove the salt shaker from the table. Taste food before salting.
■ Avoid high-sodium menu items. Recognize them by description (smoked or in broth). Keep your order simple (without sauces or fillings) and request that it be prepared without added salt.

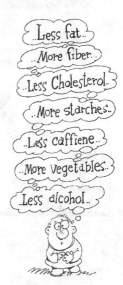

I have gastroparesis. What changes do I make in my diet?

▼
TIP:

Your stomach has lost the ability to churn food into small pieces, and food stays in the stomach too long. Symptoms include nausea, vomiting, weight loss, and a feeling of bloating and fullness. Your blood glucose level may be difficult to control because food is not delivered to the small intestine for absorption in time to match the diabetes medication you take. You may need medication that stimulates your stomach to contract and empty.

As for your diet, you may need to

■ Eat small meals over the day rather than one or two large meals
■ Avoid fatty foods because fat slows stomach emptying
■ Avoid foods that are difficult to digest such as legumes, lentils, and citrus fruits

Because high blood glucose levels can also slow stomach empty-ing, getting blood glucose levels under control is an important part of treatment. If you are taking insulin, your diabetes team may suggest intensive insulin therapy (an insulin pump or three or more injections a day) and frequent blood glucose monitoring. You may need to take your insulin after you eat because of the unpredictability of food absorption.

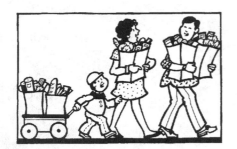

My father has type 2 diabetes and I'm worried I will get it, too. Is there a diet I can follow to prevent getting diabetes?

▼
TIP:

Yes, a healthy diet with regular exercise. Type 2 diabetes is probably caused by a hereditary defect that reduces a person's sensitivity to insulin. You can't change that, but you can change the lifestyle (high-calorie diet and being inactive and sedentary) habits that can lead to obesity, which is the most important environmental trigger of type 2 diabetes. This is why diet and exercise are the major part of prevention and treatment.

Government research studies (the Diabetes Prevention Program) are studying the effects of lifestyle changes and medication in preventing or delaying the development of type 2 diabetes. Participants in the intensive lifestyle group follow a healthy low-fat diet and regular exercise habits to achieve weight loss.

Until the results of this study are available, it's best to change your lifestyle to achieve or maintain a healthy weight. Talk with your health care providers about starting a low-fat diet and increasing your physical activity. An RD can help you learn about healthy eating and your exercise program.

101 WEIGHT LOSS TIPS
FOR PEOPLE WITH DIABETES

▲

A project of the
American Diabetes Association

▼

Written by

Anne Daly, MS, RD, BC-ADM, CDE
Linda Delahanty, MS, RD, LD
Judith Wylie-Rosett, EdD, RD

101 WEIGHT LOSS TIPS FOR PEOPLE WITH DIABETES

TABLE OF CONTENTS

▼

Chapter 1
THE BASICS

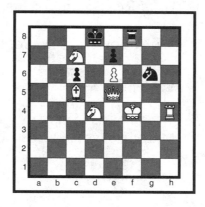

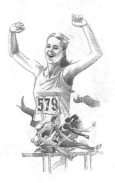

W*hat are my health benefits if I lose weight?*

▼
TIP:

If you lose weight, you can reduce your risk of getting diabetes, heart disease, high blood pressure, gall bladder disease, and breast and colon cancer. If you already have any of these health problems, losing weight improves them. When you lose weight, you'll spend less time and money on doctor's visits and health problems.

People who lose even small amounts of weight—5–7% of their starting weight (usually 10–20 pounds)—improve their health by reducing high blood pressure, high blood sugar, high cholesterol, sleep apnea, arthritis, and depression. And their self-esteem grows. Even without weight loss, you start getting health benefits just as soon as you take steps to improve your lifestyle with a meal plan and more physical activity. Just do it.

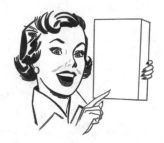 *W*hich weight table should I use to find my healthy body weight?

▼
TIP:

Since being overweight is associated with increased risk of death, the life insurance industry has been making the public aware of it. The 1959 and 1983 Metropolitan Life Insurance Company tables of ideal body weight are still among the most popular in use, but they are very strict. In 1990, the federal government issued an updated table of suggested weights for adults based on height and age—the BMI table, which lists reasonable body weights. There is no "ideal" body weight.

Body Mass Index (BMI) Values

BMI

Height	Good Weights							Increasing Risk														
	19	20	21	22	23	24	25	26	27	28	29	30	31	32	33	34	35	36	37	38	39	40
										Weight (in pounds)												
4'10"	91	96	100	105	110	115	119	124	129	134	138	143	148	153	158	162	167	172	177	181	186	191
4'11"	94	99	104	109	114	119	124	128	133	138	143	148	153	158	163	168	173	178	183	188	193	198
5'	97	102	107	112	118	123	128	133	138	143	148	153	158	163	168	174	179	184	189	194	199	204
5'1"	100	106	111	116	122	127	132	137	143	148	153	158	164	169	174	180	185	190	195	201	206	211
5'2"	104	109	115	120	126	131	136	142	147	153	158	164	169	175	180	186	191	196	202	207	213	218
5'3"	107	113	118	124	130	135	141	146	152	158	163	169	175	180	186	191	197	203	208	214	220	225
5'4"	110	116	122	128	134	140	145	151	157	163	169	174	180	186	192	197	204	209	215	221	227	232
5'5"	114	120	126	132	138	144	150	156	162	168	174	180	186	192	198	204	210	216	222	228	234	240
5'6"	118	124	130	136	142	148	155	161	167	173	179	186	192	198	204	210	216	223	229	235	241	247
5'7"	121	127	134	140	146	153	159	166	172	178	185	191	198	204	211	217	223	230	236	242	249	255
5'8"	125	131	138	144	151	158	164	171	177	184	190	197	203	210	216	223	230	236	243	249	256	262
5'9"	128	135	142	149	155	162	169	176	182	189	196	203	209	216	223	230	236	243	250	257	263	270
5'10"	132	139	146	153	160	167	174	181	188	195	202	209	216	222	229	236	243	250	257	264	271	278
5'11"	136	143	150	157	165	172	179	186	193	200	208	215	222	229	236	243	250	257	265	272	279	286
6'	140	147	154	162	169	177	184	191	199	206	213	221	228	235	242	250	258	265	272	279	287	294
6'1"	144	151	159	166	174	182	189	197	204	212	219	227	235	242	250	257	265	272	280	288	295	302
6'2"	148	155	163	171	179	186	194	202	210	218	225	233	241	249	256	264	272	280	287	295	303	311
6'3"	152	160	168	176	184	192	200	208	216	224	232	240	248	256	264	272	279	287	295	303	311	319
6'4"	156	164	172	180	189	197	205	213	221	230	238	246	254	263	271	279	287	295	304	312	320	328

BMI ≥27 are highlighted because health risk escalates rapidly above this level.

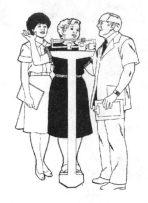

*W*hat is reasonable body weight?

▼
TIP:

Reasonable body weight is a term that appears in the *1994 Nutrition Recommendations for People with Diabetes*. This is defined as the weight that you and your health care team agree that you can probably achieve and maintain for the rest of your life. This weight turns out to be very different from ideal body weight, but it does reduce your health risks. For instance, a female who is 5'5" tall has an ideal body weight on the outdated table of 120 lbs. In real life, however, if her current weight is 220, a reasonable body weight for her might be 160 lbs.

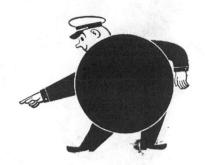

*H*ow do I know if I'm overweight or obese?

▼
TIP:

Overweight and obesity are related but do not mean the same thing. Overweight refers to an excess amount of body weight for your height that includes all tissues, such as fat, bone, muscle, and water. For example, a football player with a lot of muscle might weigh a lot but it isn't fat that makes him weigh so much. Obesity refers to an excess of body fat. You can measure obesity using the body mass index (BMI).

Category	Body Mass Index
Underweight	<18.5
Normal	18.5–24.9
Overweight	25.0–29.9
Obesity	30.0–34.9
Severe Obesity	35.0–39.9
Morbid Obesity	≥40.0

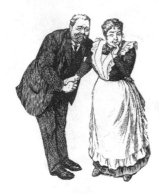

*H*ow do I calculate my BMI?

▼

TIP:

Body mass index or BMI is a way to measure overweight or obesity based on weight and height.

BMI = weight in kilograms / height in meters². To calculate your BMI, you need to know your height and your weight.
Your weight in pounds divided by 2.2 = your weight in kilograms.

For example, if you weigh 200 pounds, then you weigh 90.9 kilograms.

$$\frac{200}{2.2} = 90.9$$

Your height in inches × 2.54 = your height in centimeters. Divide your height in centimeters by 100 to get your height in meters.

If you are 68 inches tall, then you are 172.7 centimeters or 1.727 meters tall.

$$68 \times 2.54 = \frac{172.7}{100} = 1.727$$

$$\text{Your BMI would be } \frac{90.9}{1.727 \times 1.727} = 30.5$$

This BMI says that you meet the criteria for obesity, and you may have some serious health problems.

*H*ow does BMI relate to health risk?

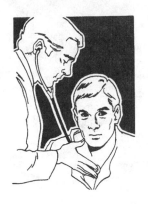

▼
TIP:

The health problems that come along with obesity are coronary heart disease, stroke, high blood pressure, sleep apnea, diabetes, gout, high cholesterol, arthritis, and gallstones. All overweight and obese adults (ages 18 years or older) with a BMI of 25 or higher are at risk for developing these health problems. Those with a BMI of 30 or higher have serious health risks, especially for heart disease. When you lose weight, you improve your health in many ways!

BMI	Health Risk Based on BMI	Risk if You Have Other Health Problems
<25	Minimal	Low
25–<26.9	Low	Moderate
27–<29.9	Moderate	High
30–<34.9	High	Very high
35–<39.9	Very high	Extremely high
≥40	Extremely high	Extremely high

Obese people may be limited in how agile they are, so they have a higher risk of having accidents. They may have difficulty getting pregnant and difficulties with pregnancy and delivery. You and your doctor should consider all of your health problems when choosing a weight loss program. NOTE: You are more likely to have health risks when your body fat is concentrated in your belly rather than in your hips. To check the location of your body fat, use the waist-to-hip measurement (page 610).

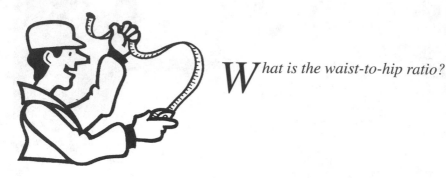

What is the waist-to-hip ratio?

▼
TIP:

The waist-to-hip ratio (WHR) is the comparison of your waist measurement to your hip measurement. It is a way to see whether your weight is primarily in your hips and buttocks (in what is known as a "pear" shape, common in females) or in the abdomen (making an "apple" shape, common in males). Measure your waist with a non-stretchable measuring tape at the smallest point (between the rib cage and navel), and measure your hips at the widest point (around the buttocks). A WHR of more than 1.0 in males and 0.8 in females suggests that you have increased health risks. As an example, a woman who weighs 300 lbs has a waist measuring 53 inches and hip measuring 60 inches.

$$\frac{53}{60} = 0.9$$

The waist-to-hip ratio is 0.9.

The risk is higher for women with a waist measurement of 35 inches or more and higher for men with a waist measurement of 40 inches or more.

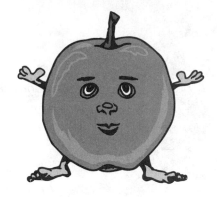

I *tend to have a belly. Is being*
shaped like an apple bad?

Yes, because where your body stores fat makes a difference in your health. People who have a larger waist are more likely to develop heart disease, high blood pressure, and diabetes. Health risks seem to come with having a waist measurement of greater than 35 inches in women and greater than 40 inches in men. Abdominal fat is worse than fat on your buttocks or thighs, because that extra fat surrounds important organs such as the liver and pancreas. When you have fat in this area of the body, your body can't use the insulin produced by your pancreas very well. This is called insulin resistance, and it causes high blood sugar levels. High blood sugar levels put your organs at higher risk.

If you lose weight, the amount of fat stored around your waist and important organs will decrease, and they will all work better.

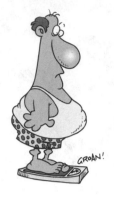

*E*verybody in my family is heavy. How can I ever expect to be thin?

You may not ever be thin, but you can certainly lose weight and get fit. It may help to think of your family's gift this way: you may have inherited genes that make you more energy efficient. People who survive a famine are likely to have a "thrifty gene" that allows them to get by on fewer calories. When the food supply is more plentiful, people who are more energy efficient gain weight.

The second thing you inherit from your family is your lifestyle. When the Pima Indians, who had low rates of obesity until 50 years ago, adopted the "Western" lifestyle, food was plentiful and they exercised less. They now have an epidemic of obesity and diabetes.

Families pass on habits that may lead to weight gain. Your parents played a strong role in the development of your food preferences, physical activity habits, and eating habits. But you can make new habits. And pass them on to your children, too.

Chapter 2
WEIGHT LOSS

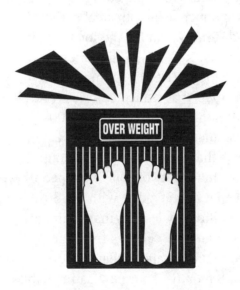

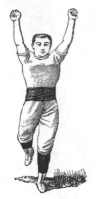

Is one method of losing weight better than the other?

▼

TIP:

Yes, eating fewer calories than you burn is the key. There are a variety of weight loss therapies ranging from nutrition therapy (low-calorie diets and increasing physical activity) to behavior therapy, drugs, and surgery. But for the long run, it's burning the calories you eat that counts. Recently, at the direction of NIH, the U.S. Department of Agriculture (USDA) completed a study on popular diets and found the diets that reduce calories result in weight loss. If you don't exercise, eating approximately 1,400–1,500 calories a day is recommended, no matter which foods you eat.

It is also appears that the easiest way to control calories is by cutting back on how much fat you eat. Most people who succeed at weight loss and keep it off eat a diet with 20–30% of their calories from fat. This is significantly less fat than is in the average American diet, which is more than 36% calories from fat.

What you need to understand is that you don't follow a diet for 8 days, 8 weeks, or 8 months. Your new eating habits are the basis of your everyday food choices for the rest of your life. Healthy meal plans are high in vegetables, fruits, and other carbohydrates such as whole grains and low-fat dairy products. This is a moderate-fat, low-calorie way of eating that stops weight gain, leads to weight loss, and keeps it off. It is fast, convenient, and inexpensive. So—why are people still looking for a magic pill? This tastes better!

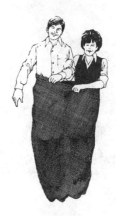

Why do I need to be physically active?

▼
TIP:

To burn the calories you eat. We gain weight when we take in more food energy than we use up. Being physically active makes you healthier because all your systems—heart, lungs, circulation, and digestion—get exercise, too. But being active is particularly helpful to people who want to lose weight, because it burns calories. You get a 1-pound weight loss for every 3,500 calories burned. Exercise also helps you build muscle. Building muscle is good because it burns calories even when you are at rest. People with diabetes benefit from exercise because it lowers blood glucose, too.

Exercise benefits are many and include

- More energy
- Weight loss
- Improved mobility and range of motion
- A better attitude and self-esteem
- Better blood glucose control
- Reduced chance of heart attack or stroke
- Improved blood pressure
- Improved cholesterol levels

Please remember muscle weighs more than fat. While you are building muscle and losing fat, don't wail at the scale. Measure the inches you're losing on waist, thigh, and biceps to see your progress at weight loss.

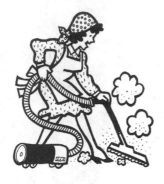

*H*ow can I burn more calories?

▼

TIP:

Y̲ou may be surprised at how many of your daily activities burn
   calories. This table shows the calories burned by a 150-pound
person doing 30 minutes of each activity. If you weigh more than 150,
you will burn more calories.

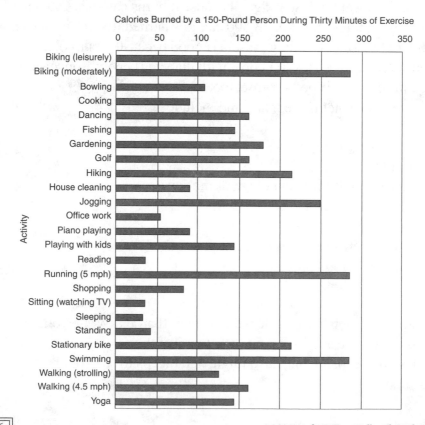

Calories Burned by a 150-Pound Person During Thirty Minutes of Exercise

1,001 Tips for Living Well with Diabetes

W*hat about the popular fad diets—*
do they work?

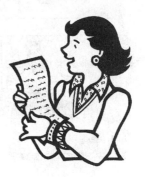

▼
TIP:

Not really. At the beginning, these diets may produce some weight loss, but you are losing water weight. The other reason they work at first is that these diets are, basically, low-calorie diets in disguise. When you follow them closely, these diets typically provide 1,000–1,600 calories daily. For most Americans, this is fewer calories than they usually eat. However, the problem is maintaining the weight loss. These diets are hard to stick with. You soon miss carbohydrate foods and wander back to old eating habits. Almost all the popular diets promote eating high protein and low carbohydrate. The authors claim that you can eat unlimited amounts of high-protein and high-fat foods, but they severely limit fruits, vegetables, legumes, whole-grain and milk products, breads, cereal, and crackers. Hey folks, those are the healthiest foods! There is a long list of serious health risks associated with these diets, such as poor nutrition, increased blood pressure, increased blood cholesterol, cancer, osteoporosis, gout, and kidney stones. For people with diabetes, these diets are particularly bad because eating lots of saturated fat puts you at risk for heart attack and stroke.

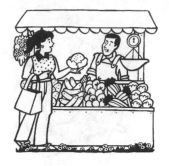

What can I do instead of the popular diets to lose weight successfully?

▼

TIP:

There are no quick fixes to losing weight. Simply put, you need to burn more calories than you take in. To help you do that, follow these guidelines:

- Eat a varied diet—include all food groups.
- Include at least 5 servings of fruits and vegetables daily.
- Limit sugary foods.
- Eat smaller servings.
- Limit fat, especially saturated (animal) fat and trans fats (in hydrogenated oils).
- Be physically active at least 30 minutes 3–5 days of the week.

Seek help from a registered dietitian (RD), preferably one who is a certified diabetes educator (CDE), if you have diabetes, to develop a meal plan based on your likes and dislikes, daily schedule, and health concerns. This is a very important step in creating a healthier lifestyle.

*W*hat should I consider when choosing
a weight management program?

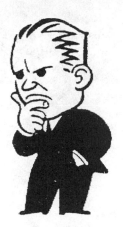

▼
TIP:

*A*sk yourself these questions about the program:

- How often do I go and how long are the sessions?
- Is the program conveniently located and does the time fit my schedule?
- What are my short-term and my long-term goals?
- Do I have high health risks?
- Is my health checked at the beginning and monitored throughout the program?
- Is the staff trained and experienced in treating my medical condition(s)?
- What method(s) are used for weight loss? Are there expensive foods to buy?
- Does the program include instruction in healthful eating, increasing physical activity, and improving self-esteem?
- Once I lose the weight, what services are provided for long-term maintenance?
- Do they have records to show their success with both weight loss and maintenance?
- What medical standards does the staff follow to care for my health conditions?
- What type(s) of ongoing support do they provide me?
- Are there any possible health risks or side effects for me to be aware of?
- What are the costs, and are any covered by insurance?

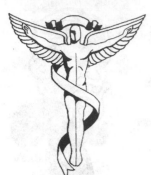

*W*hat is a "state-of-the-art" weight
management program?

TIP:

The best program is like the lifestyle-change one used to prevent
diabetes in the Diabetes Prevention Program (DPP). Lifestyle-
change patients had a daily goal for grams of total fat. If meeting that
goal did not help them lose weight, they worked on eating
1,200–1,800 calories a day, with less than 25% of calories from fat.
Patients were asked to do 30 minutes of moderate physical activity,
such as brisk walking, at least 5 days a week. For support and education, they attended 16 individual sessions over 6 months and group
sessions with 10–20 others. The lifestyle-change staff was a team of
professionals, including RDs, exercise physiologists, and behavior-
ists. Participants kept daily records of calories and physical activity
(minutes or calories burned). Most patients completed the
3-year study, reaching their lifestyle goals. The results were dramatic:
58% of those in the lifestyle-change group prevented diabetes, compared to 31% of those who just took medication. The state-of-the-art
program gives you goals for daily fat grams, calorie range, physical
activity, and record keeping, and provides you with professional support, in both individual and group sessions.

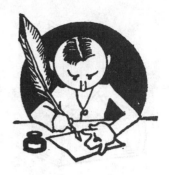

*A*re food records really necessary— *if so, why?*

▼
TIP:

Yes. This is one of the best weight loss techniques. If you write down what you eat and drink, you are more likely to succeed at weight loss and weight maintenance. Food records give you the history of what you've eaten, so that your weight loss—or weight gain— is no mystery. Besides that, food records give you something real to work with. You can identify problems, and you can begin to problem-solve. Without records, you won't even know what the problems are. Record keeping helps you monitor your progress and skill level, and identify patterns in your weight management behavior. The feedback from your records strengthens your skills for weight management. Write down foods within 15 minutes of eating. Most successful record keepers total their numbers at the end of the day or the first thing the next morning on a weekly summary sheet. Keeping good records is a skill that takes lots of practice to develop. There will be stops and starts, and most people do not enjoy keeping records, because they take work. But it is really worthwhile work. You will benefit from it!

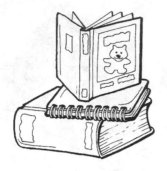

*W*hat do food records look like and what do I do with them?

▼
TIP:

Y ou can keep your records in a spiral notebook or on cards or however you want to do it. Your records need columns or places to write the name of the food, the serving size (ounces, cups, tablespoons), and the calories or fat grams or carbohydrate grams of servings or exchange groups, depending on which meal-planning method you use. For weight management, you can track the number of servings of vegetables and fruits you eat per day—and aim for 5 or more (3 veggies, 2 fruits). At the end of a week, you can add up your weekly totals of calories, vegetable servings, fruit servings, etc. From those totals, you can figure your average daily calorie, carbohydrate, and fat intake. Make a column for anything else that has an impact on your food choices or eating behavior during the day. You should note the time you eat, where you are, whom you're with, and if anything is causing tension around you. You should note your daily exercise—even if it's just climbing the stairs, it all counts. If you take diabetes medication, you can list that, too. The food you eat interacts with the pills or insulin and with exercise, so put that in your record, too.

*W*hat about very-low-calorie diets—
are they recommended for people with
diabetes?

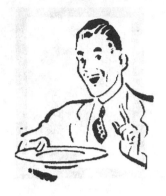

▼
TIP:

Very-low-calorie diets (VLCDs), with less than 800 calories a day, have been used in the treatment of high-risk overweight patients and, in particular, people with type 2 diabetes. On this weight loss program, you drink at least 5 servings of a commercial formula product daily plus generous amounts of calorie-free beverages, and perhaps some very-low-calorie food such as lettuce. The formula has vitamins and minerals to meet the recommended dietary allowances, because when you eat less than 1,200 calories, you cannot meet your nutritional needs from food alone. Many VLCDs do not include regular foods that you could buy in the grocery store. VLCDs appear to be safe if you are evaluated beforehand and closely monitored by medical professionals. VLCDs produce significant weight losses and improve your blood glucose levels, cholesterol, and blood pressure. Unfortunately, using a VLCD alone, without a behavior-change program, means you probably won't be able to maintain the weight loss. Some studies report that 5 years later, most people had maintained only 5% of the amount of weight they initially lost. More recent reports, however, show that weight maintenance after a VLCD program is improving. If you have a strong lifestyle-change program that emphasizes calorie balancing with increased physical activity, reducing fat calories, and keeping records, you can keep the weight off. It is important to continue to have contact with the medical professionals to improve your long-term maintenance of weight loss, too.

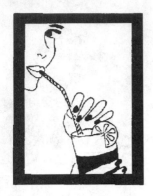

What is a meal replacement?

▼
TIP:

A meal replacement is a portion-controlled food or drink containing 100–300 calories and is used to replace a meal or snack to reduce total calories to lose weight. Meal replacements may be shakes, soups, prepackaged entrees, or snack bars. Meal replacements can be eaten instead of higher-calorie foods. They meet the demands of today's lifestyles for quick and easy dining, while avoiding high-fat, high-calorie choices from fast food chains. Only use meal replacements along with generous servings of fruits and vegetables daily, such as a fruit smoothie with a shake product or one entree plus 2 cups of vegetables. Snack bars offer convenience and variety, and most people like them.

	Calories	Nutrition Value
Formula shake (one serving)	100–300	1 serving carb 1–2 oz protein Trace fat
Entrees (one)	200–300	2–3 oz protein 2–3 servings carb Less than 5 g fat
Snack bar (one)	125–250	1 oz protein 1–2 servings carb Less than 5 g fat

1,001 Tips for Living Well with Diabetes

*W*hat are the benefits of using meal replacements?

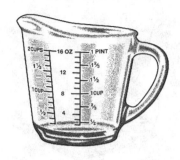

▼
TIP:

Peole who use them have significantly greater weight loss than people using standard low-calorie diets. The caloric content is consistent and accurate, so if you use meal replacements, it's easier to reduce your calorie and fat intake and your blood sugar levels if you have diabetes. They are easy to purchase, usually cost less than the meal they replace, are easy to store, and require little or no preparation. They simplify your food choices and help you avoid foods you might overeat. Most weight loss programs that use meal replacements recommend you replace 2 meals and 1 snack a day to lose weight. Replace 1 meal and 1 snack a day to maintain weight.

	Conventional Meals	Meal Replacements	Calorie Savings
Breakfast	Muffin 500 cal	Shake 100 cal	400 cal
Dinner	Meat, starch, vegetable salad 1,000 cal	Entree and 2 cups veggies 350 cal	650 cal

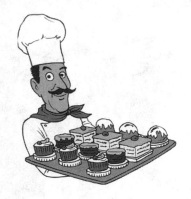

What are the pitfalls of using meal replacements?

TIP:

Meal replacements are not for everyone. Some people don't like the taste. If you eat meal replacements in addition to all the other foods you usually eat, you'll take in more calories than usual—and not lose weight. Another problem is overeating meal replacements in the mistaken idea that they are healthy, so eating more is okay. Think of a person who buys a case of 24 snack bars and eats them all in a very short period of time. As you well know, you can get too much of a good thing.

Over time, using meal replacements can become monotonous. You may feel deprived, have food cravings, or start binge eating. Meal replacements should be used only with other healthy foods, especially generous amounts of fruits and vegetables. They were made to help you limit foods that can be problems, such as starchy foods, snack foods, and sweets.

Critics of meal replacement argue that meal replacements are simply a crutch, and do not teach you how to eat foods in the real world. You need to be aware of that to use them correctly.

*H*ow do I select a weight loss program?

▼
TIP:

*F*irst, decide if you are ready to devote the time, attention, and effort that is necessary to succeed at weight loss. Then, select your short-term and long-term weight loss goals. Try to find a program that will help you meet those goals. Choose a program that focuses on healthy eating, increased activity, improved self-esteem, and maintaining the weight loss. Look for programs that help you change your eating habits through information, guidance, and skills training. Ask for program literature listing the credentials and training of the staff and factual information about the successful results of the program, not just personal stories. A safe and sound program will inform you about any possible risks of the program (especially if it includes very-low-calorie diets, medications, or surgery). It should monitor your weight and continue to work with you on your meal plan and activity habits over time. Discuss with your health care provider how the program will work for you in light of your medical history and weight loss expectations. Make a plan for regular check-ups to measure the changes in your health after you begin the program.

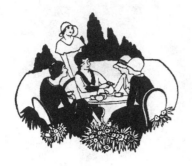

*O*nce I start losing weight, I seem to sabotage myself. What can I do about this pattern?

▼
TIP:

First, identify the ways that you might be sabotaging yourself. Evaluate both your food environment and the way you think about food and dieting. Is your food environment set up for success or sabotage? (See pages 699-704.) If the way you think about food and dieting is sabotaging you, then it is important to change your thoughts and attitudes about eating and losing weight.

1. Try to become aware of any negative thoughts that may set you up for failure.
2. Evaluate these thoughts. Do they make sense? Are they logical, reasonable, or helpful to your goals?
3. If your thoughts do not make sense or are not helpful, try challenging these sabotaging thoughts and substitute a more helpful positive message to think to yourself.
4. Set realistic goals for yourself, so that you are more likely to succeed and have positive thoughts. Give yourself permission to fail. It is unrealistic to think that you can meet all of your goals 100% of the time. If you meet your goals most of the time, you will see progress. Tell yourself that you can do it. Speak well of yourself.

*C*ould skipping breakfast help
  me lose weight?

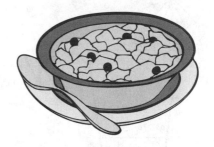

▼
TIP:

No. You may think you are saving calories by not eating breakfast, but what you are really doing is depriving yourself of a steady supply of glucose, which is your energy source, and setting yourself up for a pattern of overeating at night. If you distribute your meals and snacks evenly throughout the day, you are more likely to avoid periods of over-hunger and overeating. If you have diabetes, this helps you have better blood glucose control.

Ask yourself why you aren't hungry in the mornings. Some people eat so many of their daily calories at supper and in the evening as snacks that even the next morning they still don't feel hungry. This pattern of eating provides your body with a large supply of glucose just in time to go to sleep. If you have diabetes, it can also cause a pattern of high blood sugars overnight. Some people are just not hungry early in the morning. This doesn't mean that you need to skip breakfast. You might be able to eat a small breakfast later if you are not very hungry.

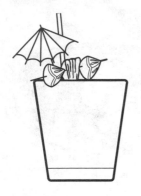

*W*hat effect does alcohol have on weight loss?

▼
TIP:

Alcohol has 7 calories per gram and is metabolized like fat. It has no vitamins or minerals, so those are "empty" calories. Many alcoholic beverages contain calories from sugar, carbohydrate, or fat. Alcohol can also reduce your self-control, leading to overeating. If you have diabetes, alcohol can contribute to problems with hypoglycemia (too low blood glucose). So, if you have diabetes and are on insulin or medications that can cause hypoglycemia, eat a meal or snack with the alcohol to prevent hypoglycemia. All of these factors can lead to too many calories and slow down your weight loss or contribute to weight gain. If you are trying to lose weight by reducing your food intake, it is better to choose foods that are a good source of vitamins and minerals and not the "empty" calories from alcohol. The lowest calorie alcoholic beverages are a 12 oz light beer, 1 oz of liquor mixed with diet soda or water, or 5 oz of wine—each contain about 100 calories. Some of the highest calorie alcoholic beverages are made with cream. A 6 oz serving of a White Russian or a Grasshopper contains 450–500 calories. If you also have snacks or extra food with the alcohol, it is easy to see why alcohol can make it more difficult to lose weight!

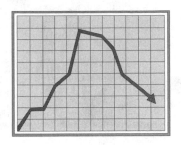

How do I know how many calories to eat each day to lose weight?

▼

TIP:

The number of calories to eat each day depends on your starting weight and the amount of weight you want to lose each week. Experts recommend a weight loss of 1–2 pounds each week. The chart below lists the number of daily calories to lose 1 pound per week and 2 pounds per week. Don't go below 1,200 calories. You do not need to eat exactly the same number of calories each day. For example, you weigh 210 pounds, so you could start with 1,300–1,500 calories per day to lose 2 pounds per week or 1,800–2,000 calories to lose 1 pound per week. You might decide to be more flexible and let your calories range between 1,300–2,000 calories each day, realizing that on some days you will consume closer to 1,300 calories and on other days, 1,800–2,000 may be more realistic.

Suggested Calorie Goals for Weight Loss

Your current weight (lb)	To lose 1 lb/week	To lose 2 lb/week
Less than 150	1,200 calories*	Not advised
150–200	1,400–1,600 calories	1,200 calories
More than 200	1,800–2,000 calories	1,300–1,500 calories

*If you don't lose weight at this level, it is better to increase your physical activity than to reduce your calories too much.
Wylie-Rosett et al. *The Complete Weight Loss Workbook,* American Diabetes Association, 1997.

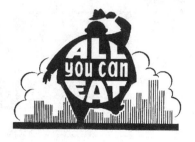

I always feel hungry. Can that really be true?

▼
TIP:

Yes, but it may not necessarily be hunger that you are feeling. You need to learn to distinguish between hunger and appetite. Hunger is a physiological response to the lack of food, and appetite is the desire to eat. Many things can trigger the desire to eat—even when you've just eaten. You can become easily conditioned to think of the desire to eat as hunger. If you find yourself feeling hungry but fairly picky about what you want to eat, ask yourself if it is truly hunger that you are feeling. On the other hand, if you try to cut calories by skipping meals, you are going to feel hungry. Unfortunately, your appetite may be so great that it will be difficult to control how much you eat to satisfy that hunger.

If you go on a very-low-calorie diet of less than 1,000 calories, you will feel very hungry much of the time. It is better for you to eat more calories—say 1,200 to 1,500 calories—for a slower but long-term weight loss. In the long run, severely restricting your calories can backfire if you are hungry all the time. And you still have to learn to eat at a higher calorie level to maintain your weight.

Chapter 3
MAINTAINING
YOUR WEIGHT

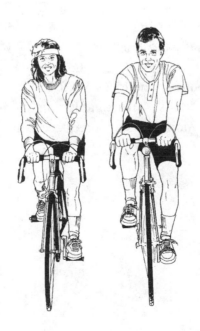

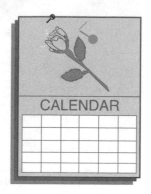

What is "significant" long-term weight loss?

▼ TIP:

The National Academy of Sciences defines significant weight loss as 5% or more of your initial body weight. This is the amount of weight loss necessary to improve your health—to lower blood glucose and blood pressure and improve cholesterol levels. In practical terms, you might aim for a weight loss of 10% of your body weight to actually achieve a 5–7% weight loss. Another method to express significant weight loss is as a reduction of your BMI by one of more points. Long term means one year or more. For example, a person who weighs 200 pounds, who loses 5–10% of his or her body weight, would lose 10–20 pounds. A reasonable timeline for reducing body weight by 10% is 6 months, using a reduced-calorie diet. (See page 614.)

*I*s anyone successful with maintaining
weight loss over the long term?

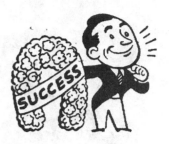

▼
TIP:

Yes, even though maintaining weight loss is the most difficult part
of the process. Research study results have been disappointing,
but be careful whose statistics you use. Health care professionals
often cite a statistic from 1959, which reports that of those who manage to lose weight, 95% will regain all of the weight lost. While we
acknowledge the difficulties of weight maintenance, we KNOW there
are individuals who are successful. And the number is growing. One
problem with statistics is that since research typically reports group
averages, the success of individual patients is often lost in the data. To
capture data on successful weight maintenance, The National Weight
Loss Registry was created in 1993 by two well-known and -respected
obesity researchers, Rena Wing, PhD, at Brown University and Jim
Hill, PhD, of Colorado Health Sciences Center in Denver. The Registry now includes more than 3,000 people who have maintained at
least a 30-pound weight loss for one year or more. In fact, the average
person in the Registry has lost an average of 60 pounds and kept it off
for an average of five and a half years. Yes, you can do it, too.

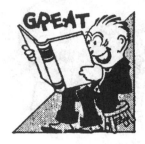

*W*hat are we learning from participants
in the National Weight Loss Registry?

▼
TIP:

The majority (89%) of participants in the Registry report using a combination of diet and physical activity, while 10% use diet alone. One half of them were enrolled in commercial weight loss programs or were under the guidance of a dietitian or psychologist, and half reported losing weight on their own. Of particular interest is that there were no striking differences between how people lost weight and how they were maintaining their weight. The most common method to regulate food intake was to avoid eating certain foods. Most reported eating smaller servings of foods. While they reported a variety of meal-planning methods, the most frequently used was counting calories. Most of them report eating less than 30% of daily calories from fat, while some eat less than 20% of calories from fat. Other behaviors that help them succeed are:

- Eating an average of 5 small meals per day
- Eating breakfast daily
- Eating out 3 or fewer meals a week
- Weighing themselves regularly, at least once a week
- Writing food records
- Daily physical activity

*H*ow can I predict if I will be able to maintain my weight loss long term?

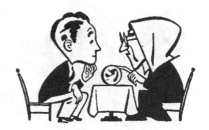

▼
TIP:

Of course, you are an individual and can succeed at maintaining the weight loss on your own. However, research has shown that it helps to participate in a structured program with frequent attendance—weekly or monthly—and if you do, you are likely to be more successful than those who have no follow-up program. We're not sure why so many people regain weight after weight loss. The answers are not simple. Keeping weight off—given the abundance of food, especially high-fat foods, and the limited opportunities for physical activity in the average American's lifestyle—is very difficult. Research supports the following positive and negative predictors of weight maintenance success:

Positive Predictors	Negative Predictors
Physical activity	Negative life events
Record keeping	Family dysfunction
Positive problem-solving attitude	
Continued contact with support	
Normal eating patterns	
Reduction of other health problems (pages 648–649)	

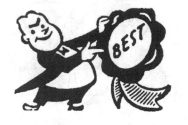

Are there words of encouragement to help me get started and to keep me going on my weight management?

▼

TIP:

Ann Fletcher, RD, has authored two books about "masters of success" with weight loss. She has interviewed hundreds of people who have successfully kept off at least 30 pounds for one year or more. In fact, the people featured in her books have kept off an average of 64 pounds. The average length of time they have kept off 20 (or more) pounds is more than 10 years. Her books tell very familiar stories of people who have struggled with their weight, and then reached a critical point where they finally believed in their own abilities to solve their problems, and how they are now managing successfully. The first volume, *Thin for Life,* is set up according to chapters that discuss ten "keys to success" used by the people interviewed. The second book, *Eating Thin for Life,* includes "food secrets" from the masters, and their favorite recipes. These books are easy reading and very encouraging for your efforts. They are much like the now-famous *Chicken Soup* series for the person who struggles with his weight.

In the National Weight Loss Registry, what "trigger" got patients to start a weight loss program?

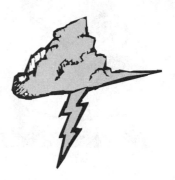

▼
TIP:

Most of the participants (77%) said their successful weight loss was triggered by certain dramatic events in their lives. The top three types of triggers were medical problems, emotional events ("my husband left me because I was fat"), and lifestyle events, such as an anniversary or wedding. Men were more likely to say they were losing weight in response to a medical event or simply for the sake of doing it, while women were more likely to cite an emotional or lifestyle event. However, no single reason was given by more than a third of the people. Each person has to find his or her own trigger. Many times these triggers were unplanned life events, but the important thing is to use the event as an opportunity to get started with lifestyle change.

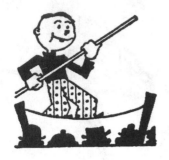

Why do so many people lose weight only to gain it back?

▼
TIP:

Recently it was discovered that genetic factors and complex biochemical systems tend to maintain body weight or return you to the weight you once were. These findings have led to the idea of obesity as a chronic disease rather than a problem simply of overeating, sedentary lifestyle, and lack of willpower. As such, obesity requires lifelong treatment, as with other chronic diseases. Once you have struggled with your weight, you will likely always feel a struggle. To succeed at weight loss and weight maintenance people probably need to see their practitioners more often and over the long term. Since weight management is a skill, it requires time and experience, and a great deal of practice, to develop new behaviors into skills. Unfortunately, many patients are not offered a program to help them maintain weight loss, or they choose not to participate in one. If such a program is offered, take it. Also ask about successful patients who have participated in a maintenance program.

*H*ow often should I weigh myself?

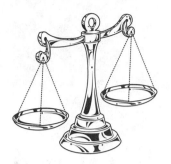

▼
TIP:

You need to weigh often enough to keep motivated while you are trying to lose weight. For most people weighing once a week is enough to see progress while avoiding playing "games" with the scale. Choose one day of the week and a time for weighing. Keep a log of your weekly weights. You can graph your progress over time.

It is tempting to weigh yourself one or more times a day, but don't. Your weight fluctuates with the amount of water in your system. When you weigh too often, you can convince yourself that you gained more weight eating a big salad and drinking a 20-oz glass of water than eating a few high-calorie extras. The salad and 20-oz serving of water may show up as a pound or two on the scale, but that weight will be water not body fat. You need to eat 500 calories extra every day to gain a pound every week.

After you get to your weight goal, monitor your weight. Set a 2- to 5-pound weight cushion. When your weight creeps up by 2 pounds, it's like the yellow traffic signal. Time to monitor your food intake and physical activity more closely and go back to the strategies that helped you lose weight.

Chapter 4
HIGH-RISK STAGES OF LIFE

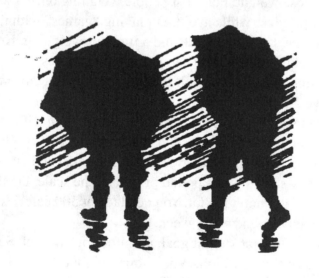

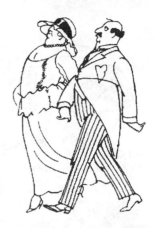

A *re you supposed to weigh more as you reach middle age?*

▼
TIP:

Most people gain about 20 pounds or about one pound per year between 25 and 50 years of age. It's not that you're supposed to, but people do. They get less daily physical activity but may eat a little more as they get older. If you eat just 100 extra calories a day, you would eat 35,000 extra calories in a year and gain 10 pounds. Unfortunately, your metabolic rate also slows down as you age, so you don't burn those extra calories. The best plan to fight middle-aged spread is to eat healthfully and to get plenty of activity. Good posture and abdominal exercises may help you feel better, but they do not reduce the health risk associated with abdominal fat. Unfortunately, much of middle-aged weight gain is abdominal fat. You may increase your waist size even if your weight does not change. Having more abdominal fat is associated with health risks such as a rise in blood pressure, triglyceride levels, insulin resistance, and diabetes (page 611). That's a vicious cycle you can stop by getting back to a younger, healthier weight for you.

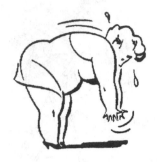

*W*hat effect does menopause have
on weight gain?

▼
TIP:

Both men and women go through midlife hormonal changes. In
men, this is called andropause. Weight gain is common during
the years of menopause and andropause; however, the reasons for the
weight gain do not appear to be due to just the hormones. The body's
metabolism slows down as we age because we lose muscle mass,
which burns calories. People tend to become less active as they get
older, which means we lose muscle mass and burn fewer calories each
day. In addition, midlife is also a time when changes in lifestyle,
mood, or health can occur, which may affect your eating habits and
activity level. The average weight gain is 1 pound a year from age 25
to 55 (or 30 pounds). Hormone changes are associated with changes
in body fat distribution and may lead to more fat in the abdomen
(page 611). So, even if you are eating the same number of calories
each day, you might gain weight if you do not maintain or increase
your activity level to preserve your muscle mass and burn extra calories. The bottom line is that if you eat less and increase your activity
level, you can lose weight no matter what stage of life you're in.

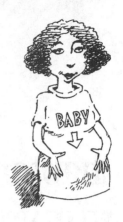

*H*ow does having children affect weight gain for women?

▼
TIP:

Many women add extra pounds because they do not lose the weight they gained after having their children. But having children does not necessarily mean extra weight after delivery. Women who gain the recommended level of weight during pregnancy have less chance of having a weight problem later. Breastfeeding helps women return to their normal body weight, too. Many women want to lose weight during their childbearing years, but few women make lifestyle changes to accomplish it. Women with young children need to find a way to focus on their health and weight. They may need to find a gym that offers programs for young children during adult exercise classes. There may be parent/child exercise programs. Being a "soccer mom" can leave little time for a "mom" exercise program. But you can walk around the soccer field while you're waiting for the kids. Be aware that buying quantities of snack foods and eating on the run can put the whole family at risk for weight gain. Keeping raw fruits and vegetables cut up and ready to eat for snacks can make it easier for you all to eat more healthfully.

Chapter 5
WHEN YOU HAVE DIABETES

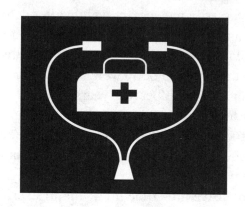

*W*hat are the health benefits of physical activity for people with diabetes?

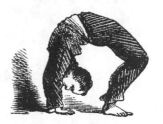

▼
TIP:

Better blood glucose control! Physical activity burns calories and lowers your blood glucose. It promotes weight loss, which lowers your blood glucose. Including physical activity in your weight management program helps you keep muscle while you lose fat, and muscle burns calories, even at rest—which lowers your blood glucose. Diabetes puts you at a much higher risk for heart disease. Exercise improves the health of your heart by keeping it strong and reducing your waist-to-hip ratio (and abdominal fat). Exercise also lowers your triglycerides level and raises your high-density lipoprotein (HDL-good) cholesterol level.

Physical activity also has powerful psychological benefits, such as improved mood, enhanced self-esteem, and a true sense of well-being. It's the best way to relieve stress. Yes, this lowers blood glucose levels, too. To get the maximum benefits from exercise for your diabetes (and keep weight off), enjoy physical activity all through your life.

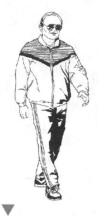

I *have a diabetic complication. Is physical activity okay for me to do?*

TIP:

Ask your diabetes care team how you can exercise safely. A graded exercise stress test is recommended if you have had type 2 diabetes more than 10 years or are older than 35. Check the following table for more about exercise and diabetic complications.

Exercising Safely with Diabetic Complications

Diabetic Complication	Caution!	Beneficial Activities
Peripheral vascular disease	High-impact activities	Moderate walking (may do intermittent exercise with periods of walking followed by periods of rest), non–weight-bearing exercise: swimming, cycling, chair exercises
Osteoporosis or arthritis	High-impact activities	Moderate daily activities, walking, water exercise, resistance exercise (e.g. light lifting activities), stretching

Exercising Safely with Diabetes Complications (cont.)

Diabetic Complication	Caution!	Beneficial Activities
Heart disease	Very strenuous activity	Moderate activity such as walking, daily chores, gardening, fishing
	Heavy lifting or straining, isometric exercises	Moderate lifting, stretching
	Exercise in extreme heat or cold	Activity in a moderate climate
High blood pressure	Very strenuous activity Heavy lifting or straining and isometric exercise	Moderate activity such as walking, weight lifting with light weights, stretching
Nephropathy (also refer to blood pressure guidelines)	Strenuous activity	Light to moderate daily activities such as walking, light household chores, gardening, water exercise
Neuropathy	Weight-bearing activities, especially if high impact, strenuous, or prolonged, such as: walking a distance, treadmill exercise, step exercise, jumping/hopping, exercise in heat or cold	Moderate activities that are low impact (e.g., cycling, swimming, chair exercises, stretching), light to moderate daily activities, exercise in a moderate climate
Retinopathy	Strenuous exercise, activities that require heavy lifting and straining, breath-holding while lifting or pushing, isometric exercise, high-impact activities that cause jarring, head-low activities	Moderate activities that are low impact (e.g., walking, cycling, water exercise), moderate daily chores that do not involve heavy lifting, straining, or the head to be lower than the waist

Hayes, C. *The "I Hate to Exercise" Book,* American Diabetes Association, 2001.

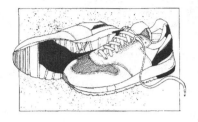

I have neuropathy. What precautions should I take with exercising?

▼
TIP:

If you have neuropathy and loss of feeling in your feet, avoid repetitive weight-bearing exercises, such as long walks or jogging. Try swimming, bicycling, chair exercises, and arm exercises. Never go barefoot except in the bath or bed. You need a good pair of running or walking shoes and socks that wick away moisture. Each time, check your shoes for nails, or pebbles, or tears to the lining before you put them on. Make sure your socks are not too thick for your shoes and that the seam in them is not too thick and putting pressure on your feet. Check your feet after every exercise session for redness, swelling, blisters, or cuts. Get them treated by your doctor promptly.

You should be evaluated regularly for cardiovascular disease. Neuropathy may prevent you from knowing you have it, because you can't feel heart attack pain or pressure. Your blood pressure must be well controlled and monitored. Always do long warm-up and cool-down periods of low intensity before and after each exercise session to ease your heart into and out of the activity.

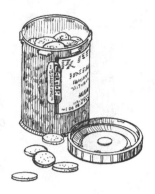

W ill taking diabetes medication make me gain weight?

▼
TIP:

Maybe. When you get better control of your diabetes, you no longer lose glucose in your urine, so your body retains those calories. Some classes of diabetes drugs are more likely to cause weight gain than others. Sulfonylureas (such as glyburide and glipizide), meglitinides (Prandin), and insulin can cause weight gain. The drug class most commonly associated with weight gain and fluid retention is the thiazolidinediones (the glitazones), such as pioglitazone and rosiglitazone. To prevent weight gain, you can intensify your lifestyle efforts (food choices and exercise). The people most likely to develop edema (retain water) are those who already have it. So, women, overweight patients, and those with kidney disease and high blood pressure are at greatest risk. Sometimes doctors prescribe diuretics to control edema and sometimes the patient must switch medications. Metformin works like the glitazones, but doesn't cause weight gain—and may help with weight loss. You can try it instead, being watchful for the side effects of gas, bloating, or diarrhea. You can't take it if you have heart problems. Alpha-glucosidase inhibitors (such as acarbose and miglitol) don't cause weight gain, either, but side effects can be gas, bloating, or diarrhea.

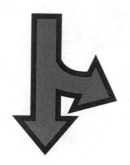

*H*ow can I lose weight and not get *discouraged by more frequent episodes of hypoglycemia?*

▼
TIP:

A ny time you reduce the amount of food you eat, your blood sugar will be lower even before the first pound is lost, which is good. Most people with type 2 diabetes won't have a problem with hypoglycemia (blood glucose below 60). But people who take insulin or diabetes pills that can cause hypoglycemia need to monitor their blood sugar levels on a weight loss program. You treat hypoglycemia by eating a snack with 15 grams of carbohydrate, but you don't want to be eating more food than is on your meal plan. Instead, it might work better to lower the dosage of your medication. As you lose weight, watch the trends in your blood sugar patterns and discuss making changes in your doses of insulin or pills with your doctor before your blood sugar levels get too low. Another way to help prevent hypoglycemia as you lose weight is to focus on lowering your fat intake and keeping your carbohydrate intake about the same at the same meal each day. If your carbohydrate intake at meals and snacks varies widely from day to day, then you are more likely to have erratic blood sugars and possibly more hypoglycemia.

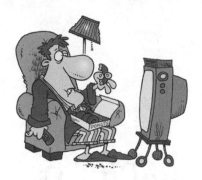

*W*hat are the recommendations for exercise for people with diabetes?

▼

TIP:

Do it. You need aerobic exercise and strength training to make your heart and lungs strong, gain muscles and strength, lower blood pressure, improve circulation, and lower blood glucose. Blood sugar is lower for 12–24 hours. How low depends on how long and how hard you exercise, the blood glucose level before exercise, and how fit you are. Some people notice higher blood sugar levels after exercise. This may be caused by hormonal changes in response to exercise or because blood sugar was high (more than 300) before exercise in people with type 1 who are not taking enough insulin. People with type 2 diabetes should exercise at least every other day and, ideally, most days of the week. This helps control blood sugar, which could be higher on days that you are sedentary and lower on days that you are active. Drink water before, during, and after exercise. It helps you keep going. If hypoglycemia is a problem for you, instead of eating too many snacks, work with your health care team to reduce your insulin or diabetes pills, so your blood sugar won't drop too low (below 70) during or after exercise. Carry a snack in case you need one.

Chapter 6
PREVENTING DIABETES

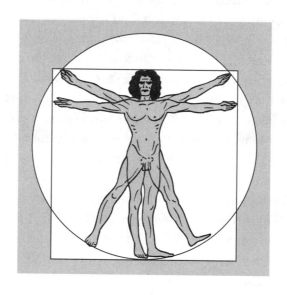

*W*ill losing weight help me prevent getting diabetes?

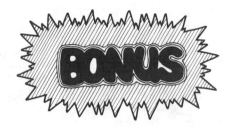

▼

TIP:

Yes, the DPP shows that people with impaired glucose tolerance (IGT) who lose 10–15 pounds reduce their risk of getting type 2 diabetes by more than 50%. If you are older than 60, the DPP found that losing this amount of weight reduced the risk of diabetes by 71%. Good news—these effects were the same for men and women and all minority groups. In addition, one-third of the people who lost the weight and exercised at least 150 minutes per week (30 min × 5 days) improved their blood sugar levels from IGT to normal. (If you have impaired glucose tolerance, your body isn't taking the glucose out of your blood as efficiently as it should.)

So, not only does losing weight help prevent diabetes, it also helps bring blood sugar levels that are above normal back to normal! The Finnish Diabetes Prevention study had similar results. A weight loss of 11% of body weight (more than 15 pounds) was associated with more than an 80% reduction in risk of getting type 2 diabetes. These results strongly suggest that the more weight you can lose, the better chance you have of preventing type 2 diabetes.

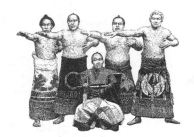

*H*ow do I know if I am at risk for diabetes?

▼
TIP:

S ome people have diabetes and do not know it. You should be screened every 3 years beginning at age 45 and perhaps more frequently if you have risk factors for diabetes. The risk increases with age, weight gain, and inactivity. The major risk factors are:

- Family history of diabetes (parents or siblings)
- Overweight (BMI ≥25)
- High blood pressure (≥140/90)
- HDL cholesterol ≤35 mg/dl
- Triglyceride level ≥250 mg/dl
- Diabetes during pregnancy or a baby weighing more than 9 lbs
- Polycystic ovary syndrome
- Ethnic groups (African American, Latin American, American Indian, Asian American, Pacific Islanders)

What's the difference between IGT and
diabetes?

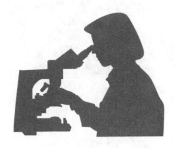

▼
TIP:

The difference is in your blood sugar levels. The most common
test for diabetes is a fasting blood sugar level (taken after at least
8 hours without food). If your fasting blood sugar is less than 110, it
is normal. You do not have diabetes. If it is 111–125, you have
impaired fasting glucose or IFG (pre-diabetes). If it is 126 or greater,
then you have diabetes.

Another screen for diabetes is an oral glucose tolerance test. This
involves getting a fasting blood sugar test, drinking a sweetened
drink, and getting a second blood sugar test 2 hours later. If the 2-hour
blood test is less than 140, it is normal. If it is 141–199, you have
IGT, meaning that your body is not using glucose the way it should.
This is also called pre-diabetes. If the result is 200 or greater, you
have diabetes. To confirm the diagnosis using either of these testing
methods, you need to have a second test on another day.

	Normal	Pre-Diabetes	Diabetes
Fasting blood sugar	110	111–125	>126
2-hr blood sugar	140	141–199	>200

When you have pre-diabetes, it may be because you are insulin
resistant. Your body may make plenty of insulin but cannot use it correctly, so your glucose levels are too high. Being overweight is one of
the causes of insulin resistance.

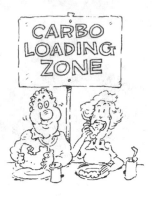

Does insulin resistance lead to weight gain?

▼
TIP:

Scientific evidence suggests that it is being overweight that causes insulin resistance rather than insulin resistance causing weight gain. Most Americans are gaining weight instead of losing because we are eating more total calories (100–300 extra calories per day) and exercising less. Many overweight adults eat too many calories from carbohydrate-rich foods as they try to cut back on fatty foods. If you eat too much carbohydrate and you are insulin resistant, then it will cause higher blood sugar levels as well as contribute extra calories. Too much is too much. To lose weight successfully and reduce insulin resistance, reduce your calories by decreasing the amounts of both carbohydrates and fats that you eat. Any diet with fewer calories than you usually eat will help you lose weight and reduce insulin resistance. The key is to find a pattern of eating that has a healthy balance between all the food groups and is lower in calories than your usual diet.

1,001 Tips for Living Well with Diabetes

D*oes exercise help prevent diabetes?*

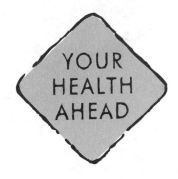

YOUR
HEALTH
AHEAD

▼

TIP:

Yes, research shows that increasing your activity level is an important lifestyle change for preventing diabetes. In the DPP, participants in the lifestyle-change group were asked to exercise at least 150 minutes a week. Most of them chose brisk walking, and others started swimming or biking. The average activity level was 208 minutes in the first year and 189 minutes at the end of the 3-year study. Another study in China showed that increasing physical activity can reduce the risk of developing diabetes by 46%. Participants in this study were asked to increase their exercise level by 2 units (see chart) a day for those over 50 years old who had no problems with heart disease or arthritis. The average activity level was 4 units per day. The clear message is that activity alone—even without weight loss—is a powerful diabetes prevention strategy.

Activities Required for One Unit of Exercise

Intensity	Time (minutes)	Exercise
Mild	30	Slow walking, traveling, shopping, housecleaning
Moderate	20	Faster walking, going downstairs, cycling, doing heavy laundry, ballroom dancing (slow)
Strenuous	10	Slow running, climbing stairs, disco dancing for the elderly, playing volleyball or table tennis
Very strenuous	5	Jumping rope, playing basketball, swimming

The Da Qing IGT and Diabetes study. *Diabetes Care.* 1997; 20(4): 537–544.

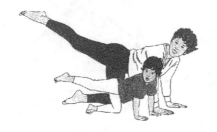

Why are so many teenagers overweight?

▼

TIP:

Today almost half of the children and teens in the United States are overweight. There has also been a dramatic increase in type 2 diabetes among these children. Environmental changes are the cause of this epidemic of obesity and diabetes. Children are bombarded with food advertising and have fewer opportunities for physical activity than in the past. This is a toxic environment with respect to diabetes risk. Kids who watch too much TV or play computer games for more than 2 hours a day, drink lots of sugared beverages, eat large portions of snack foods, and eat under stress gain lots of weight. The government and volunteer health organizations, including the American Diabetes Association (ADA), are working to reduce obesity through research and public health campaigns to promote healthier habits. Parents and kids need to make some changes: decrease the amount of time watching TV, increase after-school recreation programs, and be more physically active. They need to stop making a daily habit of eating fast foods and drinking sugared beverages. The government is making an effort to change the way foods are packaged and marketed to children, but parents and family members have to help the kids make the changes they need.

Chapter 7
WEIGHT LOSS SURGERY AND MEDICATIONS

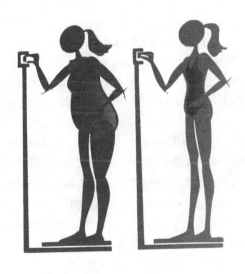

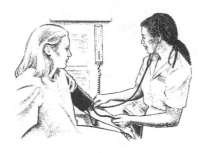

A re weight loss drugs beneficial?

TIP:

Weight loss drugs that have been approved by the Food and Drug Administration (FDA) for long-term use can be beneficial— along with lifestyle changes—for some patients with a BMI of 30 or more but no other health conditions, and for patients with a BMI of 27 or more with health problems. The health problems important enough to justify use of drugs are high blood pressure, high cholesterol, coronary heart disease (CHD), type 2 diabetes, and sleep apnea. Your health must be monitored the whole time you are taking the drug.

At the present time, two drugs are available for long-term use: sibutramine and orlistat. Sibutramine enhances weight loss and can help with weight loss maintenance. Potential side effects with drugs must be kept in mind. With sibutramine, increases in blood pressure and heart rate may occur. So, sibutramine should not be used if you have high blood pressure, heart disease, congestive heart failure, arrhythmias, or a history of stroke. With orlistat, you may need fat-soluble vitamins because you can't absorb them as well. You should be carefully monitored for any side effects.

*S*hould I have surgery to lose weight?

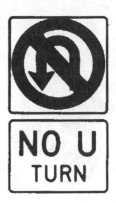

▼
TIP:

M aybe, if you have a BMI of 40 or greater. People with a BMI between 35 and 40 may be considered for surgery if they have medical conditions such as diabetes, high blood pressure, or arthritis and problems moving around. Surgery is considered for people between 18 and 65 years old who have made many unsuccessful attempts to lose weight in supervised programs. The types of weight loss surgery are vertical banded gastroplasty (VBG) and gastric bypass (GB). VBG uses stainless steel staples or a plastic "belt" to create a small pouch separate from the rest of the stomach. The pouch holds only a small amount of food, limiting how much you can eat before feeling full. Gastric bypass creates a small pouch and causes food to bypass the first part of the small intestine to reduce food absorption, producing more weight loss than VBG. For both surgeries, there are risks of the pouch stretching and the staples rupturing if you overeat. Gastric bypass has higher risk for nutritional deficiencies and dumping syndrome. (Your stomach contents "dump" too rapidly through the small intestine and cause nausea, weakness, and diarrhea.) Even with surgery, you still need to make lasting lifestyle changes.

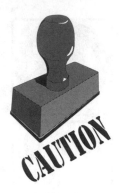

*W*hat should I consider before having surgery for weight loss?

▼
TIP:

Surgery to lose weight is a serious undertaking. You should clearly understand the benefits and the risks.

Benefits: Most people lose weight rapidly. After the first 6–9 months, the rate of weight loss usually slows down, but some people lose weight for 18–24 months. Weight losses of 60% have been reported 5 years after gastric bypass surgery. This surgery can help control type 2 diabetes without medications, because the weight loss often leads to normal blood sugar levels and also improves, or resolves, other obesity-related health problems such as high blood pressure, high cholesterol, and sleep apnea.

Risks: Approximately 10–20% of people require follow-up surgery to correct complications or side effects. The most common are hernias and vitamin B12 deficiency (corrected with supplements or monthly B12 shots). Serious complications are rupture of the staple line or a stretched stomach pouch caused by overeating. One-third of the patients develop gallstones. Another possible side effect is dumping syndrome. It occurs after eating foods with concentrated sugar and results in sweating, nausea, weakness, abdominal pain, and diarrhea due to the rapid passage of sugars into the small intestine. Dumping syndrome can be managed with attention to your diet. Any surgery under a general anesthetic also carries some risk to the patient's life.

1,001 Tips for Living Well with Diabetes

*W*hat happens after weight loss
surgery?

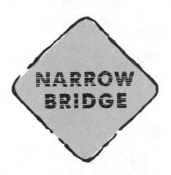

NARROW
BRIDGE

▼
TIP:

You get full faster, and you don't absorb foods as well. This can
cause nausea, abdominal pain, diarrhea, and vomiting if you eat
too much food at once or foods high in fat or sugar. Most people take
3–6 months to go through the 4 diet stages from no-added-sugar clear
liquids to 3 meals and 1–2 snacks a day. It is common to have lactose
(milk) intolerance and vitamin and mineral deficiencies. Anemia can
result from poor absorption of vitamin B12 and iron in menstruating
women. Decreased calcium absorption may increase your risk of
osteoporosis. You must take iron, calcium, and vitamin B12 supplements daily for the rest of your life. Some people have difficulty with
certain foods, such as red meat, bread, or pasta. Other people can eat
all foods, including sweets, while others have taste changes. An experienced health care team must oversee your transition to whole foods
and find the right levels of vitamin and calcium supplements. If you
drink high-calorie beverages and graze on small portions of food all
day, you can gain weight back. You need to take responsibility for
your eating habits for a lifetime if you want to keep the weight off.

Chapter 8
THE BASICS

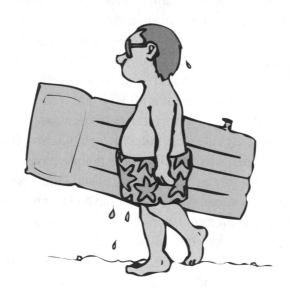

*H*ow can I get started being physically active?

▼
TIP:

C hoose an activity you enjoy to increase the chances you'll stick with it. Walking is most popular and most frequently recommended for overweight people. Start out slowly, walking about 10 minutes 5 days a week. Gradually increase to walking 30 minutes 5 days a week. You can also take the stairs, mow the lawn, and run the vacuum. Most weight loss programs encourage you to do many types of activity to burn the most calories.

You don't need to sweat or join a gym, but having a trainer at the beginning helps you succeed. Keeping records of your physical activity (minutes or calories burned) in your food record helps you identify patterns and provides good feedback on your progress. You'll be able to see the connection between calories burned and weight loss. Measure your hips, waist, biceps, and thighs. Muscle weighs more than fat, so if you don't see a change in the scale, you'll be able to encourage yourself with the changes in your measurements—and how your clothes fit, too!

While you walk, you can listen to tapes that encourage you and help you vary the pace for a better workout. Or you can get a book on tape from the library and enjoy it while you get your exercise.

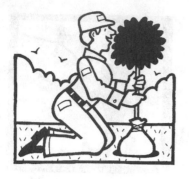

*C*an I increase my physical activity using everyday activities?

▼

TIP:

Yes. The Lifetime Activity Model encourages using types of activity that are already part of your everyday routine activities. These activities might include vacuuming, mowing the lawn with a push mower, house painting, car washing, yard work, gardening, taking the stairs, parking the car further away and walking, and just walking more. (Get a pedometer!) These activities can be done at various speeds and for varying lengths of time.

Activity Benefits of Household Chores and Yard Work

Activity Category		Average Calories Burned/ 30 minutes*
Light Household Chores		90 to 100 calories
Cooking/baking	Light carpentry	
Dusting furniture	Sweeping floors	
Laundry	Washing dishes	
Moderate House and Yard Work		130 to 190 calories
Gardening	Carrying out trash	
Mowing the lawn/	or recycling	
hedging and trimming	Vacuuming floors	
Raking leaves	Washing cars	
Scrubbing floors	Washing windows	
Hard House and Yard Work		over 200 calories
Digging light earth	Home repair	
Shoveling snow		

*Calories burned per 30 min are for an individual who weighs 150 pounds. Actual calories burned are slightly less for people who weigh under 150 pounds and are slightly more for those who weigh over 150 pounds.
Hayes, C. *The "I Hate to Exercise" Book,* American Diabetes Association, 2001.

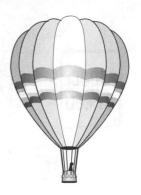

*W*hy do I need to warm up and stretch
before I exercise?

▼
TIP:

The warm-up helps get the blood flowing a little more quickly,
which helps your body prepare for more vigorous work. You
should warm up gradually by walking slowly, doing light calisthenics,
or dancing. You want to gradually increase your heart rate to within
20 beats of your target range (page 673). The warm-up also gives
your muscles and joints a chance to loosen up. End your warm-up
with stretching each part of your body. No single stretch can take care
of your whole body. Begin at your neck and work down to the ankles.
Start with neck rotations, move to shoulder rolls and arm swings, do a
gentle knee bend, and finish with ankle rotations. Stretch the tendons
that support your major joints to the point of tension, but not to the
point of pain. Do NOT bounce as you stretch because it is hard on
joints and muscles. Breathe deeply and relax into the stretch. Each
joint and muscle group should be stretched for 5–30 seconds. You are
prepared now to get the full benefit of your aerobic exercise without
injury.

Why do I need to cool down and stretch after I finish exercising?

▼
TIP:

A cooldown helps slow your heart rate down and helps muscles and joints return to an inactive state. You reduce your chances of injury and sore muscles if your brisk walks and other aerobic activities include the warm-up and stretch before you start and cooldown and stretch after you finish. You can slow down your aerobic activity or walk slowly for 5–10 minutes after aerobic activity to cool down. The cooldown should end with stretching. Again, the stretching includes neck rotations, shoulder rolls, arm swings, gentle knee bends, and ankle rotations. Your stretches should be smooth, fluid movements. As you do in yoga, you can hold a stretch, but do not make jerky, sudden movements or bounces. After the cooldown and stretching, your body should feel relaxed and more flexible. Your heart rate should have returned to its normal pre-exercise rate by the end of the cooldown and stretch.

*W*hy do I have leg pains when I walk?

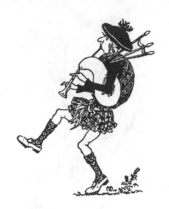

▼
TIP:

S ore muscles can hurt when you walk, but pain can also be a symptom of poor circulation. If you have diabetes or other cardiovascular risk factors such as high blood pressure, your doctor should evaluate the pain. You may have intermittent claudication or poor blood flow. Intermittent claudication feels like cramping or aching. The pain occurs because the blood vessels leading to the lower leg have narrowed, and the muscles cannot get enough blood. The pain usually occurs after you walk a short distance. Your physician may recommend that you walk until you begin to feel pain, stop to rest, and walk some more. You gradually increase the distance walked and improve circulation to your leg, relieving the pain.

Leg pain can also be due to sore muscles. If you are out of condition and try to walk quickly, you may feel discomfort in your legs. You may be stretching muscles that are not used to stretching. If you run or exercise vigorously, you can get shin splints, or tendonitis on the front of the lower leg. Walk more slowly or do a different activity for a few days until the soreness goes away.

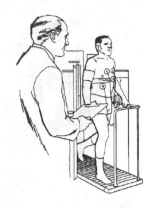

*W*hat is a stress test?

▼
TIP:

The purpose of an exercise stress test is to find out how much exercise you can safely do. An exercise stress test may also be used to develop a cardiac rehabilitation program for people who have had a heart attack or as a tool for evaluating heart disease. You may be asked to exercise on a treadmill or on a stationary bike for the test. Your blood pressure, electrocardiogram (ECG), and heart rate are measured throughout the test, which usually lasts less than 30 minutes. Exercise stress testing provides a controlled environment for observing the effects of increasing demand for oxygen by the heart. An ECG can provide evidence of damage to the coronary arteries that supply blood to the heart muscles. Blood pressure changes also provide information about the fitness of the heart. If you have an exercise stress test, you may be asked to report symptoms such as fatigue, chest pain, or shortness of breath to provide a more complete picture of how well your heart functions. A stress test may tell you your maximum heart rate. You use this to figure your target heart rate during exercise.

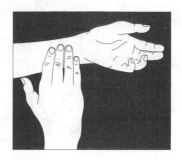

*W*hy should I check my target heart rate?

▼
TIP:

The target heart rate is usually 60–80% of your maximum heart rate (which can be determined by a mathematical formula or a stress test). You need activity levels high enough to increase blood circulation and your heart rate. However, you should not put too much stress on your heart. Your target heart rate keeps you in the safe but effective range. You have probably exceeded your target heart rate if you have difficulty catching your breath or talking while exercising. Consult with your provider if you have diabetes or heart disease. If you take medications such as beta-blockers, your heart rate may not increase with physical activity.

You can take your pulse at the arteries on either side of your windpipe or the artery 1/4 inch inside your wrist below the thumb. Do not use your thumb to take a pulse.

Target Heart Rates for Healthy People

Age	Beats per minute 60%	Beats per minute 80%	Beats/6 seconds range
20	120	160	12–16
30	114	152	11–15
40	108	144	10–14
50	102	136	10–14
60	96	128	9–13
70	90	120	9–12
80	84	112	8–11

Wylie-Rosett et al. *The Complete Weight Loss Workbook,* American Diabetes Association, 1997.

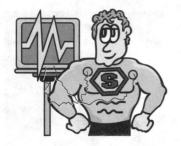

Do I need an exercise stress test?

▼
TIP:

Ask your physician. You may need an exercise stress test if you are increasing the intensity of physical activity. If you have diabetes or heart disease, you may need a stress test. In addition to being used in cardiac programs, exercise stress tests are often used as part of fitness planning. If you join a fitness center, you may need an exercise stress test to make sure that you can safely participate in various activities and to help you set exercise goals.

Good Reasons to Consult Your Physician before Beginning Exercise

- You are a male over age 40 or a female over age 50
- You have diabetes and are over age 35
- You have had type 2 diabetes for more than 10 years
- You have had type 1 diabetes for more than 15 years
- You have high blood triglycerides, high blood cholesterol, or low HDL cholesterol
- You have heart disease
- You have high blood pressure
- You take heart or blood pressure medications
- You have retinopathy, nephropathy, or autonomic neuropathy
- You have experienced chest pain or pressure, faintness, or dizziness

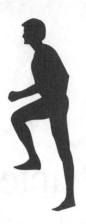

*W*hy do you recommend walking and step
counters?

▼
TIP:

Walking is inexpensive, easy, and convenient. More than 60% of
adults in the United States get less than the recommended level
of physical activity of 30 minutes 5 days a week. Inactive people take
an average of 2,000 to 4,000 steps per day. Moderately active people
take 5,000 to 7,000 steps per day. Active people take at least 10,000
steps per day. People who have diabetes are more likely to be inactive
than other people. High blood sugars can make you feel tired and
sluggish, so you don't exercise. But, studies have shown that a walking program can increase your insulin sensitivity for up to 72 hours—
lowering blood sugar and giving you more energy.

Pedometers can help you count (and increase) the number of steps
you take each day. You can purchase an inexpensive pedometer in
most stores with sporting goods. Slightly more expensive pedometers
measure distance as well. You can estimate the distance from your
number of steps. Walking 2,000 steps is about one mile. Awareness of
the number of steps helps you think of creative ways to take more.
You can even purchase a "talking" pedometer to boost your motivation while you walk.

Chapter 9
PLANNING FOR SUCCESS

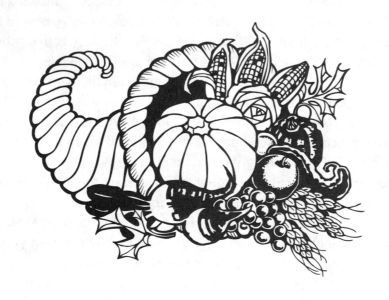

At a certain point my weight gets stuck at a plateau. What can I do when the scale won't budge?

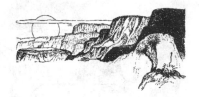

▼ TIP:

When this happens, ask yourself some questions:

1. Am I keeping track of calories and fat grams?
2. Are my serving sizes correct? Am I eyeballing portions, or actually weighing and measuring to be sure they are correct?
3. Based on my current weight, do I need to reduce my calories to continue to lose weight?
4. Have I been active enough?

If you answer "no" to any of these questions, you have a possible cause of the plateau. If you answer "yes" to all of the questions, take a look at your weight loss pattern over time. Not everyone loses the same amount each week. Some people lose 2–4 pounds in one week and then don't lose any weight for 2 weeks despite healthy eating and activity. Other people retain fluid from time to time that masks their true body weight. If you know that your eating habits and activity are on target, then weight loss will usually follow. The key is to find ways to stay motivated while the plateau lasts. Find other ways to chart your progress, such as measuring your waist or thigh with a tape measure, so you can see the inches you've lost.

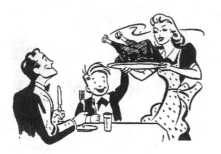

How can I deal with vacations and holidays so I don't regain weight?

▼
TIP:

Vacations and holidays are the times when most people let go and enjoy food and relaxation. So you need to set reasonable goals for your weight and activity. It may be more reasonable to expect to maintain your weight rather than lose any during vacations. Resume weight loss once the holiday is over. Plan ahead for eating out. You might decide to limit the number of times you eat out and spend the extra time and money on other activities. When you go out, eat what you want, but you can limit calories by eating smaller servings. Set up your food environment for success by bringing low-calorie food choices with you. Think ahead about what you might like to do to stay active. Before you go, discuss your eating and activity goals with family and friends and ways that they can support you. If you plan, you are more likely to meet your goals. But remember it takes 3 or 4 holidays before you get the plan just right. Learn from your experiences. See what helped you and what stopped you. Adjust your strategy the next time. Don't get discouraged, be patient, and keep trying!

How can I learn to manage binge eating, so I can succeed with weight loss?

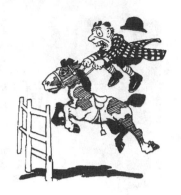

▼
TIP:

Binge eating is overeating that feels out of control. Binge eating is associated with higher body weight, more difficulty losing weight, and higher blood sugar levels. If you want to manage problems with binge eating, the first step is to keep food records. Then you can clearly see your patterns with binge eating and how they change as you try different strategies. Look at your food records to find:

- What you eat during binges (forbidden foods?)
- When binges occur (evenings, weekends, weekdays?)
- Triggers for binges (emotions, stress, loneliness?)
- Reasons for binges (to relieve tension, distract from problems?)

It is also important to check your weight once a week around the same time of day to evaluate your weight trends over time. Once you have a system to track your eating patterns and weight trends, then you are ready to try out different strategies to manage binge eating. As you try a strategy, check your food records for changes in the number of binge eating episodes, the types of food that you eat, the timing of binges, the triggers for binges, and the functions that binges serve.

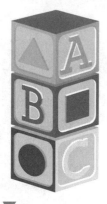

*W*hat strategies can I try to reduce
binge eating?

▼

TIP:

S ome of the strategies to manage binge eating are:

1. Keep food records.
2. Establish a regular pattern of eating with 3 meals and 2–3 snacks. Do not skip meals.
3. Eat every 3–4 hours. Most people binge when they are either over-hungry or have too much free time.
4. If you eat or binge between planned meals and snacks, go right back to your regular pattern as quickly as possible.
5. Eat more slowly and focus on savoring each bite. Enjoy the sight, the smell, the taste, and the texture of your food. It is easier to do this if you sit down, and you don't watch TV, read, or work while eating.
6. Rearrange your food environment (page 703).
7. Rearrange your emotional environment (page 708).
8. Make a list of activities you enjoy that help distract you from the urge to binge or make it difficult to binge (exercise, visit friends, work on a hobby).

Remember it takes time, patience, and practice to find the combi-nation of strategies that works best for you.

How do I know if a slip from healthy eating is a problem or not?

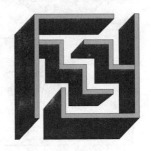

▼
TIP:

Everyone who is trying to eat healthy to lose weight is going to slip. Some people call it cheating, but it's okay. It's normal. It is usually not the slip that is the problem, rather it is the way we react to slips when they happen. The truth is that no one slip can ruin your overall progress. Slips are part of the process of changing your eating habits. One slip is not a pattern. However, if you notice a series of slips and that you are returning to old habits, losing your overall focus, and have gained back more than 3 pounds, then take steps to refocus and seek help. Try to make a list of the "clues" that show you are dealing with more than just a slip. For example, clues on your list might include a weight gain of more than 3 pounds, more than one week without exercising, certain clothes are too tight, or an old habit that you had worked hard to break comes back.

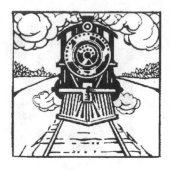

*O*nce I slip from healthy eating and
gain weight, how can I get back
on track?

▼
TIP:

W e learn from mistakes, so they are valuable. Make sure
your reaction to slips or cheating on your diet doesn't work
against you.

1. Don't engage in negative self-talk or blame. Talk positively to
   yourself and *about* yourself. Instead of thinking, "I blew it," try
   thinking, "One slip won't ruin everything. I can get back to eating
   better right now." Your positive thoughts affect how you feel and
   what you do.
2. Look for why the slip happened and try to learn from the experience. Everyone who tries to eat healthy and lose weight has their
   own list of high-risk situations that cause slips. This is your chance
   to learn more about the situations that put you at high risk. Then
   you can think about how to avoid a slip the next time.
3. Talk to someone. Family, friends, coworkers, and others can be a
   real source of support. Talk about what caused you to slip, what
   you have learned from the situation, and your ideas for handling
   this high-risk situation in the future. Consider regular appointments with a dietitian or counselor for more professional help.

I *know how to lose weight, but how do*
I get the willpower to do it?

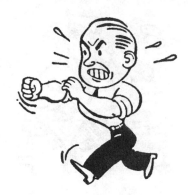

▼
TIP:

Willpower is the ability to resist eating tempting foods in your environment. If you rely only on willpower for success with weight loss, your success will probably be short-lived because the motivation to resist eating tempting foods can wax and wane over time. To lose weight you learn the best food choices, but you also shift away from relying on willpower to making a habit of self-control. You build self-control when you rearrange your food environment and change the way you think about food and dieting, so your desire to eat arises less frequently and less intensely.

There are several ways to rearrange your food environment for success.

1. Keep away from problem foods by not buying them or putting them out of sight.
2. Keep a variety of healthy low-calorie food choices around you.
3. Don't go long periods (more than 4–5 hours) without food, as this can lead to over-hunger, food cravings, and a greater tendency to overeat.
4. Choose lower-calorie foods.
5. Engage in activities away from food.

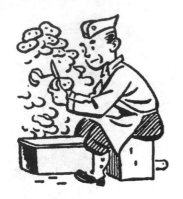

I get bored eating the same foods, and crave foods I shouldn't eat. How can I manage this problem?

▼
TIP:

You need to introduce new healthy foods into meals and maybe change the times you eat, too. Mix it up. Variety is important. When you notice you are feeling bored, ask:

- Do I sacrifice variety for convenience or speed in the lunches I carry or the dinners I make? What other foods could I use?
- What meals, snacks, or foods am I most bored with?
- How can I vary this part of my eating and still lose weight?
- Would changes in taste, texture, or temperature make my meals more satisfying and interesting? Do I want something spicy, instead of sweet or bland? Something hot, cold, or at room temperature? Something crunchy, chewy, or smooth?

When you answer the questions, you see ways to vary meals and snacks, so you are not bored or craving unhealthy foods. At the library, you can search food magazines and healthy cookbooks for quick meal recipes and new foods to meet your personal needs for taste, texture, and temperature. Have fun with your meal plan. It's one of the most important things you do each day.

*S*hould I take vitamin supplements while I'm cutting back on food to lose weight?

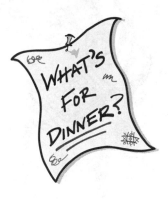

▼
TIP:

If you cut back on food to lose weight and you're not eating a healthy diet as described in the Food Guide Pyramid, then you may need a multivitamin supplement. The Food Guide Pyramid recommends eating a variety of foods and a daily minimum of:

- 6 servings of bread, cereal, rice, or pasta (a serving is usually 1 slice or 1/2 cup)
- 3 servings of vegetables
- 2 servings of fruit
- 2 servings of dairy (milk, yogurt, or cheese)
- 2 servings of meat, fish, poultry, eggs, or legumes

If your diet does not include this number of servings from each of these food groups, then it is possible that you are not getting enough protein or the vitamins and minerals that you need. A registered dietitian can help you determine the nutritional quality of your diet and tell you if it is lacking any vitamins or minerals.

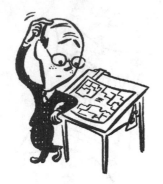

*H*ow does food-combining really work?

Several popular weight loss diets recommend avoiding specific combinations of foods to improve digestion and metabolism. They say that starchy foods are to be eaten alone to improve weight loss. People who go on these diets often do lose weight, but it's because they eat fewer calories. The food-combining approach encourages people to eat a lot of fruits and vegetables, a modest amount of starches, and limited portions of meat. This is okay, but milk and dairy foods are not permitted at all. Each type of food is basically eaten alone, which reduces the tendency to overeat. This structured approach does help avoid the added calories that come from unplanned eating. But you need very careful timing and planning to allow the recommended time before eating a food that should not be combined with a previously eaten food. The dietary plan tends to be low in calcium, vitamin B12, vitamin D, zinc, and protein.

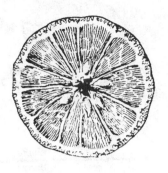

*D*oes grapefruit help you burn fat and
lose weight?

The answers are "no" to fat burning, but "yes" to helping you lose
weight. Many popular weight loss diets promote grapefruit with
claims that the acid in the grapefruit will burn fat. And people who rit-
ualistically eat grapefruit before their meals are likely to lose weight.
The reason is that grapefruit is filling and relatively low in calories, so
you are likely to be satisfied with less food when you eat the meal.

There are no research studies that support the claim that grapefruit
burns body fat, speeds up metabolism, or causes weight loss by any
other type of miracle. While grapefruit is not a miracle food for burning fat, it is a great option for filling up on more wholesome foods.
The bottom line is that you may find eating grapefruit helpful, but you
have to do more than just eat grapefruit to lose weight.

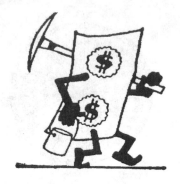

Diet food and all those fruits and vegetables seem so expensive. How can following my meal plan cost less?

You can budget money as you are budgeting calories. You do not need to buy high-priced diet foods. Fresh vegetables and fruit and foods that you prepare yourself are always the less expensive choice. You can choose to spend some time and save some money.

Low-calorie frozen entrées tend to cost more than the regular versions. Ones that have more meat cost more than the pasta-based frozen entrees. Cutting down on high-priced meat can help save money that you can use to buy vegetables and fruits. Store brands of frozen vegetables are usually lower priced than national brands. When buying vegetables, compare the bagged ones with the ones you buy by the pound. Buying fruits in season can help save money—apples in the fall, citrus fruits in the winter, and berries in the spring. Another way to save money is to buy produce directly from the farmer. The web site for the United States Department of Agriculture (*www.nal.usda.gov/afsic/csa*) provides information about the Community Supported Agriculture (CSA) program, which links local farmers to consumer buying groups whose members buy a share of the weekly harvest during the growing season.

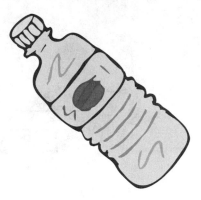

*D*oes drinking water help you lose weight?

Yes, drinking water can help you lose weight. Water contains no calories, and it helps you feel full. Experts recommend that we drink 8 glasses of water a day for good health. A growing number of weight- and health-conscious people have increased their daily water intake by carrying a bottle of water with them wherever they go.

Unfortunately, many people drink too many soft drinks instead of water. The obesity epidemic in our country is linked to the popularity of drinking bigger sizes of sugar-rich sports drinks and soft drinks. If you drink these instead of water, you should know that a 20-oz soft drink contains 300–400 calories and 15–20 teaspoons of sugar. That is 12–15 calories per ounce. Fruit juices also contain 12 calories per ounce. Even the sports drinks are 6–10 calories per ounce. These calorie levels make water a very attractive option, indeed. If you are not a fan of water, consider seltzer (without added sugar). Diet soft drinks are another option, but for health and variety, drink water, too.

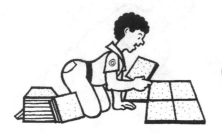

*C*an I just make up my own
  diet?

▼
TIP:

Yes. Start with the foods you like, your daily schedule, and your health needs. You can use the Food Pyramid or exchanges or carbohydrate counts in the meal plan.

1. **Limit choices.** For most people, as the variety of food increases, the amount of food eaten and calories also increase. Consider not keeping tempting foods at home and what to do when eating out. You might try some meal replacements (page 625).
2. **Identify and change behaviors leading to too many calories.** Some people don't eat all day and have an uncontrolled appetite at night. Eat breakfast, lunch, and dinner. For other people, simply eating fewer sugared beverages or snack foods makes a big difference.
3. **Become aware of your eating.** Many people are unaware of what or how much they eat. Learn more about your eating style. Slow down and chew each bite 20 times. You may need to keep a week or two of food records (page 621).
4. **Develop a positive attitude.** Many people join a weight loss program to feel they belong to a group and to get encouragement. Celebrate your ability and every success.

Chapter 10
EATING OUT

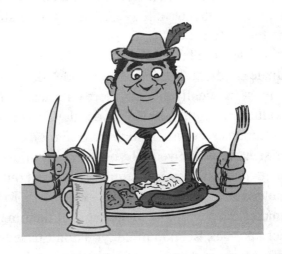

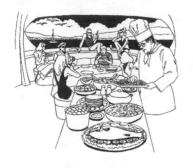

*I*s eating out in restaurants a challenge?

▼

TIP:

Yes—for everyone. Several studies show that eating out makes it almost impossible to have a low-calorie day. One study showed the group who most often ate at restaurants consumed 30% more calories per day, 5% more fat, and 36% less fiber compared to those who ate out the least often. A second study showed that those who ate in restaurants most frequently ate 228 more calories, 19 more grams of fat, more sodium, and much less fiber per day. If you go there, you will eat it. Restaurants serve many high-calorie foods, and the servings are super-sized or worse yet, all-you-can-eat buffets. Lunches are often full-course meals. The more frequently you eat out, the more you need advanced-level restaurant skills (page 693). To be successful with weight management, cook at home most of the time, and rarely eat out or order take-out. Keep in mind, you don't have to cook like Martha Stewart. Many cookbooks offer quick, easy, healthy recipes.

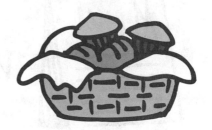

*W*hat are the restaurant skills I need for eating out and keeping on my weight loss plan?

▼

TIP:

P lan ahead. Step 1: Choose a restaurant that offers healthy choices. If you don't know what's on the menu, call ahead, stop by for a copy, or request a faxed copy. Step 2: Set a calorie goal for the meal. Use your weekly food records to see if you can afford a calorie splurge. Step 3: Ask about food preparation and serving sizes before you order. How is the item prepared (in butter, oil, fried)? Can you request special preparation (broiled, steamed, no butter)? Are low-calorie salad dressings available? What is the soup base (water, milk, cream)? What comes with the entrée (French fries, coleslaw)? Can you request items not on the menu or substitute healthier items? Can you have a child's serving?

Actions to take:

- Carry low-calorie dressings with you.
- Put half the order in a doggie bag before you start to eat.
- Split the entrée or dessert with someone.
- Remove bread, crackers, chips, or rolls from the table.
- Carry items to round out the meal, such as fresh fruit or raw vegetables to go with a turkey sandwich.
- Walk to and from the restaurant to burn some calories.

*W*hat are some tips for placing an order in restaurants?

▼
TIP:

L ook for ways to increase the amount of food and nutrition, but not the fat and calories. Try these:

■ Construct a meal without an entrée, using appetizers, soup, salad, or side vegetables. For example: shrimp cocktail, broth-based vegetable soup, baked potato, steamed vegetable.
■ Order without looking at the menu.
■ Order items not listed on the menu, such as a steamed vegetable plate.
■ Replace high-fat items with low-fat items (baked potato for French fries, tossed salad for coleslaw).
■ Request sauces on the side—dip your fork into the sauce, and then into the food.
■ Order double portions of salad and vegetable.
■ Make special requests for low-fat preparation—no added fat to fish or vegetables.
■ Order at least 2 cups of vegetables without fat with your meal. (Corn and potatoes are not counted as vegetables.)
■ Order the smaller lunch size or early-bird special portion.
■ When sharing a meal with your dining companion, order an extra potato or vegetable.
■ Ask that only one roll or breadstick be brought with your salad.
■ Become a regular customer; you'll most likely get what you request.

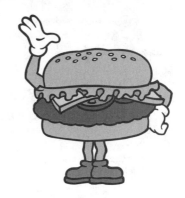

*H*ow does fast food figure into my
weight management?

▼
TIP:

I t may not fit. A recent study looked at three commonly ordered
take-out meals from three different fast food chains. The typical
meal from these fast food restaurants had more than 1,000 calories in
the meal. Authors concluded that eating even one fast food meal a
week made it extremely difficult for the participants to meet their recommended health guidelines. Another analysis has reported the calories of an average fast food meal at 1,300 calories. And that was
before you super-sized the meal for only 80 cents more. Once super-
sized, the final tally was 1,660 calories for lunch! Very few people can
afford 1,600 calories for lunch on a regular basis, yet this is the world
we live in. You have to be creative and find ways to cut calories. Don't
get super-sizes; they cost you too much. There are some lower-calorie
choices available in fast food chains, such as grilled chicken sandwiches and entrée salads with low-calorie dressings. In all fast food
restaurants, try to stay away from anything that is fried or covered in
cheese or sauce. If those are the only choices, go for smaller servings.
Making the right choice when placing your order is the key!

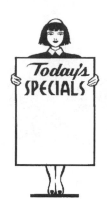

How can I work in my favorite foods when eating out?

TIP:

According to successful weight managers, "if you want it, have it." You need to break away from good food/bad food thinking. The message is simple: when you have treats, enjoy them. You don't have to feel guilty. But—plan, plan, plan. "If you fail to plan, you plan to fail." Identify the food that is important to you, and figure how many calories are in the serving it will take for you to enjoy that food. Using that calorie figure, figure what else can be included in the meal, if anything. Add up the calories you need to save up for the treat. Figure what your usual calories would be at that meal, and subtract them from the calories in the treat meal. If you usually eat 450 calories at lunch, but your favorite food is 950 calories, you have 500 extra calories to fit into your week. You need to save ahead for this favorite food. Don't try to take the 500 calories from the other meals in that same day. Better to cut some calories each day for several days before the treat. Don't forget that you can burn calories with exercise, too. It all counts.

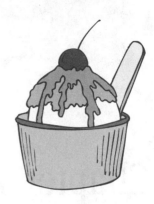

*C*an you give an example of how to save up calories for a treat?

▼
TIP:

H ere is a woman who weighs 180 lbs. To maintain her weight, her daily calorie level is 1,980. Her favorite food is a hot fudge sundae, which is made with 1 cup premium ice cream (600), 1/4 cup hot fudge sauce (240), and 1/4 cup whipped cream (200). This sundae has 1,040 calories. To create "space" for this treat, this woman is willing to eat lightly earlier in the day and to do physical activity twice that day, or also on the days before, to make this work.

Her day might look like this.

	Subtotals
Before Breakfast: Walked 2.5 miles = burned 300 calories	−300
Breakfast: 300 calories, including fruit and low-fat yogurt	300
Lunch: 2 (300-calorie) frozen entrées	
Plus 1 cup vegetables (40 calories)	640
Mid-afternoon: Walked 3 miles = burned 360 calories	−360
Supper: 600-calorie meal, not including the sundae	600
8 oz broiled whitefish with lemon (200)	
6 oz baked potato (120)	
2 Tbsp. sour cream (60)	
1 cup steamed vegetable (no oil) (40)	
1 oz roll (80)	
1 Tbsp butter (100)	
Hot Fudge Sundae	1040
Total Calories In	2580
Calories Out (physical activity) (300 + 360)	−660
Net Calories In	1920

Chapter 11
ENVIRONMENT
OUT OF CONTROL

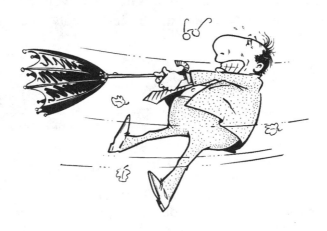

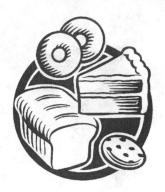

I crave carbohydrates. Am I a
carbohydrate addict?

▼
TIP:

Fresh fruit, vegetables, and beans are carbohydrates, yet no one seems to be addicted to them. It is the soft, fluffy, sugar- and fat-bearing carbohydrates that cause trouble. Write down what you crave—is it doughnuts, French fries, or candy bars? Carbohydrate craving or addiction describes how eating carbohydrate triggers your appetite and a desire for more carbohydrate. If it's an addiction, you can do something about it.

Your body breaks down carbohydrate foods to glucose. The pancreas produces insulin to help body cells take in glucose and use it for energy. Some people restrict the amount of carbohydrate they eat, thinking this reduces the craving, but you need carbohydrate to feel satisfied. Some studies suggest that choosing natural or unprocessed carbohydrates, such as oatmeal or baked beans, that have more fiber helps stop cravings. Fiber makes you feel full. There's no fiber in one (or even five) doughnuts. Raw vegetables and whole fruits, such as apples, can be filling and are rich in fiber. Get some insight on your craving by keeping a diary of how your eating pattern is related to your appetite.

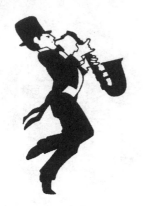

*H*ow can I lose weight when I have to eat on the run?

Plan ahead for good food choices and make use of every opportunity. It's easier to eat vegetables with ready-to-eat produce options such as prewashed bagged salad greens and peeled baby carrots. You may save time and money by bringing a frozen low-calorie entree to pop into the workplace microwave or raw vegetables and fruit from home. You can build more physical activity into each day by taking a 5-minute break to walk around.
As you go through your day, watch for opportunities to walk more. Use a pedometer and add a few extra steps each day. Many people gain weight because time for eating a balanced diet and being physically active becomes a lower priority than work or other activities. Nothing is more important than your health, exercising, and eating right. Get your priorities straight, and you can create time to take care of yourself.

To avoid confusion and indecision, set clear goals to help keep yourself organized. For example, eat an apple a day. Take the stairs. Have a salad for dinner. Make a shopping list. Cook dinner.

*H*ow can I say no to friends who push
food?

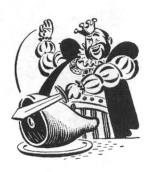

▼
TIP:

It's hard to say "no" when food is offered to you by friends and family. People can be offended when you reject the food they offer. Food has many emotional meanings. Mothers often express their love for their families by cooking favorite meals. We socialize with friends and family over foods. Say "no, thank you" firmly and clearly. Talking to others about how they can help is the first step in helping them understand that managing your weight is important to you. Sometimes you can suggest other foods. You can take a small piece. Serious food pushers may not respond to more subtle approaches. Then you have to be more firm and resort to tactics that are more direct. You may need to say, "I feel that I have trouble controlling my weight and my health when I eat with you. Please support me in my decision to avoid eating seconds" (or whatever you have decided to do). If you can get them on your side, you'll both win.

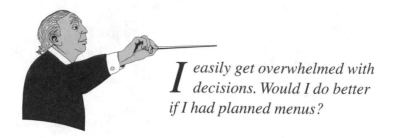

I easily get overwhelmed with decisions. Would I do better if I had planned menus?

TIP:

Yes. Studies have shown that people can achieve long-term success using menus or prepackaged foods. They help if you feel you need more structure, for example, getting started, when you are under stress, and when you have slipped or gained back some weight.

Making food choices can be difficult when you are trying to break old habits. Using menus or packaged foods can make your decisions easier. ADA publishes the Month-of-Meals series of books to provide you with millions of menus. You can choose a cuisine and calorie level suited to your needs.

If you find yourself thinking, "I cannot wait until I finish this diet," you have a high risk of going back to your old habits. You may find that you will always need menus to keep you on track. If you use prepackaged meal supplements (page 624), make sure you don't round out the meal with old high-calorie snacks. If you have a shake or bar for one or two meals a day, you may find that you are hungry. Try to satisfy that hunger with raw vegetables or a piece of fruit as snacks.

*W*hen my favorite foods are
    around, I just cannot stay
away from them. How can I stay on
my meal plan?

TIP:

*D*ealing with tempting food can be overwhelming, especially if the
food is highly visible. These techniques may help you:

- Give away or freeze tempting leftovers from special celebrations.
- Avoid buying or making the food that you find so overwhelming.
- If you buy tempting foods, get the smallest size. Get the small cup
  or cone of ice cream rather than bringing home a half gallon.
- Negotiate with household members to keep the tempting foods out
  of sight or to choose other foods that are less tempting to you. For
  example, they could choose a type of chocolate bar that you don't
  like.
- Try to learn to be satisfied with a smaller serving of the tempting
  food. Eat slowly and focus on the taste.
- Try to find some new favorite foods that are better for your waist-
  line.
- Talk, dance, laugh, or walk somewhere away from the food.

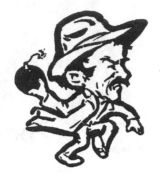

Why would my husband (or my friend) try to sabotage my diet?

▼
TIP:

If family members and friends try to lure you away or criticize your weight loss efforts, you can feel sabotaged. Let them know that you feel discouraged by their words or actions. Discuss what they can do to truly support your weight loss effort.

Think about your goals and how your weight loss may change your relationships. Sometimes the saboteur enjoys eating and wants you to be a partner in the fun of feasting. State your goals clearly to show that you are seriously trying to change the way you eat. What are their goals for you? Sometimes friends and family feel a conflict. They want your success, but may feel imposed upon if you request they keep tempting foods out of the house. You may need to negotiate an acceptable plan.

If your family and friends are aware of their ambivalent feelings about your weight loss, you may be able to talk about their views of the pros and cons. But many times the person sabotaging your effort is unaware of it. If you have difficulty talking with him or her, you might discuss the problem with a professional counselor or your health care provider.

Chapter 12
EMOTIONS AND
ROADBLOCKS

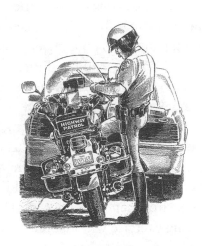

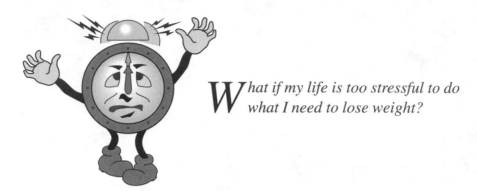

*W*hat if my life is too stressful to do
what I need to lose weight?

▼
TIP:

It is important to identify the reasons for the stress and plan ways to
reduce it or manage it. The things you can do to relieve stress—
such as exercising and making healthy food choices (for the vitamins
and minerals that help you manage stress)—are the very things you
need for weight loss, too. You can actually work on weight loss and
lowering stress at the same time. Take 30 minutes to write down the
stresses on you and some things to do to manage them. Breathe
deeply. Take a yoga class. Punch a pillow. Run around the block.
Walk every day. Read a book. You need balance in your life. Otherwise you'll do what many people do—eat more and exercise less, and
actually gain weight. If you learn to reset your goals to hold your
weight steady during high stress and then refocus on weight loss
when your stress level is reduced, you may be more successful.

If you have diabetes, any physical stress (cold, flu, infection,
or injury) or emotional stress can raise your blood sugar levels.
Overeating and skipping exercise will just raise them higher. Start
to defuse the stresses in your life today.

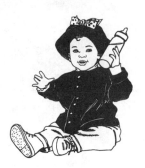

I use food to comfort and nurture myself when I'm feeling angry, depressed, or upset. Will this habit prevent me from being successful with weight loss?

▼

TIP:

Not as long as you are aware of what you're doing and can find other ways to comfort and nurture yourself. Overeating in response to negative feelings is called emotional eating. Emotional eaters use food to cope when they feel angry or upset, anxious, worried, tense, depressed, disappointed, or discouraged. Other people lose their appetite and eat less in response to these same emotions. There are several reasons people develop the habit of emotional eating; eating tends to calm mood. Children are often conditioned to associate eating with being soothed or nurtured. Eating is a quick, convenient way to temporarily distract yourself from stressful emotions. Eating food for emotional reasons is perfectly normal. The problem with eating for emotional reasons is that many people do it in a chaotic manner, often overeating in an attempt to push down or blot out feelings. This behavior pattern can make you feel numb, guilty, and out of control, which can make it difficult to manage your weight and control your blood sugars. You may need to see a counselor for help with changing this habit.

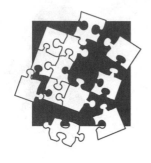

*H*ow can I change my tendency to eat in response to negative emotions, so I can make better progress with weight loss?

TIP:

*F*irst, ask yourself the following questions:

1. Is emotional eating causing me problems with overeating, weight control, or blood sugar control?
2. What kind of events, situations, people, and feelings trigger this response?
3. How does emotional eating affect my physical well-being, diabetes control, self-esteem, and mood after I've eaten?
4. What else besides eating can I choose that may also calm my mood or distract me from stressful emotions?

Share your feelings with someone else or your journal rather than stuffing them down with food. Take a walk or do some other exercise that you enjoy—this also improves your mood and distracts you. If you are tired, take a nap rather than eating to stay awake. You're likely to feel better with rest. Try to address the problem causing the negative emotions and work out a plan to deal with it. If you do eat, acknowledge how you feel and give yourself permission to eat in a positive, mindful, deliberate way. You may find that a smaller portion of food helps you feel better and still allows you success with losing weight and controlling your blood sugars.

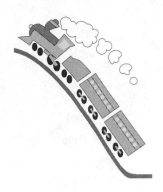

I'*ve tried so many diets and failed. How can I face weight loss again without a sense of hopelessness?*

▼
TIP:

First, work on your attitude. View your past experiences with weight loss as a wealth of information about what works for you and what doesn't. Evaluate what programs worked best for you and what in your life made you lose focus and regain weight. Make a list of things that were helpful. For example, when you exercised on the way home from work, you were more consistent, and you snacked less before dinner. Maybe a regular afternoon snack prevented you from getting too hungry and overeating at dinner.

Give yourself credit for all your "small wins." Changing your lifestyle and losing weight is not easy, and it takes a lot of time and effort. If you break your effort into smaller steps, you will set yourself up for success. For example, you set a goal to walk 30 minutes 3 times a week and decide you can do that. Give yourself credit for a small win each time you walk. If you decide to eat at least 3 servings of fruits and vegetables each day and you do it, be proud. Don't wait until you reach your goal weight to celebrate success. Each pound you lose is progress!

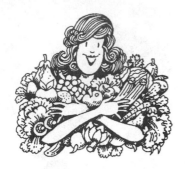

I like to eat a lot. How can I keep from feeling deprived?

▼ TIP:

If you are feeling deprived, you don't have a meal plan that can become a lifelong habit. Yours may not have enough volume of food. Other times a feeling of deprivation comes from trying to avoid favorite foods or saying "no" when others are feasting. No matter what is causing you to feel deprived, you need to develop a new way of thinking about your relationship with food and move from feeling deprived to feeling satisfied. If you need volume, focus on eating lots of low-calorie foods that are filling, such as vegetables and low-fat carbs. Salads and a broth-based soup can make you feel full and satisfied. Books that help you think about food volume as a way to feel more satisfied include *Dr. Shapiro's Picture Perfect Weight Loss: The Visual Program for Permanent Weight Loss* by Howard Shapiro and *The Volumetrics Weight Control Plan: Feel Full on Fewer Calories* by Barbara Rolls and Robert Barnett. You can plan ahead so you can eat a favorite food or meal by saving calories. Having your favorite foods is easier when you learn to appreciate small servings of them.

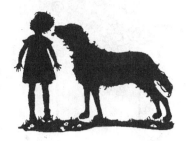

W hen I diet, I start feeling depressed. What can I do to keep from feeling this way?

▼

TIP:

Y ou need to look at what may be causing the depressed feeling. If you are feeling deprived or you are losing weight quickly but feel out of sorts and irritable, you may be eating too little. Starvation studies have shown that severely restricting the amount of food eaten can cause depression. Your body may react to a very-low-calorie weight loss diet as starvation. Increasing your calorie level by 200 or 300 calories may improve your mood. Increasing physical activity improves mood, too.

If you are not losing weight, your depressed feeling may be associated with working hard to lose weight without seeing any results of your work. Be patient and speak well of yourself and your efforts. Make this a new powerful habit for dealing with depression. No matter what the cause of your depressed mood, you may find talking to a counselor helpful. Some social workers and psychologists specialize in weight control management. Your health professional may be able to recommend one for you.

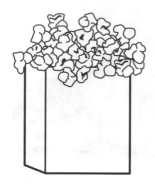

What can I do when I get the munchies?

▼
TIP:

Try a delay-and-distract strategy. Drinking a glass of water or going for a walk can keep you busy until the urge passes. Delay and distract may help with eating out of boredom. Forbidden food lists often make the food to be avoided very attractive. Eating a little serving can satisfy a craving as well as removing the temptation.

Hormones in pregnancy or PMS can trigger the munchies as can some medications or illicit drugs such as marijuana. This may occur as a craving for a specific food such as chocolate. If a medication is causing your appetite, your physician may be able to prescribe a different drug.

Food cravings are NOT your body's way of preventing nutritional deficiency. Eating a well-balanced diet and a small portion of the craved food, such as chocolate, may help control cravings that are hormonally triggered. Sometimes two foods are linked and eating one triggers a craving for the other. You can choose other foods or learn to eat one without the other. For example, if you always eat bread with butter, you can avoid both, choose a different kind of bread to enjoy without butter, or eat only a small portion.

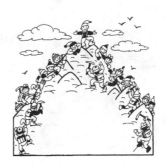

*W*hat can I do to keep motivated about eating healthfully?

▼
TIP:

*H*ere are some ideas to help you:

1. **Build your confidence that you can succeed.** You have to believe in yourself to succeed at anything you do. Talking or thinking of yourself negatively is a common pitfall. Learn from slips. Practice making positive self-statements to yourself and out loud.
2. **Build in rewards.** You need to be good to yourself. Food is not the only reward. It is easy to use high-calorie "comfort" foods to help deal with stress. Look for non-food rewards such as a new CD or a visit to a museum or park. Also, buy fresh produce, which tastes so good that it's really a treat.
3. **Think in small steps.** Set small goals that you can measure. Feel good about your accomplishments, such as going for a walk even though you were tired. Don't get discouraged by the scale. Losing 1/2 to 1 pound a week is a healthy rate of weight loss.
4. **Avoid getting too hungry.** A common pitfall is trying to go all day without food. It may be easy to skip meals during the day when you are busy, but you are at risk for a nightly food binge. Treat yourself to breakfast and lunch.

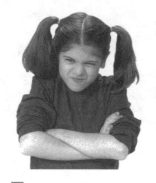

*W*hy does everybody keep nagging me when I am trying to diet? Don't they know that it makes me not even want to try to lose weight?

▼
TIP:

riends, family, and coworkers can be annoying when they provide unwanted guidance or advice. Comments such as, "You can't have that . . ." can make you feel like a child who has to get permission to eat. Even gentle reminders about your plan can make you feel resentful. You can take charge by letting people know how to change their negative support into positive support. Make a list of what you want people to do or say to help boost your motivation. For example, having a walking partner may be helpful. You may want praise for making good choices. On the other hand, you may feel you are being treated like a child. Keeping snack food out of sight may be helpful or it could make you feel left out. Some people want everybody to ignore their weight loss efforts. Only you can decide whether comments and actions are helpful or harmful. After you decide, share with friends, family, and coworkers what you want them to do to support you.

Chapter 13
INSURANCE
AND ADVOCACY

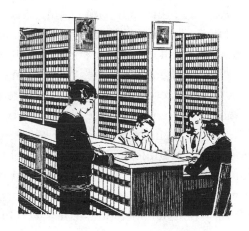

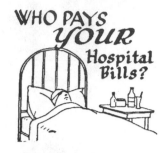

Does insurance reimburse for obesity treatment?

▼
TIP:

While reimbursement for diabetes self-management training and medical nutrition therapy in general is improving, treatment for obesity is usually not covered by third-party payers. If you have other health conditions that accompany the obesity (page 609), the chances for being reimbursed for treatment are improved. Some companies make decisions based on individual patient situations. Others have a set policy regardless of who the patient is and what their medical conditions are. Ask your insurance carriers about what coverage is available. Mention all your medical diagnoses other than obesity. For example, "My doctor has recommended I participate in this comprehensive lifestyle-change program for the treatment of my diabetes, high blood pressure, and high cholesterol." Portions of obesity treatment that are most likely eligible for coverage are physician visits and lab work. Insurance companies do not reimburse for nutritional supplements used for obesity treatment, and prescriptions are rarely covered. Coverage for the maintenance phase of a weight management program is usually not covered.

As of January 2002, medical nutrition therapy (MNT) to control diabetes is covered for patients with diabetes.

*H*ow can I become an advocate for a better environment to reduce obesity?

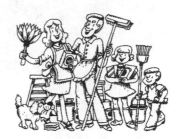

▼

TIP:

W e have an abundance of food, which is aggressively marketed in mass media. Extra-large portions of food promote high-calorie consumption. But no one gets extra portions of physical activity. We need to:

- Reduce television, video, and video game use by children.
- Lobby local schools for more fruits and vegetables and fewer high-fat foods in the cafeteria.
- Restore daily physical education classes and team sports opportunities in schools.

Changes in the community to promote physical activity may offer the most practical approach to prevent obesity. Simple changes such as improving the appearance of stairwells and adding sidewalks and bicycle trails in work, school, shopping, and residential areas will really help. Replacing automobile trips with walking or bicycling is the best way to increase physical activity in communities.

To make our communities healthier places to live we need a partnership that includes food marketers and manufacturers, public and private purchasers of health care, large employers, transportation agencies, urban planners, and real estate developers.

101 TIPS FOR AGING WELL WITH DIABETES

▲

A project of the
American Diabetes Association

▼

Written By

David B. Kelley, MD

▼

TABLE OF CONTENTS

Chapter 1
GETTING ORGANIZED

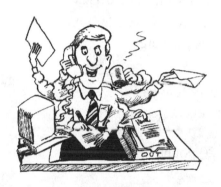

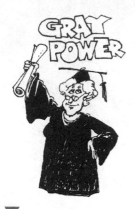

*A*s I age, how do I take care of my diabetes?

TIP:

▼

Diabetes can have a large impact on your life no matter how old you are, but with some organization and a bit of discipline to be proud of, it won't stop you from living the life you want to live. There is a plan for living with diabetes and by following it, you're on your way to a happier, longer life. The main points of this plan are:

- Acceptance and a positive attitude
- Education—at diagnosis and again every few years
- Eating in a healthy way—more fresh vegetables and fruit
- Exercising daily
- Achieving a desirable weight—even 20 pounds lighter helps
- Checking glucose levels at home
- Using medications for diabetes, if needed
- Working with health care professionals who have training in diabetes
- Getting support of family, friends, and community

Learn the skills of diabetes management. You are the expert on you. It is up to you to adapt the plan to fit your lifestyle and your needs.

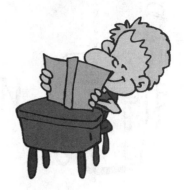

I was never good in school and that was years ago. Am I smart enough to get educated about diabetes?

▼

TIP:

Yes. It doesn't take book smarts to learn about diabetes. Here's an example. In his mid-40s, Kurt had his pancreas removed to avoid pancreatic cancer. The operation caused full-blown, insulin-dependent diabetes. Kurt also has a mental development disorder. He lives alone with supervision. His surgeons assumed that a detailed diabetes treatment plan would be too complicated and sent him home with a simpler plan. Unfortunately, the plan didn't give him enough information, and he was in blood sugar chaos.

Kurt knew his only chance for stable health was through diabetes education and fine-tuning his care plan. He rose to the challenge and has learned well. His A1C levels are great, and he seldom has low blood sugars because he heads them off before they happen. His physician ranks him at the head of the class.

It doesn't take smarts. It takes you realizing that education can help you with your diabetes. Then it takes desire, a teacher, and support from your health care provider. You can do it if you want to.

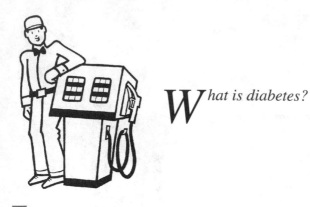

What is diabetes?

Diabetes is diagnosed when you have high levels of glucose (sugar) in your blood. Something goes wrong in getting energy from the food you eat, a process called metabolism. Food is broken down to glucose, and the glucose goes into the bloodstream to get to all the cells. Insulin, a hormone produced by your pancreas, is the key that unlocks the door to the cells.

When insulin can't do its job (type 2 diabetes), or when your pancreas can't produce insulin (type 1 diabetes), the cells can't get the glucose. You continue to eat—in fact you will feel that you are starving (your cells are)—but glucose just continues to build up in your bloodstream. Then you have high blood sugar levels all the time—diabetes.

Gestational diabetes occurs in some women only when they are pregnant. People with type 2 who lose weight and start exercising can bring their blood sugar levels back to normal, so it may appear they are healed. But their diabetes is just under very good control. Good control prevents or postpones the complications of diabetes from developing and makes you feel good every day.

W^{*hat are the differences between*}
type 1 diabetes and type 2 diabetes?

TIP:

T hey have one thing in common—high blood sugar—and treatments
are similar. People with type 1 diabetes do not make any insulin, so
they must have insulin by injection to live. Type 1 diabetes tends to
occur in younger people and comes on rather quickly. Type 1 is caused
when insulin-producing beta-cells in the pancreas are mistakenly
destroyed by the immune system.

Type 2 diabetes is the most common type of diabetes. The body
becomes resistant to its own insulin, which means it must produce more.
Over time the pancreas may just wear out, which is why it takes time to
detect type 2 diabetes—it happens gradually. People who develop it are
often quite overweight. Weight loss and exercise improve blood glucose
levels, and many people also take diabetes pills. As time passes, about
40% of people with type 2 need insulin injections to control their blood
glucose levels, especially if their blood glucose has been uncontrolled
for a long time.

Meal planning and exercise are part of the diabetes care plan for
both types of diabetes.

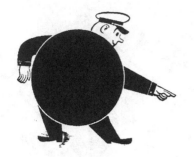

*M*y doctor told me I have borderline
diabetes. What does this mean?

▼
TIP:

It means you have diabetes. Borderline diabetes or a "touch of sugar" or any term like that means that you have diabetes—and your provider should be more up to date. If your blood glucose levels are above the cutoff point, you have diabetes. The problem is, when your blood glucose is just approaching the cutoff level, you are still at risk for the same health problems of someone who has diabetes—heart disease, nerve damage, kidney damage, and stroke.

Unfortunately, many patients and physicians don't treat borderline cases as serious, and this can lead to serious problems later on. If your blood glucose levels are close to the diabetic levels, talk to your health care practitioner about what steps to take right now to get your blood glucose nearer normal. Losing some weight—even 10 to 20 pounds— makes a considerable improvement in your blood glucose level. And exercise is the magic pill we're all looking for—try it, too. Taking action now can prevent all kinds of complications down the road.

I'm in my 70s, and I just got diabetes. How many other people my age have it?

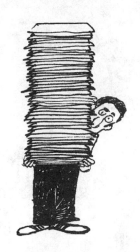

▼

TIP:

More than 16 million people in the United States have diabetes, with that number steadily increasing. The number of diabetes cases is about equal between men and women and increases with each passing decade of life. As you can see, more than 30% of people over the age of 60 have diabetes or impaired fasting glucose—meaning they have higher than normal blood glucose levels but not as high as the level for diabetes. Unfortunately, only 10 million of these people are diagnosed and under treatment, and of those 10 million, only 5 million are getting the best care!

Age	Percent of Population with Diabetes and/or Impaired Fasting Glucose
20 to 39	5%
40 to 49	13%
50 to 59	20%
60 or above	30% or more

Your ethnic background also makes a difference. African Americans and Latinos are almost twice as likely to get diabetes.

You are definitely not alone!

*W*ill I get long-term complications of diabetes?

▼

TIP:

There is no definite answer to this. Many of the complications often linked with diabetes are the same complications that come to people with advancing age, such as poor circulation or blurry vision. Others are unique to diabetes, such as retinopathy and kidney damage. Most parts of the body can be affected by high blood sugar levels over a long period of time. Too much of anything is not good, and as time passes, high blood sugar causes chemical and structural injury to delicate tissues, especially in blood vessels and nerves.

The best way to prevent complications is to keep your blood sugar under control—nearer to normal levels. Even if you already have some complications, you can slow them down and, sometimes, reverse the damage by getting your blood glucose under better control. This is your best defense against complications. Figuring out how to manage your diabetes better is an investment in time and energy that pays big dividends by making you feel better day to day and keeping you healthier over the long run.

*D*oes having diabetes mean I'm going to have a shorter life expectancy?

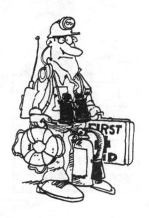

▼
TIP:

No, not necessarily. Fifty years ago, it was thought that if you had type 1 diabetes, you'd barely make middle age, and if you had mature-onset type 2, you were nearing the end. Many people have received their 50-year medals from the Eli Lilly Company, celebrating fifty years with diabetes and putting to rest the fears about life expectancy. The future is bright for people with diabetes. Technologies to help you control your blood sugar are much better, medications are better, treatments are more effective, and we know a lot more about the disease than in the past.

Still, the choice is up to you. All of the advancements in diabetes care don't mean anything if you're not committed to proper blood glucose management. If you don't take care of your diabetes, your diabetes will take care of you in ways you'd probably not prefer.

Many people live with diabetes for 40, 50, even 70 years, but it's because they stay committed to their care. How committed are you?

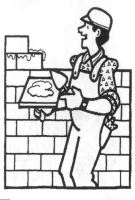

A re there target blood sugar levels for
older people?

TIP:

Y es, and you need to decide what yours are with your doctor's help.
As you age, you will probably have higher targets to guard against
hypoglycemia (extremely low blood sugar).

Here's a chart of ideal blood glucose target ranges. The blood glucose monitors and strips you use give either plasma or whole blood
results. It is important to know which result your meter gives. Plasma
results are 10–15% higher than whole blood results. These are plasma
values in milligrams per deciliter (mg/dl).

Plasma values (mg/dl)	Non-diabetes	Goal	Action suggested
Before meals	Less than 110	90–130	Less than 90 or greater than 150
After meals (1–2 hours)	Less than 140	Less than 180	Greater than 180
Bedtime	Less than 120	110–150	Less than 110 or greater than 180

*W*hat affects my blood glucose levels?

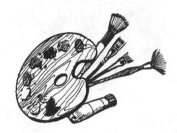

▼
TIP:

Blood glucose is never level. The ups and downs are natural and caused by several things, including:

- **Eating**. Depending on the food, glucose rises about 30 minutes after eating and will return to normal about 3 hours later. Eating large servings can raise glucose higher than you want. Lots of fat in a meal can slow the rise in blood glucose for several hours.
- **Physical activity**. Regular exercise usually lowers glucose, which makes it a valuable part of your diabetes plan. If your glucose is above 250 mg/dl and has been for some time, exercise may cause it to rise even higher.
- **Stress**. Emotional upset can cause your glucose to be high, due to a flood of stress hormones. Worrying and anxiety do it, too.
- **Illness**. Even the slightest cold can raise blood glucose.
- **Sluggish stomach function**. Sometimes food stays undigested in the stomach and is absorbed over many hours. Glucose may be up and down when you don't expect it.
- **Medications**. Some may influence blood glucose, causing it to be higher or lower than expected. Ask your doctor and pharmacist about this whenever you get a new prescription.

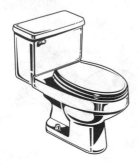

I *was recently diagnosed, and my doctor says*
I've probably had high blood sugar for years.
What are the symptoms of high blood sugar?

▼

TIP:

The symptoms of diabetes are complex, but the treachery is that with type 2 diabetes there may be no symptoms for many years. High blood sugar may cause symptoms such as poor healing of cuts and scratches, bacterial or yeast infections, fatigue, itching, or blurred vision. You may feel tired and cranky and refuse to get off the couch. This is true for people with type 1 or type 2 diabetes. Your symptoms came on gradually, so you didn't notice them.

If a person with type 1 diabetes forgets to take an insulin injection or doesn't take enough, his health suffers within hours or days. The body has to burn fat for fuel instead of the glucose it can't get. The symptoms of high blood sugar at these times are thirst, excessive urination, and weight loss. If your blood sugar level gets very high with type 2, you will probably have these symptoms, too.

If it is not treated, very high blood glucose can lead to severe problems.

M*y mother lives in an assisted living facility. Could she get problems with very high blood glucose?*

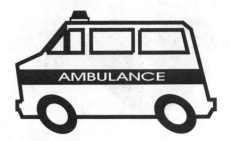

▼

TIP:

Yes. Two serious complications can happen: ketoacidosis and hyperosmolar hyperglycemia. In both conditions:

- Dehydration is caused by high glucose, because glucose spills over into urine with great "water" loss.
- Infection is the common cause. Other causes include strokes, heart attacks, injuries, alcohol abuse, stopping or reducing insulin, and medications such as cortisone.

Ketoacidosis happens to people with type 1 diabetes. Their blood glucose is usually above 250 mg/dl. Ketoacidosis usually comes on quickly, over 24 hours, so check her ketones with urine tests every 1–4 hours until her blood glucose comes back down.

Hyperosmolar hyperglycemia happens to people with type 2 over several days to weeks. Dehydration is severe. Their blood glucose is usually above 650 mg/dl, and the patient goes into a coma, which is difficult to reverse.

Make sure the staff at the nursing home know what to watch for and what to do to prevent her from developing very high blood glucose.

A m I going to have a heart attack?

▼
TIP:

Diabetes puts you at very high risk for a heart attack, so you should adopt the health practices of people who've already had one. This may prevent you from ever having one.

The things that contribute to developing diabetes, such as being overweight, inactivity, smoking, hypertension, and blood fat disorders, also put you at risk for heart disease. You can control these factors (lose weight, stop smoking, etc.) and reduce the added risk to your heart.

Because of the damage that diabetes does to nerve pathways, you may not be able to feel chest pain if you are having angina or a heart attack. Be aware of your blood pressure and pulse rate, especially when you are exercising. Be aware that your only symptoms of a heart attack may be tiredness, shortness of breath, or indigestion.

Ask your doctor about heart tests, such as a stress test or arteriogram. If you have heart problems, they can be treated.

*H*ow often should I see a diabetes
educator?

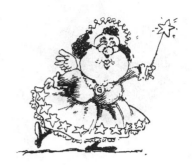

▼
TIP:

See an educator when your diabetes is discovered to learn blood glucose monitoring, how to give insulin injections, the signs and treatment of low and high blood glucose, when to take pills, and how to be
successful in lifestyle changes (such as exercise and giving up tobacco).
Follow-up visits are important, too. See an educator when you have big
lifestyle changes or problems with diabetes management. For example,
you start exercising every day and have low blood glucose too often. An
educator can help you adjust your meal plan and medication to avoid
that. Or help you adjust for other health problems, or retirement. Even if
everything is going smoothly, an educator can teach you the latest devel-
opments in diabetes care. Education can make you healthier.

Diabetes educators are key members of a diabetes treatment team.
Chances are that you can find one in your town or a larger community
nearby. Most diabetes educators are nurses or dietitians, but any health
care professional with an interest in diabetes management may become
trained as a certified diabetes educator (CDE).

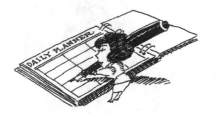

How can I organize my diabetes care, so it doesn't take so much time?

▼
TIP:

Here are some ideas for getting organized:

Get diabetes education. Know what to do, why, and what to expect.

Write things down in a daily record of blood glucose checks, food, exercise, stress, illness, or anything that affects your blood glucose. Take it with you to doctor's appointments.

Keep your glucose monitor calibrated and in working order. Use it.

Always carry everything you need for diabetes with you in a cooler, tote, or backpack.

Wear a medical ID saying you have diabetes.

Keep a list of medications, what they are for, and when you take them. Take this to your doctor's appointments.

Learn from your experiences. Observing how your blood sugar responds to activity, medication, stress, and other things, such as eating pizza or birthday cake, helps you fine-tune your treatment plan to fit you.

*S*ince I've retired, I spend a lot of time
traveling. What can I do to make sure
my diabetes is under control while I'm
away from home?

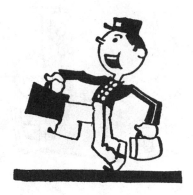

▼
TIP:

*B*e organized! Be sure you have everything you need with you. If
you're flying, make sure your medication, supplies, and extra food
are in your carry-on luggage. Bring twice the amount of medications
and supplies you think you need. Other things to bring are:

- A letter from your physician or health care provider stating that you
  have diabetes, what your insulin or medication program is, what
  medications are prescribed to you, and the contact phone numbers for
  emergencies
- A medical ID bracelet to be worn at all times
- Enough food for 24 hours
- Copies of all your prescriptions, in case you run out while you're
  traveling
- Locations and phone numbers of hospitals and pharmacies in the area
  in which you will be traveling

Keep in mind that your daily schedule will be dramatically changed
while traveling. If you're traveling through different time zones, try and
schedule your medication and eating regimen to your *home time zone*,
not the one you're flying through. Also keep in mind that you may get
more exercise than normal and be eating different foods—putting you at
risk for hypoglycemia (low blood sugar).

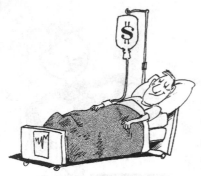

Diabetes is expensive, and I'm on a limited budget. Sometimes I just don't have the money to cover the cost. Are there resources available to help me out?

▼

TIP:

Yes, there are. If you have diabetes and you're on a fixed income, you're not alone in your struggle for good health and proper management. There are a variety of resources available to help you. To find out what resources are in your area, call the Eldercare Locator (funded by the Federal Administration on Aging) at (800)-677-1116, or talk to a certified diabetes educator (CDE) (most hospitals have them on staff). Available programs vary by area, but you might find:

- Special transportation arrangements to take you to your doctor
- Volunteers who will stop by and see that everything's all right
- Organizations that serve low-cost meals or deliver meals to your home
- Free diabetes education classes and support groups
- Information on special equipment that might help your needs

You may also contact your insurance company or Medicare office to see what diabetes services they cover.

*I*s the future of diabetes care bright?

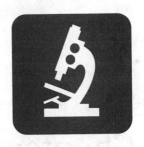

▼
TIP:

Each year brings new therapies for diabetes. The future holds great promise with new products that will make diabetes management simpler and more effective for you. Successful islet-cell transplants are now being done. New oral medications are being developed almost yearly. Exciting progress is being made in non-injection insulin delivery systems (nasal spray, inhalers, and capsules). The GlucoWatch, which checks glucose without requiring a drop of blood, is brand new. You still need to use a regular glucose monitor to check the accuracy of the GlucoWatch, but now we have laser lancets, which are nearly painless, and the ability to take a blood sample from a forearm, which is also not painful. Dietitians are updating nutrition recommendations to make them healthy for everyone and less difficult to follow. There is research being done on how to prevent diabetes, map chromosomes (genes) and predict future health conditions, and manipulate genes to avoid or alter health conditions. The future is very bright indeed. More and more help is on the way.

Chapter 2
MIGHTY MEDICATIONS

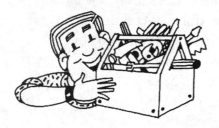

*H*ow do pills for diabetes work?

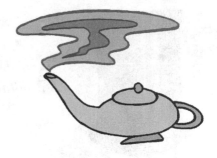

▼
TIP:

There are several types of pills for blood glucose control in people with type 2 diabetes. They include:

■ Pills that stimulate the pancreas to release insulin: sulfonylureas (such as glyburide and glipizide) and meglitinides (repaglinide [Prandin]). These medications may cause low blood glucose.

■ Pills that help body cells take in glucose: thiazolidinediones (rosiglitazone and pioglitazone) and biguanides (metformin). These do not cause low blood glucose if used alone.

■ Pills that block absorption of carbohydrate from the intestines: alpha-glucosidase inhibitors (such as acarbose and miglitol). These do not cause low blood glucose if used alone. Uncomfortable side effects, such as gasiness, limit the popularity of these medications.

Other types of medications are under study. Discuss your choices carefully with your health care provider, considering the cost, the number of times per day you have to take it, and side effects. Some people need to take more than one diabetes pill to control their blood glucose, and others need to move on to insulin for better control.

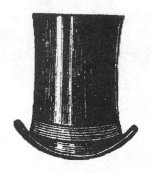

*A*re there advantages to taking one diabetes pill rather than another?

TIP:

Which pill you take depends on what is causing your high blood glucose. If you need to produce more insulin, sulfonylureas and meglitinides help. Sulfonylureas have been around longest and work well, but can cause hypoglycemia and weight gain. You can't use them if you're allergic to sulfa drugs or have kidney problems. Meglitinides (Prandin) are taken before meals, so if you don't eat, you don't take it, which is handy. It's okay with kidney problems, but weight gain is possible.

Two pills increase how much glucose gets into your cells: thiazolidinediones ('glitazones) and biguanides (metformin). You take glitazones only once a day, and they lower triglyceride levels. But they cause weight gain. Metformin does not cause weight gain or low blood glucose and improves blood fats. Side effects, however, are nausea and diarrhea, and you can't take it with kidney, heart, or liver problems, or if you drink alcohol excessively.

Alpha-glucosidase inhibitors block absorption of carbohydrate in your intestines, keeping glucose lower after a meal. There's no weight gain, but gas, bloating, and diarrhea are side effects. Talk with your doctor to decide which pill will work best for you.

Why aren't my new diabetes pills lowering my blood glucose?

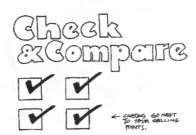

CHECKS GO NEXT
TO YOUR SELLING
POINTS.

▼

TIP:

Time is required for any new medication to start working. The time varies for the different types of pills used to treat diabetes:

■ Pills that stimulate the release of insulin from the pancreas, including sulfonylureas and meglitinides, will reach full effect in one week.

■ Pills that block absorption of carbohydrate from the intestinal tract work immediately and are used with each meal.

■ Pills that improve the efficiency of insulin action, "insulin sensitizers," include biguanides and thiazolidinediones. Metformin (currently the only approved biguanide) reaches full effect in one week. Thiazolidinediones do not start working for approximately three weeks and may not reach full effect for ten to twelve weeks. Watch for their effect to show up on your blood glucose checks at home.

Did your doctor prescribe a thiazolidinedione (insulin sensitizer)? Take these facts into consideration when starting a new diabetes medication or when considering a change in the dose of your medication.

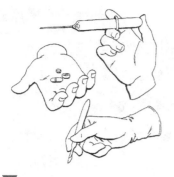

*I*t's becoming harder to control my diabetes with pills. What are the advantages and disadvantages of my taking insulin now?

▼
TIP:

Insulin does the same thing that your body's insulin does—helps you get energy from the food you eat and thrive. As you age with type 2, the chances are you will probably need to start insulin therapy at some point. When you start is often your choice. Here are some advantages and disadvantages to using insulin:

Advantages:
  Much better blood glucose control
  More flexibility in diabetes management. For example, you can make an on-the-spot increase in insulin dose to cover a large birthday meal, or be able to delay a meal
  The types of insulin have different time-action patterns. Some start to work rapidly and are gone in two hours. Some act gradually over 24 hours. Pills are not so easy to adjust

Disadvantages:
  Possibility of too low blood glucose (hypoglycemia)
  Weight gain from improved control
  Need for injections
  Reluctance from you or your physician

I recently had pneumonia, and my doctor put me on insulin. Will I have to stay on insulin forever?

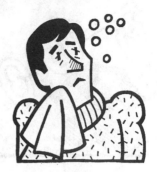

▼
TIP:

No, probably not. When you're ill, your body's under a lot of stress, and this can cause your blood sugar to go a little crazy. Insulin is the best way to get things back under control. However, once you're back up to speed, you can probably return to your regular management plan.

Temporary insulin therapy may also be used when type 2 diabetes is first diagnosed, to overcome very high glucose. Once the glucose is under control, oral medication will usually do the trick.

Some people use rapid-acting insulin occasionally when they're eating a large meal, for example, at the holidays. The insulin covers the extra carbohydrate in the meal and brings their blood sugar back to normal levels after the meal.

And now for the "probably not" part. As you age, oral medications might not control your blood glucose as well as they should. To get good control and stay healthy, you might have to start using insulin. If you're to this level, you'll have to keep using insulin from then on.

My doctor suggested I start using insulin. Will I be able to handle this regimen at my age?

▼
TIP:

You may feel scared or overwhelmed, but the mechanics of drawing the insulin dose and giving an injection are simple to do. It's learning to think like a pancreas that is the challenge. If you already have a good management plan consisting of a meal plan, exercise, and oral medications, you have experience that will help you use insulin. You will need to check your blood glucose levels more often because now they can drop too low—and you don't want that to happen. You'll need to carry snacks or glucose tablets with you at all times to bring low blood sugar back up.

Along with your regular oral medications you will probably start with a bedtime injection of intermediate- or long-acting insulin, such as glargine, to restore normal morning glucose so your oral medications will work better during the day. If blood glucose control worsens, you'll probably move on to several insulin injections a day. No one likes injections, but they keep you healthier. Once you face your fear and get some practice, you'll be amazed at how well you do.

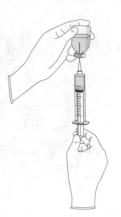

I *can't see well. How can I measure my insulin dose?*

▼
TIP:

S everal devices are available to help you draw up and measure insulin when you can't see.

■ Syringe magnifiers are magnifying glasses that attach to the insulin syringe, making the numbers larger.

■ There are several non-visual insulin measurement aides. These devices hold the syringe and the insulin bottle. A predetermined "stop" on the device halts the insulin syringe plunger at a given dose. Or, a slide moves the syringe plunger with a "click" sound that indicates each unit of insulin drawn into the syringe.

■ Needle guides hold syringe and insulin bottle in place for syringe filling or have a funnel shape that fits over the insulin bottle and directs the syringe needle tip to the insulin bottle stopper.

■ Insulin pens have an insulin reservoir, a double-ended needle (one end in the insulin reservoir, the other for you), and a dose-dialing mechanism. You can set the dose visually or by counting off the clicks. Two styles of such pens are available—disposable and refillable.

Ask your diabetes educator or occupational therapist for suggestions and help learning how to use them.

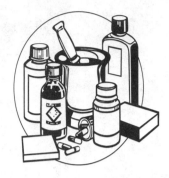

I take a lot of non-diabetes medications. Can any of these affect my blood glucose?

▼

TIP:

If you take a sulfonylurea or meglitinide, your glucose may go too low if you are also taking:

- Nonsteroidal anti-inflammatory medications, such as aspirin or ibuprofen
- Sulfa drugs and certain antibiotics
- Monoamine oxidase inhibitors (MAOs) (for depression)
- Beta-blockers (for heart problems or high blood pressure)

Anyone's blood glucose may be made higher by:

- Cold remedies, such as ephedrine or pseudoephedrine
- Phenothiazines (for nausea and anxiety)
- Phenytoin (for peripheral neuropathy or seizures)
- Diuretics (to remove fluid from the body)
- Corticosteroids, such as cortisone or prednisone
- Thyroid medications
- Estrogen medications
- Calcium-channel blockers
- Nicotinic acid (for abnormal blood fats)

Ask your doctor or pharmacist how your medications will affect your blood glucose and be alert to your own reactions to a new drug.

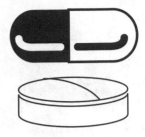

I'm retired and on a tight budget. Can I cut my
diabetes pills in half?

▼
TIP:

If you're a thrifty medical consumer, you've probably thought of
buying pills containing larger doses of medication, and then just using
the portion you need, so you can save money on prescription prices.
However, there are some things you should know.

If you just break the pill, the pieces may not contain the same
amount of medication and may not work the same way. Pills that are
"scored"—meaning they have a line cut into them—and that *do not* have
a special coating may be broken along the line, and both halves will
have the same amount of medication. However, a shiny tablet without a
line in it or a capsule might not work correctly if you break it in two.
The coating on the pill may be necessary to control how fast or where
the pill is absorbed in your body.

Leave shiny, un-scored pills as they are, unless you ask your pharmacist if it is okay to break the pills into pieces.

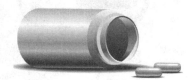

I've heard that taking an aspirin everyday
is recommended for seniors. Is this true if
I have diabetes?

▼
TIP:

Probably. As the years go by, everyone runs a higher risk of heart
attack, stroke, and poor circulation, whether they have diabetes or
not. This higher risk is caused by atherosclerosis, or hardening of the
arteries. This condition is made even worse by thromboxane, a chemical
in your blood. Aspirin helps by blocking the production of thromboxane.
So, aspirin is especially helpful for you with diabetes because you have
an even higher risk for heart attack and stroke.

As you and your physician decide whether you should take a daily
aspirin, consider the following:

■ The low dose treatment is 81–325 mg of enteric-coated aspirin per
day. This is lower than the amount you take for aches and pains, but it
gives you the benefits without many of the side effects.

■ People with aspirin allergy, bleeding tendencies, recent bleeding in
the stomach or intestinal tract, anticoagulant therapy, and liver troubles should not use aspirin.

■ Low-dose aspirin will not trigger or irritate diabetes-related eye problems.

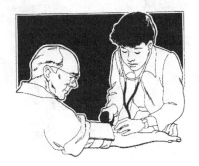

I've developed high blood pressure. What types of pills are available to control it, and how will they affect my diabetes?

▼
TIP:

There are five types of blood pressure medication. They may be started in any order and added if one or more do not get the job done. Each has advantages and disadvantages:

Thiazide diuretics are also useful in controlling fluid retention. Side effects include blood fat (lipid) abnormalities, mild elevation in blood glucose, possible low potassium, and elevation in uric acid (linked to gout).

Beta-blockers are also beneficial in reducing recurring heart problems after a heart attack. Side effects include lipid abnormalities, masking of the symptoms of low blood glucose, cool hands and feet, and making asthma worse.

Angiotensin-converting enzyme (ACE) inhibitors are also proven to reduce or protect against diabetes-related kidney problems. Side effects include raising potassium levels and reducing kidney function. Cough may be a side effect (a newer medication is less likely to cause cough).

Calcium antagonists do not affect lipids or blood glucose. Side effects include fluid retention (swelling of the feet) and constipation.

Alpha-1-receptor blockers benefit lipid levels and improve insulin sensitivity. A possible serious side effect is low blood pressure when standing, causing dizziness.

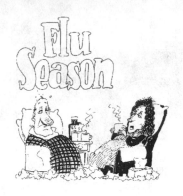

D^{o I need flu and pneumonia shots?}

▼

TIP:

W hether to have influenza and pneumonia immunizations is a
personal decision. However, people over the age of 64 will
usually benefit from the protection conferred by these injections. If flu
or pneumonia are "in the air," immunizations will prevent the illnesses
or make them less severe.

Getting a flu shot is strongly recommended in September of each
year. The vaccine should not be used if you are allergic to chicken eggs
(the vaccine is prepared in a chicken egg environment) or to other components of the vaccine, or in people with a past history of Guillain-Barré
syndrome (a rare nerve disorder occasionally linked to immunizations).

The pneumonia vaccine protects against a relatively common type—
pneumococcal pneumonia. A one-time dose of vaccine is recommended
for people over the age of 64. If you got a dose before age 65, a one-time
re-vaccination is recommended. Almost half of the people receiving this
injection will have flu-like side effects lasting up to two days.

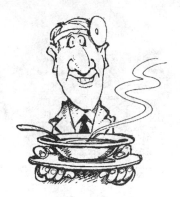

*A*re there vitamins or minerals I should be taking to help with the aging process?

▼
TIP:

If you follow a meal plan with fresh vegetables, fruit, lean meats and fish, eggs, and whole grains, there's no need for supplemental vitamins. You also need healthy fats like olive oil in your diet. Most people don't eat this well, however. Talk with your doctor or dietitian about taking vitamins or using herbal supplements. Be honest because these can interact with your other medications. Some herbs, like Siberian ginseng, have had years of research done on their benefits for older people, but most have not.

You may need a calcium supplement to keep bones strong. There are also special situations where you may need supplements:

- If you are being fed through an IV tube, you may need chromium.
- Magnesium deficiency can cause insulin resistance, high blood pressure, and high blood glucose, but deficiency is not common. Unless you have low blood levels of magnesium, don't worry about a supplement.
- If you are taking diuretics, you might need potassium. But, you may need to restrict it if it is too high from kidney problems or from taking ACE inhibitors for high blood pressure.

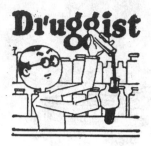

Druggist

I take so many medications that it's hard for me to keep them straight. What can I do?

▼

TIP:

Organize your medications to avoid mixing medicines, taking the wrong medications, or not taking the medicine at all. Try these tips:

Get a plastic pill organizer with as many sections as you need to keep track of what you're taking and when you're taking it. Refill it at the same time each week.

Keep an updated list of all your medications with you at all times.

Tell your doctor every medication you take (including herbs, vitamins, and over-the-counter medications).

Try to have all your prescriptions filled at the same pharmacy.

Make sure you understand the instructions and dosages. If you can't read the label, have someone read it for you.

Mark off each medication as you take it on a calendar.

Label the caps of your pills with big letters, so you can see which is which. For example, a big, yellow "BP" for blood pressure pills.

Put bright stickers or tape on each bottle, so you can tell them apart.

Be aware that some diabetes pills look like artificial sweeteners—don't confuse them. One woman put three in her husband's oatmeal, causing very low blood sugar!

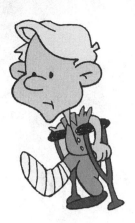

I've recently had my toe amputated and doing
day-to-day activities is a big challenge. What
can I do?

▼
TIP:

Ask your doctor for a referral to an occupational therapist. In fact,
anyone who has trouble with daily activities for any reason
whatsoever (such as arthritis or poor vision), probably should see an occupational therapist for help. Don't let the name fool you. An occupational
therapist isn't someone who just helps you with challenges at your job.
The therapist provides you with physical therapy to increase your
strength and mobility and training— often in your home—in better ways
to deal with a variety of physical ailments. He or she can show you the
nifty inventions that can help you and how to use them. If you've had an
amputation, you'll need to learn to do things differently and safely to
prevent further injury to that leg and to the rest of you, too! You may
need to learn to use a cane or a wheelchair, or need grab bars to get onto
the toilet, and into and out of the bathtub. The therapist can do a survey
of your home and suggest adjustments that will make things easier for
you.

Chapter 3
FOOD, GLORIOUS FOOD

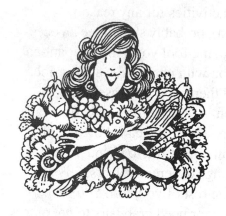

*H*ow can I eat healthy?

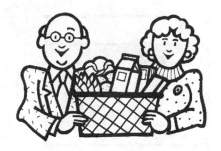

▼
TIP:

Ask your doctor to refer you to a registered dietitian (RD) who can design a meal plan for your food likes and dislikes and your cooking ability. Try these tips:

- Eat more fresh (or frozen) vegetables and fruit daily.
- Eat more greens, like romaine, watercress, spinach, and arugula every day.
- Drink 6–8 glasses of water a day.
- Eat breakfast (try oatmeal).
- Eat an egg. It's a perfect food.
- Use olive oil to cook and add nuts to your oatmeal—for healthy fat.
- Stop eating processed foods. (Read the ingredients—partially hydrogenated oil is an unhealthy fat).
- Measure your servings with a measuring cup or food scale.
- Try 5 or 6 small meals a day.
- Use herbs and spices instead of salt and fat.
- Buy a healthy cookbook.
- Stop smoking to improve your sense of taste and smell.
- Think about the energy the food brings you and what you intend to do with the energy. Participate in the dance of life.

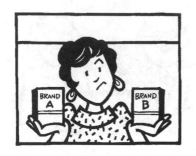

*W*hy would I learn to "count carbs"?

▼
TIP:

It is the carbohydrate in food that raises your blood glucose. If you count how much carbohydrate (carb) is in your meal, you'll know how much to eat. Carbohydrate is in grains, beans, fruits, milk, and sweets. You can look up how much carbohydrate is in a serving of food on food labels and in "carb count" books. Make sure the serving you eat is the same size as the one on the label or in the book. Add up the carb in your meal and write it in your record. Check your blood glucose two hours later and record that, too. After a week or two you'll see how high certain amounts of carb raise your blood sugar. If you try to eat about the same amount of carb at the same times each day, you may get better diabetes control.

Carb raises blood glucose. Exercise and diabetes medication lower it. If you exercise after eating, record that. If you are going to eat more carb than usual—at a birthday party for example—then you know you need to take a walk afterwards or adjust your diabetes medication to bring the blood glucose level back down. You can adjust insulin to the carb you eat and some of the diabetes pills. Ask your doctor or diabetes educator for help with this.

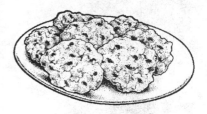

*F*or years I've heard that people with diabetes can't eat sugar. Is this true?

▼
TIP:

No, it's not true. Twenty years of research have shown that sugar is just another carbohydrate. As far as your blood glucose is concerned, a brownie and a baked potato have about the same effect.

It is the carbohydrate in foods that raises blood glucose. Carbohydrate—whether in grains, beans, fruit, milk, or sweets—turns into glucose and is used for fuel. So, carbohydrates like potatoes and bread raise blood glucose the same way that table sugar (another carbohydrate) does. Don't focus on the sugar; focus on the total amount of carbohydrate in the meal.

Table sugar is considered a "bad guy" because it gives you calories but no vitamins or minerals—these are empty calories. If you want a natural sugar that is packaged with vitamins and minerals, you can choose a piece of fresh fruit! But if you want to eat dessert, go ahead and try just 2 or 3 bites. You can trade the carb in the bites of brownie for a piece of bread or serving of rice in your meal plan.

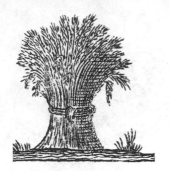

*W*hy should I eat more fiber?

Fiber makes your body work better. It improves your digestion and prevents constipation. It is found in whole grains, beans, fruits, and vegetables. It's on the food label, too. Try to eat 20–35 grams of fiber a day. There are two types of fiber:

- Insoluble fiber is in whole-grain cereals and breads. It grabs onto liquid as it travels your gastrointestinal tract. That's good because the combination of fiber and liquid pushes food through more quickly. Insoluble fiber promotes a bulkier and softer bowel movement and gives you other health benefits—preventing hemorrhoids, diverticulosis, and colon and rectal cancer.
- Soluble fiber is in beans, peas, oats, and barley. It can prevent your body from absorbing cholesterol and glucose. But to lower your blood cholesterol or glucose with it, you would have to eat a very large amount.

If you count carbs and there are more than 5 grams of fiber in the serving you eat, subtract the number of grams of fiber from the grams of total carbohydrate. Use that number for the carb count in the food. The carb from fiber will not raise your blood glucose.

*W*hy do I have to drink 6–8 glasses of water a day?

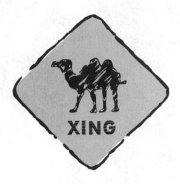

XING

▼
TIP:

Water is vital to every process and system in your body. It keeps you healthy. When blood sugars run high, you're at risk of getting dehydrated because your body tries to flush out the extra glucose in your blood through urination. The flushed-out fluids need to be replaced. If they're not, you get sick.

Be sure to drink water throughout the day. Why not get a measuring cup and check the amount of water that your favorite drinking glass or water bottle will hold? You can make this the week you add more water to your routine.

Coffee and tea with caffeine and carbonated sodas are diuretics and can remove water from your system. Drinking plain water is the best way to get the fluid you need.

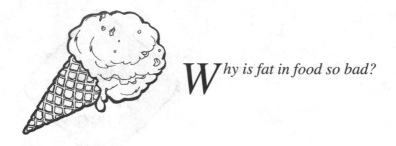

*W*hy is fat in food so bad?

▼
TIP:

Fats are not the root of all evil. In fact, fats

- Help your body and brain work
- Transport essential vitamins (A, D, and E)
- Make skin and hair look healthy
- Reduce hunger feelings
- Make food taste good

It's just that too much of a good thing is bad. Excessive amounts of fat in your diet are linked to a variety of health issues. This is especially true as you age. Excessive amounts of fat in your bloodstream can stick to your arteries, causing them to become smaller. When you have diabetes, these fats become stickier and cause even more buildup. As you age, you get more and more buildup, narrowing your arteries, too. When the space inside your arteries shrinks, you develop high blood pressure (hypertension), and a higher risk for heart attack and stroke.

When you eat wisely, choosing healthier fats such as olive oil instead of butter or margarine (or even dark chocolate instead of milk chocolate), and cut some processed or fried foods out of your meal plan, you're seriously reducing the risks to your health.

*H*ow much fat should I have in my diet?

▼
TIP:

Y ou need a little fat every day—but only a little because fat has so many calories. One gram of fat has 9 calories. If you read food labels, you'll see the calories from fat add up quickly. Fat should only make up about 30% of the total calories you eat in a day (if you eat 2,000 calories a day, then 600 of those can come from fat).

There are actually three types of fat in the food you eat—monounsaturated, polyunsaturated, and saturated fats. The healthiest are monounsaturated, found in olive oil and nuts. Polyunsaturated are the next healthiest (found in canola and corn oils). Saturated fats in meat and dairy products are the least healthy.

If your blood fat levels are too high, you may need to eat different amounts of the fats, and you might need prescription medication. If you need to lose weight, pay attention to how much fat you eat because fat has more calories than protein or carbohydrate. Get the help of an RD who can help you make a meal plan with healthy amounts of the three kinds of fat.

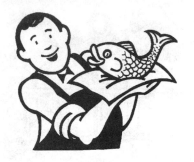

I'm confused about fats. Which ones can I eat?

▼
TIP:

The healthiest fats are found in olives, olive oil, and canola oil. The fats in nuts, seeds, and avocados help protect your heart and improve your health. Butter is okay in small amounts for taste! Eat whole grains and legumes like soy.

Probably the worst fat is trans fat. It is in most processed foods, such as crackers and cookies. Look for it on the list of ingredients as partially hydrogenated oil. Liquid oil is treated with hydrogen to make it solid at room temperature. Hydrogenation makes a liquid fat—which is usually healthier—into a saturated fat, which takes away the health benefit, as with margarine. Foods that are fried in most restaurants also have trans fats, which is why you choose a baked potato instead of French fries. If you want fries, fry them at home and discard the oil afterward or make oven-fried potatoes with less oil.

Research is showing that eliminating trans fats from your diet dramatically improves your health by lowering your risk of cancer and heart disease.

Chapter 4
EVERY BODY IS BEAUTIFUL

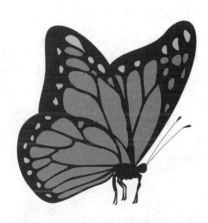

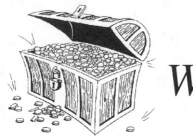

*W*hat does exercise do for me?

▼
TIP:

The benefits of exercise are many, and they include:

Strong muscles
More energy
One-pound weight loss for every 3,500 calories burned
Improved mobility and range of joint motion
Enhanced quality of life and independence
A better mental attitude and self-image
Improved blood glucose control
Reduced chance of heart attacks and strokes
Improved cholesterol and lipids
Improved blood pressure
Improved blood flow (reduced chances of conditions such as phlebitis)
Improved appetite
Improved enjoyment of sex
Improved ability to play with your grandchildren
Respect from your children

Exercise keeps you young and healthy. Are there any good reasons not to exercise?

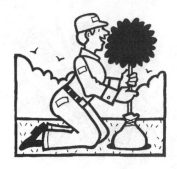

I'm not the young pup I used to be. What kinds of exercise are best for me?

▼

TIP:

The best exercise is one you will do regularly. Aerobic exercise (exercise that raises the heart rate and feels like work) is best, but just about any physical activity is a step in the right direction.

There are three basic approaches to exercise and all are beneficial:

- **Lifestyle approach.** Stand rather than sit. Take the stairs. Lift everyday weights (groceries, bottles of water, bags of flour). Garden. Bend and stretch.
- **Non-competitive activity.** Compete against the clock rather than other athletes. Organize a walking group. Take a yoga class. Lift weights. Swim. Bicycle.
- **Competitive sports.** Just that. Everything from golf to running a marathon.

Exercise regularly, three to four times a week. Aerobic sessions can be 20–60 minutes, but start with 5 minutes if you've never exercised. Mix up your workouts with yoga twice a week and lift light weights once or twice a week, too. Ease your way into it. The benefits are many. For example, yoga increases your flexibility, strength, coordination, and balance, and it reduces stress. It can lower blood glucose levels, too.

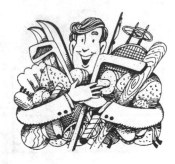

*W*hy *do I need to burn more calories?*

TIP:

B urning calories is how you lose weight. You lose one pound for every 3,500 calories you burn and don't replace with more calories. The table shows the calories burned by a 150-pound person doing 30 minutes of each of the activities.

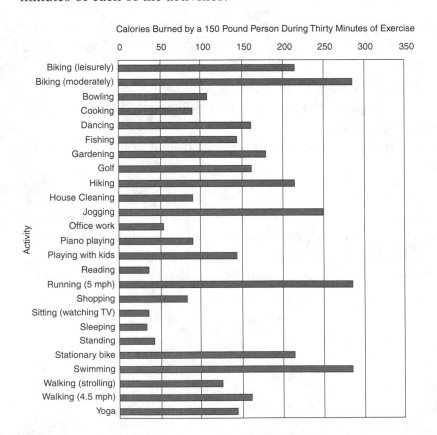

Calories Burned by a 150 Pound Person During Thirty Minutes of Exercise

This year I'll be celebrating my 75th birthday. Am I too old to exercise?

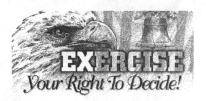

EXERCISE
Your Right To Decide!

▼

TIP:

The answer to that question is always going to be "no." You're never too old to exercise. The benefits you receive with regular exercise are always there. Start walking, swimming, gardening, or doing something you enjoy now, and you'll benefit every system in your body and reduce all your health risks. You won't get frail, and you won't have to depend on others to do things for you. Now that's a birthday present!

Recent studies have shown that strength training in 90-year-olds produces muscle mass just as it does in 20-year-olds. Now, this doesn't mean you'll be winning any bodybuilding competitions—even though we know of an 83-year-old lady who is—but it does mean that you can get benefits from strength training no matter how old you are. Weight lifting—even 1-lb weights—increases muscle and bone, which keeps you stronger and gives you endurance. And muscle burns calories even at rest—keeping weight and blood glucose levels in control.

So grumble if you will, but do it. Strong muscles mean improved health, well-being, and longevity.

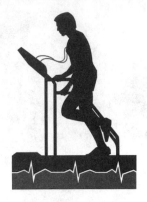

*H*ow do I know that I'm healthy enough to exercise?

TIP:

Before starting an exercise program, you should have a health evaluation, especially if you

- Are over 35 years old
- Have had type 2 diabetes for more than 10 years or type 1 diabetes for more than 15 years
- Have diabetes-related eye or kidney problems (retinopathy or nephropathy)
- Have poor circulation in your legs
- Have neuropathy preventing an increase in heart rate with exercise
- Have high blood pressure
- Smoke

Your doctor can help you determine whether you have any conditions that would limit the way you exercise. If you have eye problems, don't do jumping or jarring exercise or lift heavy weights. If you have lost feeling in your feet, be careful not to injure your feet, and you may find swimming preferable to jogging. An exercise tolerance test is important if you have heart disease.

Exercise will improve your diabetes control, your blood pressure, and your circulation.

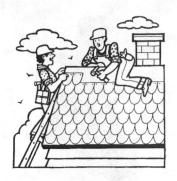

I *take insulin. Do I need to take special precautions when I exercise?*

▼

TIP:

If you take insulin, sulfonylureas, or a meglitinide, you need to watch that your blood sugar does not drop too low during and for hours after exercise. If the exercise is unusual, vigorous, or long-lasting, you may need to check your blood sugar during it and after. Have plenty of snacks to eat. In general:

- If your glucose levels are below 100 mg/dl, you need to eat 15–30 grams of carbohydrate.
- Always have carbohydrate food close at hand. You can carry glucose gel or tablets, peanut butter crackers, or a bike bottle filled with fruit juice.
- You may be surprised by lower than usual blood glucose levels during the night or the next day! You need to adjust your diabetes treatment for this.
- Avoid exercise if your blood glucose level is above 240 mg/dl and ketones are present in your urine, or if blood glucose is above 300 mg/dl without ketones in the urine. Under these conditions, exercise may actually raise your blood glucose.

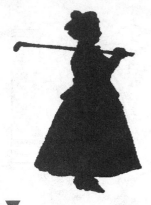

I've had type 2 diabetes for 20 years and want to start exercising. What do I need to know?

TIP:

S tart slowly with walking or a yoga or tai chi class. Begin like this:

Before any physical activity, warm up your bones, joints, and muscles for 5–10 minutes, by swinging your arms and marching, for example.

After you are warmed-up, gently stretch for another 5–10 minutes. Never stretch cold muscles. Don't bounce.

After exercise, spend 5–10 minutes cooling down—moving slower and slower. Try some yoga stretches.

You need to move quickly enough to get your heart and lungs working.

Protect your feet. Wear good walking or running shoes with cushioned innersoles that fit well. Wear socks made of a fabric that keeps your feet dry.

Inspect your feet regularly for blisters or injury.

Drink water before, during, and after exercise.

Lift some light weights. Even 1-lb cans of soup can build muscle—and muscle burns calories even when you are at rest! Don't carry weights while you're walking because that can damage your wrist, elbow, and shoulder joints. Never wear ankle weights while walking! Keep your knees slightly bent, not locked.

I *have arthritis and neuropathy in*
my feet and legs. How can I
exercise?

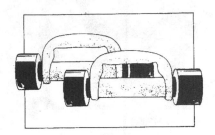

▼
TIP:

Where there's a will, there's a way. Swimming is good, but you need weight-bearing exercise to protect your bones. You might try yoga or tai chi for no-impact exercise. You can lift weights and do yoga stretches sitting in a chair or on the floor. Wave two long scarves up, down, and around while listening to music to increase the range of motion in your arms and shoulders and get your heart rate going. Write the alphabet in the air with your pointed toes. There are exercise books and videotapes especially for people who have to exercise sitting down. If you start looking for ways to accomplish your goal, you will find them.

If you have other complications, such as retinopathy or high blood pressure, don't lift heavy weights or bend way over with your head hanging down.

After exercise, massage your knees with peanut or olive oil. Arnica oil (found at health food stores) is good for muscle and bone aches, too. Make sure you are getting enough calcium and magnesium in meals or supplements. Be sure to check your feet for redness, bruises, or blisters every time you exercise.

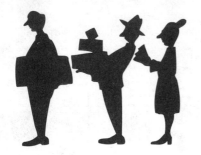

F rom middle age on, what is a realistic weight goal?

▼

TIP:

This is a hard question to answer because no two bodies are built exactly the same. Your body type is strongly influenced by the genes passed down from your folks, and if you have a large body type, you're always going to be bigger. Just because you weigh more or less than other people your same height, does not mean that you're over- or underweight. People are just built differently.

Don't take models or movie stars as a proper gauge. The average woman in the United States is 5'4" and weighs 152 pounds. The best way to gauge your ideal weight is to recall what you weighed at age 18–20 and add another 20 pounds "for the years." This, of course, is not completely accurate, since what you weighed at age 19 may not have been an ideal weight (especially now, as obesity among young people rises) and 20 extra pounds might be a little generous on a small body frame. But this is a pretty good working number.

To be more accurate about your ideal weight, talk with your physician. For most people, losing 20 pounds will improve their blood glucose numbers.

*D*oes diabetes have an impact on
osteoporosis in men and women?

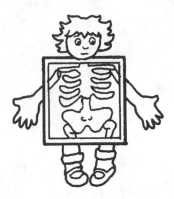

▼
TIP:

People with diabetes tend to have a higher rate of osteoporosis, so
taking steps to prevent it would be worth your while. Osteoporosis is
a loss of bone mass causing the bones to weaken and eventually break.
Osteoporosis is caused by many things, including

- Not doing enough weight-bearing exercise
- Not getting enough calcium (1,000–1,500 mg) and vitamin D (800 IU) daily
- Reduced levels of estrogen or testosterone, as happens later in life
- An overactive thyroid
- Using certain medications such as cortisone
- Smoking
- Drinking too much alcohol

There are medical tests to measure bone mass and see whether you
have osteoporosis. You may want to include more calcium in your meal
plan or take a supplement. You can lift light weights and benefit your
bones. Walking is good. Women's bones may be helped by estrogen
therapy at menopause, and men's by testosterone therapy.

Chapter 5
WHAT'S COMMON, WHAT'S NOT

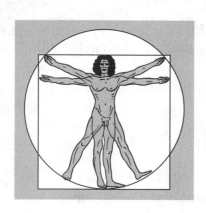

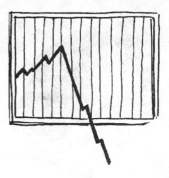

*H*ow do I recognize low blood glucose,
   and how do I treat it?

▼
TIP:

When glucose drops below 60–70 mg/dl, you will probably have symptoms, such as anxiety, sweating, headache, hunger, numbness, heart pounding, shakiness, or weakness. Learn what your symptoms are.

You must eat or drink carbohydrate as soon as you get the warning signs! If you ignore them, your glucose may fall below 30–40 mg/dl, and you may fall into a coma. To treat low blood glucose:

- Eat or drink food or liquid containing 15 grams of carbohydrate. Examples are 4 oz fruit juice or regular (not diet) soft drink, 3 graham crackers, 4 teaspoons sugar, or 1 tablespoon honey.
- Wait 15–20 minutes and check your blood glucose. If it's still below 70 mg/dl, eat 15 grams of carb and check it again in 15–20 minutes.
- Repeat until your blood glucose is above 70 mg/dl.
- If the next meal is more than an hour away, eat some cheese and crackers or half a meat sandwich (protein and carb) to keep your glucose level up.
- Do not eat or drink too much carbohydrate. You don't want your glucose level to go too high.

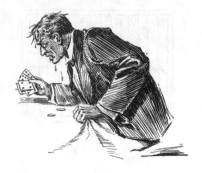

Is hypoglycemia (low blood sugar) more dangerous in seniors?

▼
TIP:

Yes, severely low blood sugar can cause you to pass out and fall down. For 12-year-olds, that's not too bad. When their blood sugar rises, they hop up and move on. For you, however, falling down can break bones. The danger of breaking a hip or leg is much greater as we age. And the injury may not heal properly. There is also danger with passing out when you're driving a car, mowing the lawn, or operating any kind of machinery.

If you're older, hypoglycemia can also cause a stroke. You want to do whatever you can to avoid hypoglycemia. Check your blood sugar, don't guess what it is. Eat on schedule, and if you get exercise, eat a snack. Keep a carbohydrate food, such as a juice box, with you all the time. You might want to keep your blood sugar level slightly higher than the suggested levels for younger people. Talk with your doctor about the best target levels for you and about how to adjust your diabetes care plan to reach them.

*D*oes my risk for complications
increase with age?

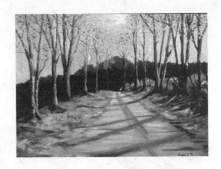

▼
TIP:

The longer that you have high blood glucose levels, the higher your risk for developing complications from diabetes. In some ways, that means it doesn't matter how old you are or even how long you've had diabetes. What does matter is how long your diabetes has been out of control and how far out of control it has been. A 50-year-old man who has let his blood glucose run high for 10 years may be at a greater risk for diabetes-related complications than an 80-year-old woman who has controlled her glucose well for more than 30 years. As a rule, however, the older you get, the more at risk you are for developing complications.

The good news is that the better you control your blood glucose, the smaller your risks for serious complications. Every bit of improvement in blood glucose control will yield benefits in long-term health and well being. It's worth the time and the effort to do it!

My vision fluctuates between blurry and clear. My eyesight hasn't been good for a long time, but it's never done this. Is this retinopathy?

▼
TIP:

If your vision improves on its own, it's not permanent damage or retinopathy. This does indicate, however, that your diabetes is out of control. The changes in your vision are due to wild swings in blood glucose, which then trigger ebb and flow of fluid in the eyes. When the level of glucose in your blood increases, the body requires more fluid to maintain a healthy balance elsewhere. Some fluid can come from your eyes, which will affect the function and structure of the eye. Blurred vision results.

The cure? Focus on diabetes control. Postpone an eye exam until you've brought some order to your blood sugar levels, which can take several weeks. Don't buy new glasses every time your vision changes because the shifting blood sugar will keep changing the way your eyes work. Spend some time on planning your meals and getting some exercise to bring your blood glucose levels nearer normal. This symptom is just another way that your body shows you when your system is out of balance.

Get a dilated eye exam every year to check for retinopathy.

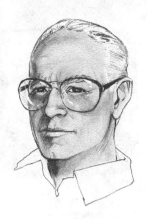

I cannot see well anymore and thought it was because I was getting older. Could this be caused by diabetes?

▼

TIP:

Yes, over time, high levels of blood glucose can injure blood vessels in your retina, the "screen" on the back of your eye that sends images to the brain. The damage is called retinopathy, and it's common. Many new blood vessels grow on the retina and some break, leaking blood that obscures vision and scarring the retina, which affects your vision, too.

In early stages, the only symptom may be blurred vision or no symptoms at all. This is why it's so important to have yearly dilated eye exams with an ophthalmologist. Your ophthalmologist can detect retinopathy early and begin treatment, which is how you save your eyesight. Laser surgery may be required, and it is effective, so don't be afraid to try it.

Like all diabetes-related complications, the best way to treat and prevent retinopathy is to control blood sugar. By managing it and getting regular eye examinations, you can drastically reduce any chances of serious vision problems.

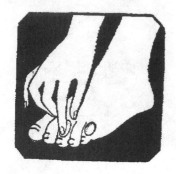

I have heard horror stories about diabetes and amputations. What can diabetes do to my feet?

TIP:

Diabetes can put you at risk for serious injury to your feet for several reasons.

- **Peripheral neuropathy** (nerve damage) causes numbness, burning, tingling, weakness, and decreased sweating. The numbness is perhaps most important, because you can't feel pain or changes in temperature. This is why a person can walk around with a nail poking through his shoe and not know it, or burn her feet on hot sand at the beach. You have to learn to "feel" for your numb feet. Never go barefoot, and always look inside your shoes for nails or foreign objects.
- **Bone and joint deformities** (bunions, arthritic bumps, or toes that turn downward) rub against shoes and pressure points develop. These can wear through the skin, causing foot ulcers. Make sure your shoes fit, and see a doctor immediately if you get a sore on your foot. Don't wait until it's infected.
- **Reduced blood circulation** interferes with healing of foot ulcers. White blood cells and antibiotics that fight infection can't get where they need to go.
- **Infection** is more likely to happen in the dry, cracked skin that diabetes can cause. Keep your feet clean and dry and apply a good moisturizing cream every day (but not between your toes).

1,001 Tips for Living Well with Diabetes

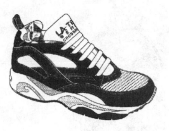

*A*m I going to have to have my foot *amputated?*

▼

TIP:

Not if you take care of yourself. Learn to think for your feet. You can:

- Never go barefoot, not even in your house.
- Have your feet checked at least once a year by your doctor. Get a "monofilament" test for loss of feeling.
- Check your feet daily. Use a mirror to see the bottoms of your feet. Run your hands over them to feel any changes.
- Wash your feet daily in warm soapy water and dry them thoroughly.
- Check inside your shoes before you put them on for nails, rips, and foreign objects.
- Only wear shoes and socks that fit. Our feet get larger as we age, so don't wear old shoes you've saved for special occasions.
- Trim toenails carefully. Get help from a podiatrist if you cannot see well or you've lost feeling in your feet.
- Avoid burns from hot water, sand, or pavement.
- Don't do bathroom surgery on your feet. Let the doctor do it.
- If you get a callus, find out what's causing it. Have your feet changed shape, so your shoes don't fit? Do you need to see a specialist to evaluate the changes in the shape of your feet?

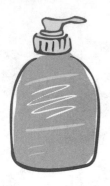

*I*s it safe for me to use creams and lotions on my feet?

▼
TIP:

When buying over-the-counter products, keep these points in mind:

- Dry skin benefits from moisturizing creams. Apply it daily after your bath or shower to prevent skin cracks and infection that may creep in through such cracks. Cost doesn't show how good the cream is—start low. You can use olive or peanut oil and wear socks to bed.
- Do not confuse dry skin with skin infection—let your doctor see it. Infections require special therapy, but some, such as athlete's foot, can be treated with over-the-counter medicines. Just make sure your physician approves of your choice. If there is redness, heat, or swelling anywhere on your feet, see your doctor immediately.
- Do not cut on corns and calluses. Better to soften them with moisturizing lotion and file them down with an Emory board. Find out what's causing the callus—a change in foot shape? A poorly fitting shoe?
- Never use over-the-counter products to remove corns or calluses! Many contain acid, which burns away tissue, causing inflammation, and that may lead to infection.

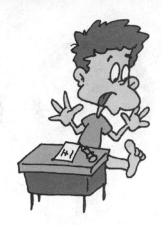

*M*y feet hurt, and I think I'm developing
neuropathy. What can I expect and how
can I treat the symptoms?

▼

TIP:

What you can expect is discomfort—discomfort in your feet, hands,
or perhaps throughout your body. Unfortunately, this is the hard-
est part of neuropathy to treat. There are many medications available to
help keep the pain under control, from antidepressants to capsaicin
cream made from hot peppers. Physical therapy to stretch sore muscles
may also be useful. However, pain therapy is most successful when
supervised by a physician educated in pain management. The nerve
damage may progress to the point of numbness in your feet and legs.
This is when you must take great care to protect your feet from any
injury and to wear shoes and socks that fit well.

You may develop muscle weakness, for example, weakness in your
lower leg that results in foot drop and a slapping gait when you walk.
This can be managed by using a thin, right-angled support that runs
down the back of your lower leg and into your shoes to support the bottom of your foot.

The best way to prevent and, in some cases, to heal neuropathy is to
control your diabetes.

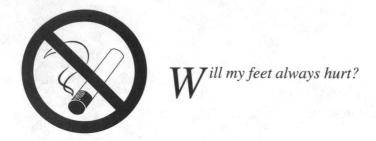

*W*ill my feet always hurt?

▼
TIP:

No, they won't. If you catch neuropathy early, you have a chance to reverse the effects it has on your body. Getting your blood glucose under control before the condition advances and your feet get completely numb is the first—and biggest—step. The next step is to control factors that are linked to the development of neuropathy. These include

- High blood fats levels
- High blood pressure
- Smoking
- Excessive alcohol consumption
- Uncontrolled diabetes

Now, you need to know that as you improve your diabetes control, pain in your feet and hands may get worse. Hang in there—this is temporary. The important thing to remember is that the earlier you start to treat the condition, the better. Once your feet have gone numb, chances are you won't get the feeling back. Don't let neuropathy get out of hand. Fight back early!

W*hat is neuropathy?*

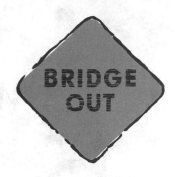

BRIDGE
OUT

▼
TIP:

Plain and simple, it's pretty scary stuff. Neuropathy is a long-term complication of diabetes that results in nerve damage. Unfortunately, the signs are often overlooked, leaving you with a bad condition that just gets worse. When your doctor starts rattling off four-syllable words, check these definitions to know what he's talking about.

- **Distal symmetrical polyneuropathy** involves your feet and hands, most often the feet. Symptoms usually involve discomfort (pins and needles, burning, or no feeling at all) or weakness.
- **Autonomic neuropathy** affects the part of the nervous system we don't control consciously, such as the nerves that regulate blood pressure, sweating, digestion, and bladder function.
- **Entrapment neuropathy** is caused by a squeezing of the nerves, as in carpal tunnel syndrome.

The way to avoid developing neuropathy or to improve it is to get your blood glucose levels nearer your target goals.

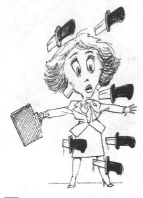

What is causing my leg pain?

▼

TIP:

Poor circulation could cause it, and walking can improve it. If your leg hurts, stop walking while the pain eases, and then walk a bit more. Your persistence causes your body to form new pathways for the blood to circulate.

In his late 50s, Ed has had diabetes for 20 years. Retinopathy and peripheral neuropathy handicap his running skills but do not diminish his enthusiasm or discipline. He is out there, a tube of glucose gel stuck in his headband, exercising regularly, doing races every month. He is fit and healthy to his limits.

In recent weeks, however, Ed has developed pain after exercise in his right calf and is not able to maintain his exercise schedule. He is worried that diabetes has caused poor circulation. Examination revealed nothing more than a pulled calf muscle. A brief course of physical therapy restored Ed's muscle, and he is back on the running circuit.

The moral? People with diabetes may be at risk for diabetes-related conditions. However, they are people who just happen to have diabetes. They are also entitled to have the common ailments that happen to everyone in the human race. Don't blame everything on your diabetes.

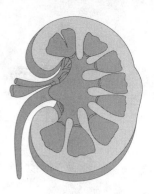

*A*m *I going to lose my kidneys?*

▼

TIP:

Not necessarily. You can do things to protect them. People with diabetes tend to overwork their kidneys when they have high blood glucose—the kidneys have to flush out the excess sugar—so uncontrolled diabetes can lead to kidney problems. Injury to your delicate kidney structures and tiny blood vessels may cause the filters to leak, which allows albumin (a protein) to pass into your urine. A small amount of leaking albumin is called microalbuminuria. This is the beginning of nephropathy.

If the overworking of your kidneys continues unchecked for a number of years, larger amounts of albumin are released into your urine. High blood pressure usually develops. Your kidneys are no longer able to keep up with their workload. Waste products build up in your blood. Your kidneys will finally stop working. Kidney dialysis or a kidney transplant are required to remove the toxins from your body.

Do your best to get your blood glucose levels nearer to normal, exercise, and choose healthy meals. Your doctor may ask you to cut back on salty foods and protein. Drink plenty of water every day. And think positive about your health and future.

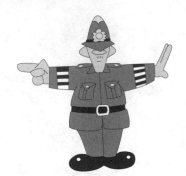

*H*ow can I reduce my risk of kidney
complications?

▼

TIP:

Keeping your blood glucose under control is the best way to prevent diabetic complications. There are ways to keep tabs on how your kidneys are doing and keep them healthy. You should:

- Have a urine test to check for microalbumin every year if you have type 2 diabetes and after you have had type 1 for more than five years. Be sure it's a microalbumin test and not an ordinary test for urine protein (this does not show microalbumin). Using 24-hour urine collection is the most accurate test, but that's not always necessary.
- If you have microalbuminuria, with or without high blood pressure, use an ACE inhibitor to protect your kidneys from damage.
- Control high blood pressure, even mild high blood pressure. The recommended blood pressure goal is 130/80. ACE inhibitors treat high blood pressure and have a beneficial effect on your kidneys.
- Follow your doctor's advice about how much protein and salt to eat.
- Don't smoke.

I've heard something about "male menopause."
Does it exist and will it affect my diabetes?

TIP:

What you've heard about is called andropause, and like menopause, it is caused by a drop in hormone levels—testosterone instead of estrogen. It also occurs in men in their 40s and 50s. However, andropause is more subtle and less predictable. Some of the symptoms include

- Low sex drive
- Fatigue or loss of energy
- Emotional, psychological, and behavioral changes
- Decreased muscle mass and loss of muscle strength
- Increased upper- and central-body fat
- Reduced bone density

Luckily, there is no direct association between diabetes and andropause. However, unrecognized and untreated andropause can cause you to gain weight and increase your risk for diabetes-related problems. The solution is to add more activity to your daily schedule and to eat wisely. You can increase your muscle mass and strength and retain bone density by doing weight-bearing exercises, such as walking or lifting small weights. This will help with your diabetes control, too.

If you think you're suffering from andropause, talk to your physician. Treatment with testosterone replacement therapy may be beneficial.

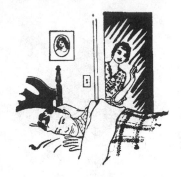

I've been having problems with impotence. Is it from getting older or from diabetes?

Yes, diabetes-related damage to nerves and circulation can cause impotence but so can aging. Impotence is not unique to diabetes. Millions of men who don't have diabetes do have impotence, and frequently the cause is psychological. Sexual enjoyment requires a healthy connection between brain and penis, and a physical shortcoming may not always be the problem. Impotence related to diabetes, on the other hand, has possible physical causes. The more common ones are

- Nerve damage (neuropathy)
- Reduction of blood flow to the penis (made worse by smoking)
- Low levels of testosterone (the male sex hormone)
- Medications—pills for high blood pressure, anxiety, depression, and peptic ulcer (Don't stop taking your medications without your doctor's approval.)
- Drinking too much alcohol

There are tests available to help determine the causes of impotence. Talk with your doctor about your concern and your options for treatment. Get your blood sugar under control now to keep your sexual health in top form.

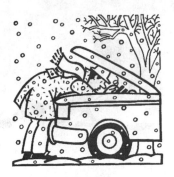

*I*f I have impotence caused by diabetes,
how can I treat it?

▼

TIP:

The best way to prevent diabetes-related impotence is with good
blood glucose control, with exercise, and by not smoking. But diabetes may not be the cause. Treatments depend on the cause and include

■ Working with a therapist to overcome impotence based on psychological issues
■ Medication injected or inserted into the penis
■ A cylindrical vacuum pump into which the penis is placed, and from
which air is pumped out, creating a negative pressure and pulling
blood into the penis (Placing a rubber band at the base of the penis
maintains the erection.)
■ Testosterone therapy, if testosterone levels are low
■ A variety of oral medications, such as Viagra and Levitra, intended to
create an erection
■ Checking to see which of your other medications, such as pills for
high blood pressure or anti-depressants, could be causing impotence
and seeing if another drug will work better for you

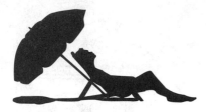

*W*ill menopause affect my diabetes?

▼

TIP:

Yes. Unpredictable swings in hormones (estrogen and progesterone) affect your blood glucose levels during puberty, pregnancy, menstruation, and menopause. Menopause is when production of estrogen and progesterone slows and finally stops. It usually occurs between the ages of 45 and 55 but may be sooner or later in life.

Estrogen and progesterone counteract the effects of insulin in your body, so when they are high, your blood glucose may also be high. When levels of these hormones fall, your blood glucose may be lower than you expect, and you may be surprised by hypoglycemia. If you use insulin or diabetes pills, you may need to decrease the dose. You may need to check your blood glucose levels more often than usual when you are going through a time of hot flashes and other symptoms of menopause.

Be aware that estrogen provides protection to your heart, and you lose that protection during menopause. Take care to take care of your heart (see tips on pages 736 and 797).

*S*ince I have diabetes, should I take hormones at menopause?

▼
TIP:

Maybe. Hormone replacement therapy (HRT) is a controversial treatment right now. Diabetes puts you at high risk for heart disease, and that risk increases when your body stops making estrogen. It was thought that HRT with estrogen and progesterone would be beneficial, though this is still being determined. HRT is not advised if you have a history of breast or uterine cancer, blood clotting problems, severe eye disease, or kidney disease. If you take HRT, your doctor must monitor your blood fats closely. Another point is that women who take hormones are more likely to have gallbladder problems, which is also a common problem for people with diabetes.

On the plus side is that HRT helps with vaginal dryness, loss of desire, and other menopause-related sexual problems. Weigh the pros and cons of HRT with your doctor. Newer forms of estrogen and progesterone may have fewer side effects and fewer health risks for women with diabetes. Also, you may want to add soy foods to your diet because they contain natural estrogen for your heart and your uncomfortable symptoms.

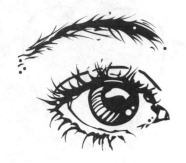

*D*oes diabetes affect a woman's ability to enjoy sex?

It may, but all women share the following common problems at any and all ages. Here are the problems and some suggested remedies:

- **Vaginal dryness.** Restore hormone levels if they are low. Use vaginal lubricants if you choose not to use HRT.
- **Pain accompanying sexual intercourse.** Speak to your physician about muscle exercises. Try different positions for intercourse.
- **Vaginal yeast infection.** Control your blood glucose and use medication for the infection. Don't use anything but water to wash your vagina.
- **Nerve damage** in the genital area. A gentle touch or vibration in touch may help.
- **Bladder weakness** (or neurogenic bladder). Always empty your bladder before and after sexual intercourse. Do kegel exercises by stopping the flow of urine midstream and tightening those same muscles at other times (50 kegels a day). Ask your doctor if you should use antibiotics after intercourse to prevent bladder infection.
- **Limited mobility or discomfort** (from neuropathy or arthritis). Vary position or use pillows for support.

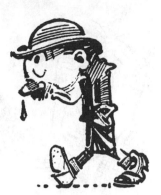

I've been feeling very depressed lately.
Someone mentioned that this could be caused
by my diabetes. Is this true?

▼
TIP:

Yes. If your blood sugar is not being controlled properly, you can suffer from mood swings, confusion, forgetfulness, and most dramatically, depression. Unfortunately, many seniors with diabetes suffer from depression but don't attribute it to their diabetes. If you have any of the following symptoms, talk to your doctor about how to improve your mood:

- Persistent feelings of sadness and emptiness
- Change in sleeping patterns—too much or too little
- Change in appetite
- Lack of desire to do the things you once enjoyed, such as reading, hobbies, and visiting with friends and family
- Extreme fatigue or lack of energy
- Feelings of worthlessness or undeserved guilt

Fortunately, depression can be helped, and if your diabetes is at fault, getting your blood sugar under control can bring some very positive changes. Exercise will improve your mood. There are medications that can make you feel well enough to get up and go—don't wait.

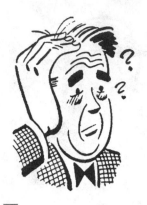

C *an diabetes cause me to be forgetful and*
confused?

▼

TIP:

Yes it can. A lot of seniors with diabetes think that being absent-minded and forgetful is just part of the aging process. While some short-term memory loss is expected with aging, there's also a good chance your diabetes is playing a part. High blood sugar can cause you to be, among other things, forgetful, confused, and disoriented. Before blaming a little senility on the years, talk with your doctor about the possibility of high blood sugar.

Try to keep your wits in shape by doing crossword puzzles or playing games, such as Scrabble, chess, or bridge. Research shows that bridge is especially helpful! Try to keep learning new things, such as how to play a musical instrument or speak another language. Every time you learn something new, you create new pathways in your brain that improve your memory and thinking. It makes your life more interesting and you a more interesting person, too.

Chapter 6
CHECKUPS THAT COUNT

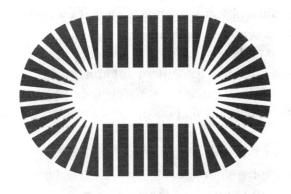

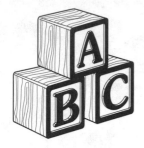

*W*hat do I need to do now that my diabetes has been discovered?

▼
TIP:

The ADA recommends the following medical help for you:

■ A complete medical history and a physical examination that focuses on body "parts" affected by uncontrolled diabetes.
■ Laboratory tests: fasting blood fat levels, creatinine (a blood test of kidney function), urinalysis, a urine test for "microalbumin" (trace amounts of protein), a urine culture if infection is suspected, a thyroid function test (for people with type 1 diabetes), and an electrocardiogram.
■ A management plan—the key to success with diabetes. This plan takes all things into consideration—your age, lifestyle, daily schedule, physical activity, personality, cultural factors, family, friends, the presence of other health conditions, food preferences, how often you want to check blood glucose, and what your goals are. This plan is the product of discussion between you, your family or friends, and your physician. But you have the final say.
■ A schedule for your periodic return visits.

*W*hat is my A1C level?

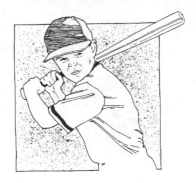

▼
TIP:

Hemoglobin is a protein in your blood that carries oxygen from the lungs to tissues. A1C is a type of hemoglobin (type A) with glucose attached to it (it's also called HbA1c). So why is it important to you? Because your A1C level tells you your average blood glucose level for the past two to three months. It's your blood sugar "batting average," and it lets you know how well you're managing your diabetes.

Hemoglobin is packaged in red blood cells. Red blood cells live for 100–120 days, and during this period, the hemoglobin gets a coating of the glucose that's circulating in your blood. By measuring the percentage of sugar-coated A1C cells in your blood, you can determine the average amount of glucose that has been in your blood for the previous two or three months.

A normal A1C is 4–6.4%. The goal of diabetes management in most people is to have an A1C closer to normal levels—about 7%, depending on your health and age. Research has shown clearly that this is the way you can prevent or slow development of long-term complications of diabetes. Check with your doctor to see what yourA1C is.

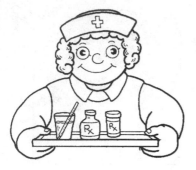

Who can teach me how to use a blood glucose meter?

▼

TIP:

To be sure, individual or group instruction is the best way to learn. Consider the following possibilities:

- A doctor with interest in diabetes management usually has an assistant skilled in meter education.
- The local hospital may have a diabetes teaching program.
- There may be a diabetes nurse educator working alone or with a physician in your community.
- The pharmacist who sells meters or test strips may have a special knowledge and interest in meter use.
- If all else fails, ask for advice from the nearest American Diabetes Association office.
- Blood glucose meters all have an instruction booklet. Everything you need to know is there. You can also call the company for guidance. Company resources are available online, too.

And remember—experience is the best teacher. You will learn much in doing it. After a year or two, take a refresher course, just to be sure you're still doing it right.

*H*ow often should I check my blood glucose?

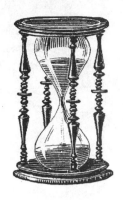

▼
TIP:

It depends on how stable your diabetes is. People with type 2 diabetes usually have smaller swings in glucose than people with type 1 diabetes. If you are challenged by wide swings in glucose, you might want to check four to eight times daily. People on tight control do. If you have a stable glucose pattern, you would check perhaps every two or three days.

It is important to check not only in the morning or before meals, but also 1–2 hours after meals, and perhaps during the night. You could spread these checks out over the week so that you always do a morning fasting check and one other at a different time each day.

Routines in life help you have a stable and healthy existence. Checking your glucose level is an important part of your routine. It gives you information and confidence and security.

Many meters store the results. But you also need information about the date, time, meals, events, exercise, and medication. You would benefit from keeping a log book of this information that you can take to doctor's appointments. You use this information to decide when to eat, how much to eat, when to exercise, and how much diabetes medication to take.

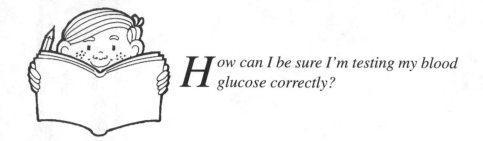

*H*ow can I be sure I'm testing my blood glucose correctly?

▼
TIP:

*T*he top testing tips are:

Use the instruction manual to check your technique.

Select a meter that meets your needs, say with a larger display screen or audio readings.

Use the side of any finger. Do not use the center of the fingertip because it will hurt more. Some use areas other than a finger, for example the forearm.

Keep the sensor and strip areas of the meter clean.

Be sure that the meter is properly calibrated on a schedule.

Periodically check your meter's accuracy (and your technique) with a control solution.

Your meter should be accurate to within 15% of your doctor's laboratory results, and this is okay for your use.

If blood flows slowly, warm your hands before taking the sample.

Make sure your hands are dry with no soap still on them.

Don't fret about the number. Just use it to decide what to do.

I can't see well. How can I test my glucose?

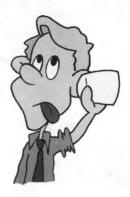

▼
TIP:

S everal glucose meters can be equipped to give step-by-step verbal instructions for testing and to report the results audibly. English is the standard language, but other languages are available. Additional features available with selected talking meters include cassette instructions, Braille identification of controls, plug-in ports and earphones, and large-print instructions. At least one device reads the bar codes on the insulin bottles and verbally identifies the insulin contained in the bottle, so you don't make a mistake getting the right one. In all cases, the synthesized voice is considerate and non-judgmental. Ask your doctor, diabetes educator, or pharmacist for help finding a system that is comfortable for you.

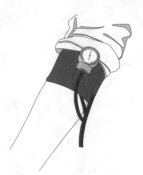

*W*hat should my blood pressure be?

▼
TIP:

For good health, blood pressure should be no more than 130/80. Setting the goal at 130/80 or below is a reasonable and safe objective. Controlling your blood pressure is the way to reduce your risk of developing diabetes-related complications and other serious health conditions, such as having a stroke.

The first and most important steps to take control of high blood pressure are lifestyle changes. These include losing weight, exercising more, reducing the amount of salt (sodium) you eat (read the food labels), and limiting the amount of alcohol you drink.

If lifestyle changes do not bring your blood pressure down, your doctor will prescribe medication for it. If one medication doesn't do the job, another, and perhaps another are added in a stepwise fashion (see page 753). Blood pressure pills have side effects, so be sure you understand what they are.

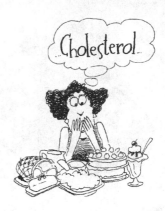

W*hat is a lipid?*

▼
TIP:

L ipids are blood fats. There are different kinds of lipids, and they form important structural parts of the human body. However, several kinds of lipids are linked to hardening of the arteries (atherosclerosis). If you eat meals that are high in saturated fat, and are very overweight and physically inactive, you have the ingredients for lipid problems.

There are three kinds of blood fats that affect blood vessels—HDL cholesterol (good cholesterol), LDL cholesterol, and triglycerides. To maintain health, try to keep your lipid levels as follows:

■ HDL cholesterol protects against atherosclerosis. Blood test values less than 35 mg/dl are unhealthy. Values above 45 mg/dl in men and above 55 mg/dl in women are healthy.

■ LDL cholesterol should be at low levels to reduce the risk of athero-sclerosis. Levels above 130 mg/dl carry risk. Values below 100 mg/dl are healthy.

■ Triglycerides should be at levels below 200 mg/dl. Increased levels are linked to inflammation of the pancreas (pancreatitis), and are likely involved in atherosclerosis.

Have your lipids tested every year to make sure you're maintaining healthy levels of blood fats.

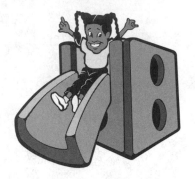

*H*ow do I control my lipids and why?

Y̵ou control lipids to save your heart. You reduce your chance of developing coronary heart disease (heart trouble from "hardening" of the arteries that nourish the heart). If you already have coronary heart disease, lipid control will reduce the chance of it getting worse.

There are four cornerstones of lipid control:

- A meal plan. A meal plan for glucose control will improve certain lipid disorders. Fats in a meal plan are more unsaturated fats (olive or canola oils) than saturated (animal products). Too much alcohol may cause irregularity of certain lipids, so it's wise to cut back.
- Weight reduction. When you cut back your total daily calories by eating less fat (the high-calorie foodstuff), you lose weight.
- Physical activity. Increasing your physical activity will, by itself, improve lipid levels and aid in successful weight loss.
- If your lipids are not in good control after 3–6 months of cornerstone therapy, you may need a medication—the type depends on the type of lipid disorder.

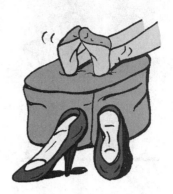

I *can't move much. How can I take care of my feet?*

▼
TIP:

Try these tips:

- Get a bench or stool for your bathtub or shower, so you can sit to clean your feet.
- Have grab bars installed in your shower, so you can support yourself when you bend over.
- Buy or make a long-handled sponge or bath brush, so you can wash your feet.
- Lay a towel on the floor, and rub your feet across the towel to dry them (try to dry well between the toes).
- Have another long-handled sponge or brush to apply lotion (do not use the same one you use in the shower).
- To inspect the bottom of your feet, lay a mirror on the floor and hold your foot above it to see underneath.
- Ask your spouse or a friend to inspect the bottom of your feet for you.
- Never go barefoot, unless you are bathing or sleeping.
- If you lose feeling in your feet, have your doctor look at them at each visit.

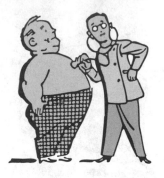

*W*hat medical tests should I get
to take care of my diabetes?

TIP:

Continuing care is important. The ADA recommends:

Making doctor visits whenever needed. If you need changes in treatment, visits may be daily or weekly. If all is stable, then your visits
are every 3–6 months.

At each visit, give a recent medical history and get a physical
examination.

At each visit, your diabetes plan should be reviewed and adjusted, if
it's not working for you.

Every 3–6 months, A1C should be measured (how often depends on
how stable your diabetes control is).

Yearly, have a complete eye examination, with eye drops to dilate the
eyes, performed by an ophthalmologist or optometrist trained in
diabetes care.

Yearly, have a complete foot examination. If you have a risk of foot
problems, this examination should be done at every visit.

Yearly, have a fasting lipid blood test if your lipids are in control. If
you are at low risk, every two years is okay. You need blood tests
more often when lipids are out of control.

Yearly, have a urine test for microalbumin. If your urine contains
albumin, and therapy is prescribed to control it, you may be tested
more often.

Chapter 7
DOCTORS, NURSES, AND YOU

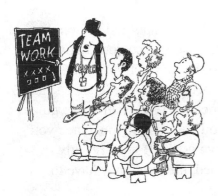

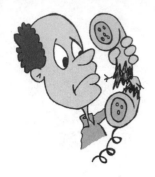

*M*y doctor acts like she doesn't have time to talk to me. What can I do?

▼

TIP:

Your doctor is your teammate. To win you must communicate with respect, genuineness, good manners, and unconditional acceptance. Beware the pitfalls that stud the playing field for both of you. Does your doctor want to control the conversation by asking questions that let you make only "yes" or "no" answers? Or does she just not have any time?

With a chronic disease, you are the one in charge, and you need the benefit of your doctor's knowledge, both clinical facts and personal expertise. Write down your questions before you go so you are organized and use the appointed time well. Ask her to refer you to a diabetes educator, so you can learn more about diabetes in a more relaxed setting.

Learn to speak up for yourself. The doctor serves as an active guide, but she needs the information that only you have about you. Once you have been fully informed, you set your own goals. If you are truly frustrated that you are not being heard or helped, then you may have to change doctors.

H *ow can I make a doctor's visit go smoothly?*

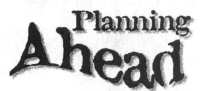
Planning Ahead

▼
TIP:

☐ Be sure you understand what your doctor is saying! If you have trouble hearing, say so. Ask him or her to speak up or write his directions for you.

■ Respect the time allowed for your visit. There is a limit to the number of issues you can discuss. Prepare a list of the most important issues.

■ Inform the doctor's secretary of insurance changes or need to have paperwork done.

■ Bring a list of your medications and doses (or bring the bottles). Have your glucose log book open for review.

■ Inform the doctor of lifestyle (exercise, for example) or meal plan changes.

☐ Wear clothing that is easy to remove.

☐ Don't bring the family. A friend or your spouse may be important, but a group of people spreads chaos.

☐ Request help from the doctor's staff with removal of clothing or getting on the examining table.

■ Be sure to get lab tests done far enough ahead so that results are available at the visit.

☐ You may call or email between appointments, but don't discuss major issues that way.

☐ Accept that your doctor is human, too. Smile.

☐ Not working? Change doctors.

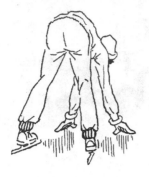

Who should make the final decisions—the patient or the doctor?

▼

TIP:

It is your life. It is your decision.

Forty years ago, Bill developed diabetes at age 36. At 76, he has enjoyed a rich quality of life, but time has taken its toll. Kidney malfunction has required kidney dialysis three times weekly over the past five years. Strong in mind, he is physically enfeebled by years and circumstances. Although his physician is anxious to carry on with dialysis, Bill wants to stop and spend the final days at home with his family.

There is a beginning and there is an end to all things. Reaching the older side of age often brings dilemmas in what to do and how much to do for health care. Advances in technology have brought amazing treatment options. But what do you do when continuing treatment no longer brings quality of life? An informed person of sound mind has the privilege of deciding what is best. Final days spent with family and other loved ones, spent on unfinished business, spent in peace, can be the most meaningful days of a person's life.

Bill will be making his decision soon. It's the right one.

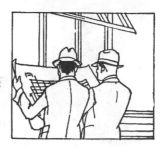

*W*hat should my medical insurance cover in diabetes care?

▼

TIP:

Your insurance should cover the checkups and tests you need to stay healthy. You should be able to see your doctor regularly (four times a year for type 1 and one or two times a year for type 2) and get your A1C, blood pressure, and blood fats (if necessary) checked. You should also have yearly dilated eye exams. These checkups benefit your health and well-being, reduce the complications of diabetes, and significantly reduce health care costs. ADA believes that health insurers must cover the following:

- Health care visits
- Diabetes education by a trained team
- Laboratory tests as needed
- All medications and supplies for complete diabetes care

However, not all insurance will cover all these areas. In recent years, progress has been made on state and national levels, both in government and private insurance companies. But as you know, reimbursement is spotty. The health care dollar is only so big. Join the cause to make others more aware! Lobby your lawmakers and insurance company for what we believe is your right. Be in touch with the ADA and find out how you can help in securing proper reimbursement for all people with diabetes.

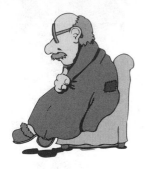

I *live in a nursing home and seem to catch a lot of colds. How do I manage diabetes when I am sick?*

▼
TIP:

Your doctor or educator should help you make a sick-day plan ahead of time. Glucose levels vary during illness but usually are high. Key points are:

- Peform frequent blood glucose checks, four times or more daily, to see where your glucose level is.
- If glucose is above 240 mg/dl, check your urine for ketones. Ketones alert you to developing ketoacidosis.
- If you take diabetes medications, continue to take them on schedule. Insulin, or extra insulin, may be required temporarily if your glucose is too high. Take a little even if you can't keep food down. This is important.
- If you're nauseated or vomiting, drinking small amounts (2–4 oz) of regular (not diet) soda or juice every 2–3 hours is usually easier on your stomach. Getting some carbohydrate is important for energy. Eat food that is easy on your stomach, such as crackers or broth.
- Manage the illness as well as the diabetes.
- Set guidelines ahead of time for when to call your physician. Be able to tell him what your blood glucose level is, your temperature, and your ketone level.

Chapter 8
SHARPENING YOUR WITS

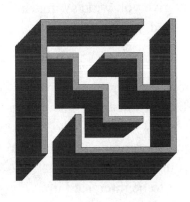

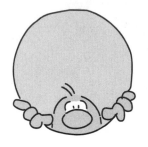

I'm not as hungry any more, and I eat less often. Will this affect my diabetes control?

▼

TIP:

Yes. This is a change in your meal plan. If you use insulin, sulfony-lureas, or Prandin, not eating can put you at risk for very low blood sugar (hypoglycemia). Eating at odd times may give you wide swings in blood sugar and malnutrition. We do need less food as we age, but we still need to eat to stay healthy.

Perhaps you cannot taste or smell the food. Try brushing your tongue as well as your teeth before you eat. Stop smoking to improve your senses. Eat more fresh foods and use herbs and spices for flavor instead of salt.

Could you be depressed? Clinical depression is common in diabetes and certainly affects your appetite. Talk with your doctor about your symptoms. When you are depressed, it's difficult to be interested in doing things for yourself or staying healthy. It can keep you from getting up and going for a walk.

Getting exercise will help build your appetite, improve your mental outlook, and give you more energy.

*H*ow do I let go?

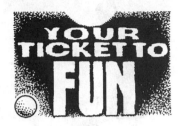

▼
TIP:

Realize that, "He who laughs, lasts." Yes, diabetes is hard work and frustrating at times. There are situations and events that just cannot be explained or resolved. In tough times, humor can be the great healer. It releases tension, lowers your blood pressure, and makes you healthier all over.

Jane received a Lilly 60-Year Medal at age 78. She has outlived two husbands—who were worriers, far too serious. She was using intensive therapy 60 years ago. Insulin was available only in rapid-acting murky brown solution, and she injected it four times daily with large re-sharpened hypodermic needles attached to glass syringes that she boiled periodically and stored in alcohol. She has developed some complications of diabetes over the decades, but she is knowledgeable, proud, and graceful. What has supported her is humor. She jokes about her limitations and puts her physicians at ease if they are struggling to figure out her diabetes care plan. Her appreciation for and use of humor allows her to live a full and productive life.

Work hard, and let go just as hard. Try to laugh at least once every day!

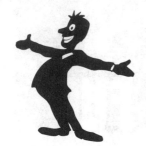

I'm in my 70s. Should I be concerned about target blood glucose levels?

TIP:

Yes. Effective glucose control improves health at any age. However, you may need to have higher target glucose levels. They should be higher if you

Take diabetes medications, including insulin, at incorrect times. Your blood glucose levels could go dangerously low.

Eat at irregular times

Have had a stroke or reduced brain circulation. You may not recognize the symptoms of falling glucose and get into trouble.

Live alone. It may be hard to get help when you have falling blood glucose.

Have gastroparesis. This fancy word means "sluggish stomach function," and is a type of neuropathy. The food you eat may not be processed speedily and your glucose levels may be up or down at unexpected times.

Have neuropathy. In this condition, you may no longer have any symptoms of falling glucose.

Exercise. Exercise lowers glucose during and for hours after the activity, so you may have a higher level before (not above 250 mg/dl), so you don't go too low afterward.

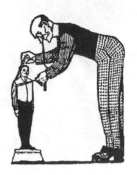

*H*ow much weight do I have to lose to control diabetes?

▼

TIP:

If you have type 2 diabetes, you probably weigh more than you should, or did when you were diagnosed. If this is the case, the first thing your physician probably told you was, "Lose some weight!" It's a tough job, but it's essential to getting your diabetes under control.

So, how much weight is enough to see results? 2 pounds? 10 pounds? 150? Actually, any weight you lose will be beneficial. But to see real results, a loss of 10–20 pounds can do wonders and can be accomplished in 3 to 4 months. Not only will your blood glucose levels drop (meaning less medication, which means less expense), but you'll also feel better, and your risk for other serious health problems will drop, too.

Losing weight means doing some exercise and changing the way you eat. It may be as simple a step as measuring—with a measuring cup or a scale—each serving that you eat. Even if it's healthy food, too much is still too much.

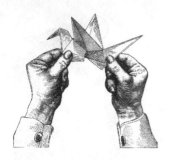

I'm retired. Isn't it time to just sit?

▼
TIP:

It isn't healthy for anyone of any age to just sit. For example, Sharon expected an enriched life when she retired from nursing in her early 60s. But she found herself adrift, stressed, preoccupied by petty ailments, gaining weight, inactive, and lacking self-worth.

Although health care professionals are usually poor patients, she had the good sense to get a checkup. Her weight, high blood pressure, and family history of diabetes led to blood glucose tests. And in fact, Sharon had high fasting blood glucose on two occasions—diabetes.

She attacked the condition she was in. She began a program of physical fitness. She got a meal plan and followed it. Her weight dropped, and she was able to control her blood glucose without medication. She took a small dose of an ACE inhibitor to control her blood pressure.

Her success in managing the diabetes rekindled her sense of self-worth and put Sharon back on course. In fact, she returned to nursing and continues to work in an office serving the needs of other people with diabetes.

Chapter 9
FRIENDS AND FAMILY

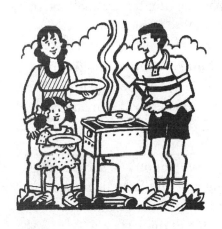

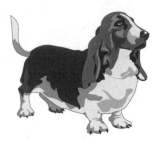

*C*an I manage my diabetes by myself?

▼
TIP:

It would be best if you would share it. Companionship and personal relationships are important throughout life and, over the years, may become necessary for help in managing your health. It may spell the difference between living independently and having to move from your home.

Companionship can include a spouse, family member, hired caregiver, hospice volunteer, Good Samaritan, or pet. Yes, pets qualify. They are not skilled at administering medications but are good at many tasks and are ideal companions (*Animals are such agreeable friends—they ask no questions, they pass no criticisms.* —George Eliot).

Encourage a companion in your life. A companion can serve many functions beyond the delights of socializing and intellectual stimulation. It is no accident that you are encouraged to bring a companion to most diabetes education programs. With knowledge of diabetes, the companion can help prepare meals, monitor glucose, give medication, and participate in all your activities of daily living. Diabetes is safer.

And remember, the way to have a friend is to be a friend. Encourage and keep good friends. Your life will be much richer and your diabetes easier to manage.

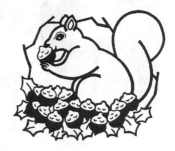

*H*ow can I make things easier for myself
and my family if I get very ill?

▼
TIP:

Plan ahead and get the documents, such as a will, written now. Sherm was a fire inspector—he did things by the book. At age 68, he developed a raging bone infection in his left foot. Thirty-four years of diabetes has marked him with neuropathy and poor circulation in the legs. This bone infection had happened before and required partial amputation of the left foot. This time, he didn't want surgery and was willing to accept whatever happened.

Sherm was prepared. All adults should plan and make known their end-of-life decisions. Such planning is a service to your family and friends. Sherm had the following documents properly completed:

■ Will
■ Advance directive—stating his personal wishes regarding being given CPR, IV feedings, and other interventions, which is to be used if he is unable to make such decisions when they are needed
■ Durable power of attorney—assigning decision-making authority regarding his health care to a designated person, a person who knows his wishes and who will act on his behalf if and when he is unable to make such decisions

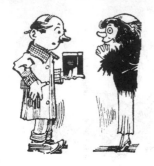

*W*hy did my wife's personality really change after she got diabetes?

TIP:

It would take a book to answer, but let's start with questions that can apply to anyone with diabetes. Personality doesn't very often change. What was her personality before diabetes? What was your relationship before diabetes? Is the household one of harmony and understanding? Diabetes causes stress and threatens stability. Has diabetes changed your expectations or lifestyle? Are you supportive and understanding? Is your lifestyle healthy, or do you resent making the changes that are important for her?

Is she keeping it all in and not talking about it? Is she overwhelmed by fear? Does she need the confidence that comes from diabetes education? Is she frustrated by her relationship with her doctors? Is she worried or guilty about the possibility of passing diabetes to your children or grandchildren? Is she afraid of letting you down? Is she clinically depressed? Is she in one of the five stages of grief—denial, anger, bargaining, depression, or acceptance?

Diabetes is a challenge, often creating emotional turmoil. But with support from you and her health care providers, she can manage her diabetes with a smile most of the time.

Try to lighten the mood every day. Compliment her. And share laughter—it's still the best medicine.

*H*ow do I manage large meals at special celebrations?

▼

TIP:

Special celebrations are an important part of our culture. Here are some tips to remain popular and avoid frustration, weight gain, and poor glucose control:

- Stay confident and in control. It's okay to be who you are.
- Remember that all foods can fit your meal plan in reasonable amounts—even 2 bites of your favorite dessert.
- Don't change your usual eating pattern, except you might omit snacks that day.
- Be proud of your discipline. Focus on the event and not on the food and drink.
- Honor the host and hostess. Smile, accept what you're served graciously, and limit the amounts of food you eat (you won't be the only one doing this).
- Ask to take a portion home to eat tomorrow.
- Be prepared. Discuss these situations ahead of time with your doctor and dietitian and have a plan. If you take insulin, you may take extra rapid-acting insulin to cover more carbohydrate in the meal. Meglitinide pills can be adjusted just before meals as needed. People using other oral medications may use supplemental insulin for situations such as this.

I don't know anything about cooking. Who's going to cook if my wife is sick?

▼
TIP:

You can do it. Sure, you could eat out every night, but a home-cooked meal is healthier and can express creativity and love. It pays back some of what you've received over the years. If you're new to the kitchen (and maybe a little overwhelmed), keep these things in mind:

- Start with some easy dishes that you like.
- Purchase an ADA cookbook and try new things.
- Watch a cooking show on television for ideas.
- Purchase some new cooking tools to replace or enhance the tools already in your kitchen (your wife may grumble over the fact that you consider hers inferior equipment).
- Take a cooking course and learn to prepare foods you never thought you could cook. You're young as long as you keep learning new things.

It can be as simple as oatmeal for breakfast, a chef salad for lunch, and roast beef with vegetables for dinner. You don't even have to "cook" much. You'll be surprised at how satisfying preparing a good meal can be. Even more rewarding will be the pleasure and appreciation you receive from your wife.

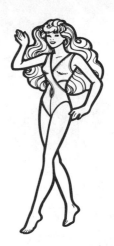

*M*y friends are going on a trendy new diet. Is it safe for me?

▼

TIP:

Most likely, the answer is "no." There are a lot of new diets that promise rapid weight loss, but most do not follow the healthy eating guidelines set up by our government nor do they follow the guidelines for people with diabetes. When you have diabetes, what you eat is an essential part of your diabetes management plan. Not following your meal plan could lead to poor health for you. In fact, many of these diets can be hard on your body and deprive you of nutrients that you need.

When all is said and done, the only diet that works is one that restricts the number of calories eaten in a day and adds exercise to your daily routine. You'll do better to design a meal plan that fits your needs and lifestyle with an RD. You take weight off slowly over time and that's the best way to do it—with a good balanced meal plan to keep you healthy throughout the process. When your friends are back to where they started, you'll be glad you did it your way.

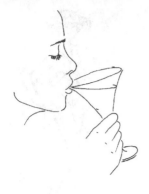

I enjoy a drink every once in awhile and have for over 50 years. Is diabetes going to force me to give up my evening cocktail?

▼
TIP:

It doesn't have to. In fact, an occasional drink, such as a glass of wine with dinner, can have health benefits both mental and physical. However, there are precautions to take when drinking alcoholic beverages:

- Limit daily drinks to two for men and one for women. One drink equals 12 oz beer, 5 oz wine, or 1 1/2 oz distilled spirits.
- Fit the alcohol into your daily meal plan. It has lots of calories. One alcoholic beverage equals two fat exchanges. Beer, sweet wines, and mixers contain additional carbohydrate and calories that will affect your blood sugar level—and maybe your weight.
- If you don't eat food when you are having the drink, alcohol can cause very low levels of blood glucose (hypoglycemia). This is especially dangerous since low blood glucose and drunkenness have similar symptoms. While people are figuring out that you are not drunk, there may be a serious delay in getting the treatment you need to raise your blood sugar.
- Never drink and drive.

101 TIPS FOR SIMPLIFYING DIABETES

▲

A project of the
American Diabetes Association

▼

Written By

The University of New Mexico Diabetes Care Team

David S. Schade, MD
Mark R. Burge, MD
Leslie Atler, PhD
Lisa Butler, BUS.
Lynda Shey, RN, CDE

101 TIPS FOR SIMPLIFYING DIABETES

▼

TABLE OF CONTENTS

Chapter 1
WHIPPING YOUR BLOOD SUGARS INTO SHAPE

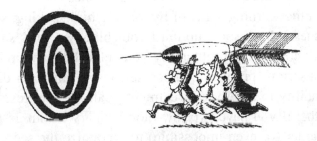

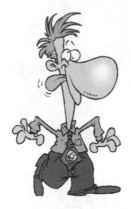

*C*an one low blood sugar put me at risk for another one?

TIP:

Frequent episodes of hypoglycemia (low blood sugar) can cause a problem called hypoglycemia unawareness. This is a condition in which the warning signs of hypoglycemia (shaking, sweating, or nervousness) don't show up until your blood sugar is so low that you can't correct the problem by yourself. Hypoglycemia unawareness is a serious problem and can seriously limit your diabetes care team's ability to meet your treatment goals. Recent research has shown that if you have two low blood sugars within 24 hours, it's much harder (or even impossible) to recognize the second episode. This is because your body's hormone response to the first episode of hypoglycemia reduces your body's hormone response to the second episode. Thus, you are at a higher risk for a severe low blood sugar for about 24 hours after experiencing an episode of hypoglycemia. One way to prevent hypoglycemia unawareness is to avoid hypoglycemia for several days or a week. Then your body will be better prepared to recognize a low blood sugar attack.

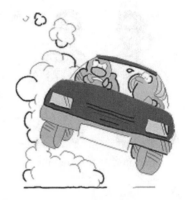

*S*hould I eat before I drive my car?

▼
TIP:

For years, researchers have tried to determine what a good blood sugar level is for someone who is going to drive a car or operate any type of heavy machinery. Until recently, the answer was unclear. A new study tried to shed light on this issue by having 37 people with type 1 diabetes operate an advanced driving simulator while various levels of insulin and glucose were injected into their veins. The patients did not know what their blood sugar level was. Driving ability was studied at four different blood sugar levels: 110 mg/dl (normal), 65 mg/dl, 56 mg/dl, and less than 50 mg/dl. Surprisingly, the patients did not recognize that they were hypoglycemic until their blood sugars were less than 50 mg/dl. However, their driving performance was worse at every level of low blood sugar when compared to the normal blood sugar test. Thus, driving ability suffered even before the patients noticed that they had low blood sugar. With this in mind, you should always determine your blood sugar level before you drive a car. If your blood sugar is below 80 mg/dl, eat a snack to avoid impaired driving ability.

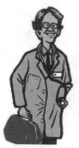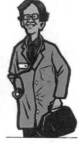

Specialist   **Generalist**

If I am hospitalized with diabetic ketoacidosis, should I be under the care of a diabetes specialist?

TIP:

For decades, the medical community has debated over who can give you the best care—a specialist or your general care physician. In debates like this, it's hard to come up with a clear answer. Often, the best solution is a mix of both. Recently, a study examined the outcome of patients who were hospitalized for diabetic keto-acidosis. They compared the care received from a general physician and an endocrinologist, a doctor who specializes in hormone diseases, including diabetes. Patients who received care from an endocrinologist had shorter hospital stays (3.3 days versus 4.9 days), lower hospital bills ($5,400 versus $10,100), and had to readmit themselves to the hospital less (2% versus 6%). Although there was no difference in death rates or complication rates between the endocrinologists and the generalists, the numbers suggest that endocrinologists are able to care for diabetic ketoacidosis more effectively in terms of time and money. However, just because you visit a specialist doesn't mean you can't still receive care from your general physician. If a diabetes specialist is available, try to coordinate the care you receive from them with the care you receive from your generalist. Working as a team will provide the best results.

*H*ow can sticking my finger for a blood
sample be less painful?

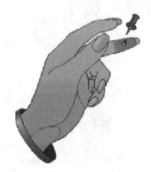

▼

TIP:

There are several ways to make getting a drop of blood less
painful.

- Do not swab your finger with alcohol. It stings, and it's not
  necessary.
- The tip of your finger is the most sensitive part. The side of your
  fingertip is less sensitive and is a better place to stick.
- "Milking" your finger for blood (squeezing your finger several
  times after you stick it) can be uncomfortable. Instead, make a
  puncture deep enough so that you don't need to squeeze your
  finger after the stick to get enough blood for the sample.
- Another trick is to trap extra blood in your finger before sticking
  it. Use the thumb of the same hand you're using to get the blood
  sample from. Slide your thumb from the base of your finger up
  to the last joint. This makes more blood available by pushing
  extra blood up into your fingertip. Also, you might try crowding
  your fingertips together. If your fingertip gets redder, there's
  more blood than usual. This makes it easier to get a drop of
  blood.
- Use another site besides the finger. See tip on page 919 for more.

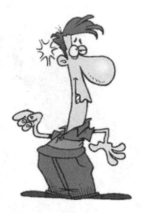

How long does it take me to recover from an episode of severe hypoglycemia?

TIP:

Low blood sugars can affect your ability to think clearly, because your brain does not work normally when it's not receiving enough sugar. The good news is that your brain function usually returns to normal after your low blood sugar is treated. Studies have shown that if you're practicing intensive diabetes management, frequent hypoglycemia does not cause any permanent brain damage. Researchers recently studied brain function before and after severe hypoglycemia. They found that brain function generally returns to normal within 36 hours of a severe hypoglycemic attack. However, they also found that patients with frequent hypoglycemia were more likely to suffer from extreme mood changes, such as depression, though whether or not frequent hypoglycemia causes these changes is still unclear. You should also be aware that prolonged or severe hypoglycemia that is untreated can cause permanent brain damage or lead to a coma.

*W*hy don't I wake up when my blood sugar gets low at night?

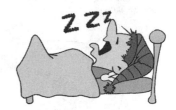

▼
TIP:

Hypoglycemia (low blood sugar) that hits while you sleep can be a serious problem. In fact, many people with diabetes are so afraid of an overnight attack they let their diabetes management slip. Their fear is understandable. Researchers have found that sleep can interfere with your body's normal response to hypoglycemia. Normally, when you have a low blood sugar, your body releases hormones that raise the blood sugar. Epinephrine (or adrenaline) is probably the most important of these chemicals. While you sleep, the epinephrine responses to hypoglycemia can be a lot lower than when you're awake, which might be why you don't wake up during the night if your blood sugar drops too low. If you think you are experiencing hypoglycemia during the night, you should set your alarm clock for 3:00 A.M. so you can check your blood sugar in the middle of the night. If your blood sugar is below 65 mg/dl, you should lower your nighttime insulin dose or take a bedtime snack in order to prevent hypoglycemia. You might also be able to change the kind of insulin you take to reduce nighttime low blood sugars.

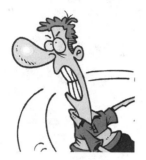

How can I help someone who has low blood sugar?

▼
TIP:

Be prepared. Low blood sugar can make people feel very irritable. Very low blood sugars can make it almost impossible to think clearly. A person with low blood sugar rarely feels like talking and may become irritated if you try to start a conversation. Instead of talking, try bringing something that will help the attack (such as a cup of fruit juice) and set it down by the person. If the person is having a low blood sugar, he will probably drink the juice. If he doesn't, you might ask if he's feeling all right. If his response is normal, tell him you think his blood sugar is low and ask him to test it. If you get a response that's not so normal (such as an angry stare or, "Why are you bothering me?!"), this may be a sign that the person needs help. Ask him to please drink the juice. If he is very confused, you might try to use glucagon. Glucagon is a hormone injection that raises blood sugar levels quickly. It is recommended that everyone who uses insulin have a glucagon kit on hand for emergencies. If the person you're trying to help is well prepared, he will probably have some available.

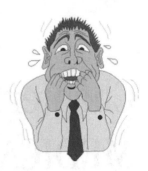

*W*hy do I feel shaky, sweaty, and have a
pounding heart when my blood sugar is
normal?

TIP:

*Y*ou could be having a panic attack. The symptoms of a panic
attack include feelings of terror, shakiness, sweatiness, and a
pounding heart. As you probably know, these are the symptoms
caused by low blood sugar. Often it is your fear of something happening that actually triggers a panic attack. If you're worried about
what might happen if "this or that" occurs, you can trigger your
adrenalin, and it's the adrenalin that causes the symptoms. The
symptoms cause your fear to further increase and you feel out of
control. For example, just the fear of having a low blood sugar reaction might be enough to trigger this vicious cycle. Also keep in
mind that if your blood sugar is usually very high, and then quickly
drops to normal levels, you can experience these symptoms.

If you think you are having panic attacks, counseling may be
helpful. If the fears that are triggering the attacks are related to your
diabetes, a few sessions of diabetes counseling should help you feel
more in control. Also, some medications have been shown to reduce
the intensity and frequency of anxiety attacks. Ask your diabetes
care team for more information.

Chapter 2
MEDICATIONS AND YOU

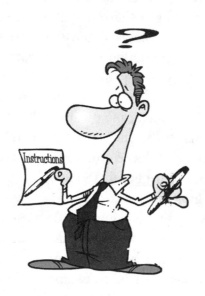

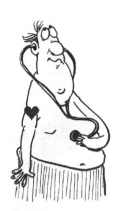

*B*esides keeping my cholesterol level low, is
there anything I can do to prevent heart
disease?

TIP:

Heart disease is the number one killer of people with diabetes.
Many of the strategies for preventing heart disease are well
known: stop smoking, control your blood pressure (less then
130/80), keep your LDL cholesterol level below 100, exercise regularly, and eat healthy. Other strategies, however, are less well
publicized, are still being studied, or are too specific to people with
diabetes to receive much media attention. For example, a recent
study of drugs called ACE inhibitors has shown that the risk of
having a heart attack or dying from cardiovascular disease was
reduced by 25% to 30% among people with diabetes who took an
ACE inhibitor. This was true even if the people did not have high
blood pressure or a history of heart disease. Since ACE inhibitors
have been shown to help people with diabetes by reducing the
progression of kidney disease, many physicians are prescribing
ACE inhibitors to reduce heart disease in their patients.

Taking a low-dose aspirin (81 mg) daily may also reduce the
risk of heart disease. To avoid stomach problems, use enteric-coated
aspirin.

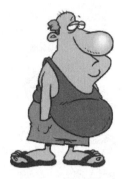

*I*s there an upper limit to how much insulin I can take for my diabetes?

TIP:

There is no upper limit to the insulin dose you can take. Most people with diabetes need between 1/2 and 1 unit of insulin per kilogram of body weight per day to control their diabetes. That means 35–70 units per day for an average 150-pound person. Needing any more than this is usually a sign of insulin resistance. Some very insulin-resistant people can require hundreds of units of insulin per day to control their blood sugars. A few medical scientists have argued that patients with type 2 diabetes and insulin resistance should be treated with insulin-sensitizing agents rather than insulin. They think that high levels of insulin increase the risk for cardiovascular disease, though there is no strong evidence to support this.

A principal side effect of using high doses of insulin is a 5% to 15% weight gain. The most important thing to keep in mind is that high blood glucose is more dangerous than an increase in medication, so talk to your doctor and do whatever it takes to get your blood glucose down.

*C*an I take my insulin without using a needle?

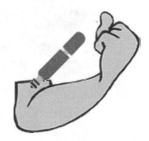

▼

TIP:

Many people prefer to inject insulin with an insulin injector. Insulin injectors have become smaller and more convenient and no longer require a prescription. They work by using compressed air to inject the insulin. You dial up the dose of insulin you want, press a button, and inject the insulin into your skin. Some individuals find that this is less painful than needle sticks. If you have a child with diabetes or a phobia of needles, insulin injectors can be an attractive choice. In addition, some studies show that insulin is absorbed more rapidly with injectors, since the insulin is more evenly dispersed than with needles.

The downside of insulin injectors is how expensive they are. Compared to needles, they're pretty pricey. You can obtain more information about insulin injectors by visiting a company's website, such as that available from Antares Pharma, Inc. for the Medi-Jector Vision, at *www.mediject.com*, or you can call toll-free at 1-800-328-3074. They will send you a free video describing the Medi-Jector Vision. Other available jet injectors include Advanta Jet (Activa Brand Products, Inc.), Gentle Jet (Activa Brand Products, Inc.), Advanta Jet ES (Activa Brand Products, Inc.), Vitajet 3 (Bioject Corp.), Injex (Equidyne Corp.), and At Last (Amira).

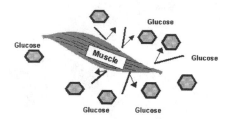

What is insulin resistance?

▼

TIP:

Resistance to insulin is a trait of type 2 diabetes. However, people without diabetes and people with type 1 diabetes can also have insulin resistance.

Basically, insulin resistance keeps your liver, muscles, and fat cells from working as they should. When working properly, insulin signals your liver that you have eaten and that it should store the extra glucose as starch. In between meals your liver makes glucose to supply the brain with energy. If you have insulin resistance, you're unable to stop the liver from making glucose, so your liver keeps making glucose even when you don't need it. In muscles, insulin allows cells to absorb glucose so that it can be used for muscle energy. If you have insulin resistance, muscles do not transport glucose into the cells well. In fat cells, insulin causes you to grow and store fat for use when you don't eat. This process is sluggish if you have insulin resistance.

To make up for insulin resistance in your liver and muscle cells, your pancreas produces too much insulin. After awhile, your body won't be able to keep up with this demand, your insulin levels drop, blood sugar levels get higher, and, eventually, you have diabetes.

*W*ill insulin analogs improve my diabetes treatment plan?

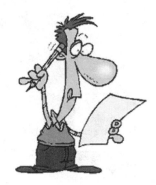

▼
TIP:

An insulin analog is a form of human insulin that is slightly different from the insulin that is secreted from the human pancreas. Surprisingly, these insulin analogs may work better than the insulin your body would normally produce. When your pancreas releases insulin, it secretes it into your bloodstream. When used to treat diabetes, insulin is usually injected under your skin, not into the bloodstream. Unfortunately, injected insulin may not be absorbed fast enough to be really effective. Insulin analogs are designed to help this process. By altering the chemical structure of human insulin, it can be more quickly absorbed, making it more effective when you eat a meal.

There are two choices of rapid-acting insulin analogs—insulin lispro and insulin aspart. Both insulin analogs are safe and can be injected 0–15 minutes before a meal. In addition, a long-acting insulin analog, insulin glargine ("glar-jeen"), is now available. It provides a steady level of background insulin throughout the day and night after one injection. This insulin does not have to be agitated before you inject it, but because of its acidity, it cannot be mixed with short-acting insulins.

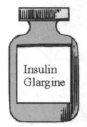

*A*re there any new insulins that could simplify *my diabetes care?*

TIP:

Yes. It's called insulin glargine. This man-made insulin is very similar to human insulin but it's designed to be more slowly absorbed from your skin. This means it only needs to be taken once a day. It gives you a very stable, effective background insulin level upon which you can add rapid-acting insulin for each meal (if you have type 1 diabetes) or no other insulin at all (if you have well-controlled type 2 diabetes). Several large clinical studies using insulin glargine have shown that it is better than NPH and ultralente insulin at providing a steady-state level of insulin in your blood.

If you are currently taking a combination of a long-acting and a rapid-acting insulin, you can substitute insulin glargine for your long-acting insulin. However, you can't combine insulin glargine with rapid-acting insulins in the syringe, so separate injections are necessary.

*C*an I premix my insulin lispro (Humalog)
   with NPH insulin and keep the syringe in
my purse until lunch?

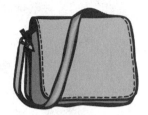

▼
TIP:

Y ou're probably aware that you can mix short-acting insulins or
   regular insulin with NPH insulin and inject them immediately
without any problem. However, some worry that if these insulins are
mixed and then kept for several hours, the NPH insulin will change
some of the regular insulin to a longer-acting form of insulin. In fact,
the package insert for insulin lispro suggests that you should not prefill the syringe with both insulins without injecting them immediately.
However, a recent study has shown that these mixed insulins are
stable for up to 28 days and can be taken without any major
problems, with one exception. If you usually mix the two insulins,
and then decide not to prefill one day (or vice versa), the short acting
insulin (insulin lispro) will act differently.

   Therefore, yes, you can mix the two insulins and keep them in
your purse until you need them, but only if you plan on doing this
every day. Be sure to mix the insulins (except with ultralente
insulin). Importantly, Humalog should not be mixed with ultralente
insulin more than 5 minutes prior to injection because ultralente will
delay the onset of activity in the Humalog.

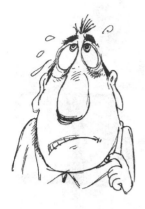

Should I be afraid to start taking insulin?

TIP:

If you've been asked to start taking insulin, you may have some initial fears. You may believe that your diabetes is not "serious" as long as you don't have to take insulin. Or you may believe that being on insulin means you have failed in your diabetes management. Or you might have a fear of needles. But your doctor has good reasons for wanting you to start insulin, some of which may include:

■ Your body is no longer responding effectively to oral medication.
■ Insulin may be more affordable.
■ You do not like the side effects of oral medication.
■ Oral medications are not safe for you. For example, if you are on dialysis, oral medications can be dangerous.

Insulin is one of the most powerful medications we have to keep blood sugars down. Nowadays, there are ways to take insulin that are very flexible, including needle-free solutions to injecting. Talk to your diabetes team and with other people who take insulin to find out the regimen that will work best for you. You will find that instead of making things more complicated and serious, taking insulin may make your life with diabetes easier.

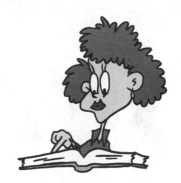

*W*here can I get more information on
insulin sensitizers?

TIP:

Insulin sensitizers are the newest oral medications approved for type
2 diabetes. They can be effectively used with other medications and
have allowed many individuals to stop insulin injections and use only
oral medications. The first medication on the market was troglitazone
(Rezulin), which was extremely popular in Japan and the United
States. Unfortunately, it was very toxic to the liver and has been taken
off the market. Currently, there are two FDA-approved insulin
sensitizers on the market—rosiglitazone (Avandia) and pioglitazone
(Actos). Neither of these have shown serious danger to the liver in
animals or humans. You should be aware that these medications
might cause you to retain fluids, which may require you to take a
diuretic (water pill). Metformin also increases sensitivity to insulin
but is not usually thought of as an "insulin sensitizer." Its primary
function is to decrease your liver's ability to make sugar.

Information on each of these medications may be obtained from
the company's web site. The website for Avandia is
www.avandia.com, or you can call (800) 282-6342. For Actos, the
web site address is *www.actos.com*, or you can call (877) 825-3327.
Ask your doctor or diabetes care team if you have any questions.

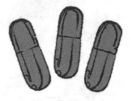

*C*an I take a pill to lose weight?

▼
TIP:

One new drug called orlistat (Xenical) has been tested in people with type 2 diabetes and can probably be used safely. This drug works by not allowing your body to absorb fats from the food you eat. As a result, dietary fats are not digested. In a study of 391 seriously overweight men with type 2 diabetes, men taking orlistat lost about 6% of their body weight, on average, over a one-year period compared to about a 4% weight loss in men taking a placebo (a "dummy pill"). This is a 4-pound difference in a 200-pound man (200 × 6% = 12 pounds; 200 × 4% = 8 pounds). Blood sugars went down in both groups and were only slightly lower in the orlistat group. Because the drug doesn't allow you to absorb as much fat, you might be at risk for low levels of fat-soluble vitamins, such as vitamin A, E, K, and D. If you're taking orlistat, you should consider taking a vitamin supplement. While orlistat can aid in weight loss, it's no replacement for healthy eating and an exercise strategy. Weigh the costs and the benefits and speak with your diabetes care team before deciding whether or not orlistat is the right approach for you.

Chapter 3
PLANNING YOUR MEALS

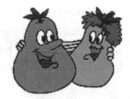

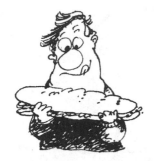

If I eat the right foods, does the amount matter?

▼
TIP:

Whether you're eating ice cream or carrot sticks, portion size does matter. Body weight increases, decreases, or stays the same based on how many calories you eat versus how many calories you burn. If the calories you eat equal the calories you use, your weight will remain the same. On the other hand, if you burn more calories than you take in, you can expect to lose weight. It is important to eat a variety of healthy foods, and even more important to eat the recommended portions. Eating too much of one type of food, or not enough of another, can be unhealthy. When the urge to eat is too strong, try eating "free foods." Free foods are items that have less than 20 calories per serving. All items must be sugar-free and should be low fat. Below is a list of some free foods.

Drinks—bouillon, diet sodas, diet club soda, diet tonic water
Fruits—1/2 cup cranberries, 1/2 cup rhubarb
Vegetables/Greens—cabbage, celery, cucumber, green onion, mushrooms, radishes, zucchini, endive, escarole, lettuce, romaine, spinach
Sweet Substitutes—sugar-free candy, gelatin, sugar-free gum, sugar-free jam, sugar-free jelly
Condiments—mustard, taco sauce, vinegar

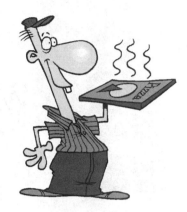

Does fast food like pizza fit into my meal plan?

▼
TIP:

Diabetes meal plans have changed quite a bit in the last decade. In the past, people with type 1 diabetes were told to follow rigid eating patterns. Rich foods like pizza and ice cream were strictly off limits. The timing, amount, and kind of food you ate were restricted, and the food you ate had to be matched to your insulin dose. Luckily, things are a little more flexible now. Since the availability of rapid-acting insulin (such as insulin lispro), people with type 1 diabetes can follow a normal, balanced diet. Insulin can be matched to your daily lifestyle, instead of the other way around. For example, a salad with chicken strips and a diet cola might require one or two units of insulin. Two slices of pizza, a glass of milk, and ice cream might require 10 units. With training from your diabetes care team and a little personal experience, you can learn how much insulin you need to control your blood sugars for different types of meals. If you are using the old style therapy of pattern control, talk to your diabetes care team about how to change your therapy to the food you eat. You may also contact the American Association of Diabetes Educators at (800) 832-6874 to find someone who can help you with your diabetes meal plans.

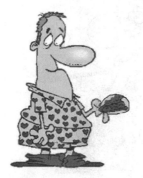

*W*hy do I eat more than I should in the evenings?

TIP:

Many people eat sensibly during the day, only to eat too much at night. This can make it hard to keep blood sugars under control. There could be several reasons why you eat too much or eat the wrong foods at night. Maybe you've been trying so hard to eat "healthy" that you are feeling deprived of some of your "comfort" foods. Perhaps you manage to ignore uncomfortable feelings like depression, anxiety, loneliness, or even boredom during the day, but these feelings surface once the sun goes down. If these reasons explain why you are eating more at night, you have taken the first step toward changing that pattern. The following is an example of small steps you might take to change your pattern:

- **Step 1**—Figure out why you overeat in the evenings. For example, you're strict with your diet during the day and you miss the cookies you usually eat for lunch.
- **Step 2**—Figure out what might be a healthier response. Have a plan for cookie cravings in the evening. Try eating one with lunch and three at night, instead of four all at once. Then, slowly decrease the amount you eat over time.
- **Step 3**—Substitute a healthier snack, such as a fruit, for the cookie.

*H*ow can I eat less fat at a fast food
restaurant?

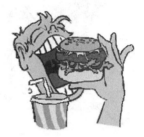

▼
TIP:

S ince most fast food restaurants have adopted the "bigger is better"
attitude, classic small, medium, and large sizes are no longer
available. Now you have large, extra large, and supersize. Because of
these larger portion sizes, the average American takes in 150 more
calories a day, and most of these calories are fat. Although an extra
150 calories a day doesn't sound like much, these calories add up
with bad results for you. There are many ways you can lower calories
and fat in a fast food restaurant. The easiest way is to choose the
smallest serving available. Just choosing a plain cheeseburger instead
of a double cheeseburger will remove more than 200 calories. Most
important is to choose low-fat items in place of high-fat items. For
example, choose a baked potato with salsa or steak sauce (instead of
butter and sour cream) to replace French fries. Order sandwiches
without fancy sauces, and order salads with low-fat dressings (or "on-
the-side" to control the amount of dressing you put on your salad).
When low-fat options are not available, leave a few fries on your
plate or a few bites of your sandwich, and skip dessert. The best way
to reduce fat in fast food? Reduce how often you eat fast food.

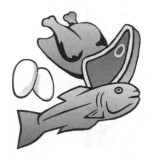

*W*ill the new high-protein, low-carbohydrate diets help me lose weight?

TIP:

Popular low-carbohydrate diets promise quick weight loss while you take in unlimited calories from protein and fat. People who support these diets claim that carbohydrates are harmful because they increase the insulin levels in your blood. They suggest high insulin levels cause obesity, which leads to many other problems, including diabetes. All of this sounds exciting. Finally, a "magic" way to lose weight. Unfortunately, it's not that simple. Severely reducing carbohydrates in your diet can give you quick weight loss, but there may be consequences. The quick weight you lose from these diets is mostly water loss. Carbohydrates are the main fuel for many of your body's systems (including the brain). If there is not enough carbohydrate coming in, your body turns to different energy sources. Your body first uses stored glucose (glycogen) and when that runs out, the protein in your muscles may be converted to sugar. Fat is also broken down for energy. This sounds good, but the breakdown can give you nausea, constipation, and low energy. If you have diabetes, you may be at a higher risk for some of the more severe consequences of a low-carbohydrate diet, such as diabetic ketoacidosis. The best way to lose weight, and keep it off, is still the "calories in" vs. "calories out" method. At this time there are no long-term scientific studies to support the claims of low-carbohydrate diets.

How can I keep from gaining weight during the holidays?

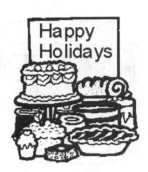

▼
TIP:

The reasons for weight gain (and high blood sugars!) during the holiday season are no mystery. People gain weight during the holidays because they eat too much and get less physical activity. This does not have to happen. The holiday season is a time for renewing family and spiritual ties through tradition. If you have diabetes, a healthy response to the holiday season may include beginning new traditions. For example, substituting pumpkin custard for pumpkin pie as the traditional dessert for Thanksgiving dinner will get rid of the piecrust (and a lot of calories). Most importantly, you should maintain your daily routine as much as possible. That means getting out of bed at your usual time, testing your blood sugar at regular intervals, eating only at mealtime, and performing your daily exercise. If you take care of yourself during the holidays, you will feel better and reduce the chance for unwanted weight gain.

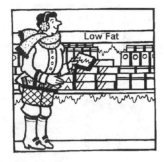

What are the advantages of a low-fat meal plan?

TIP:

Staying on a diet is difficult. Cutting down on the food you eat can result in a cycle of weight loss followed by weight gain. Fat has more than twice as many calories per gram as either protein or carbohydrate. If you cut fat, you will cut calories. A low-fat meal plan helps you

Lose weight
Lower cholesterol
Improve your blood lipids
Lower your risk for cardiovascular disease
Reduce your risk for colon cancer, since a low-fat meal plan is associated with high fiber
Eat larger portions of food without the calories
Improve your self-esteem

So do what you can to cut fat from your eating and you'll be well on your way to better health.

*H*ow can I organize my meal
preparation?

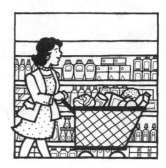

▼
TIP:

I t's hard to find the time to do anything anymore. Still, sticking with
your meal plan is important. By planning time for food chores and
cooking you can save time later. The following schedule allows you
to stick to your meal plan while cooking only once a month.

1. Sit down with your family and make a list of their favorite foods
   (1/2 hour).
2. From that list, put together menus for six days (1/2 hour).
3. Make a shopping list of the food and supplies needed to make
   these meals and multiply the list by four. Remember to include
   freezer bags (1/2 hour).
4. Shop for all the food and supplies (2.5 hours).
5. Take one whole day or two evenings and cook four meals worth
   of all the dishes you have chosen. Freeze everything in portion
   sizes big enough for one meal (6–8 hours).
6. Go out to dinner and relax.
7. You now have 24 days of meals prepared. Rotate menus each day
   for the next four weeks. The remaining days of the month are for
   eating out (remember, you still need to eat healthy).

Using this plan, it will take you about 12 hours to prepare a month's
worth of meals.

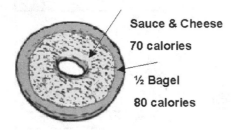

Sauce & Cheese
70 calories

½ Bagel
80 calories

*I*s it okay for me to eat snacks?

▼
TIP:

Absolutely! In fact, snacks can be a very important part of your meal plan. Many people think of snacks as the same as "junk food." This is not always the case. Snacking can be healthy and can help you avoid being hungry all the time. It can be designed to fit your needs and your diabetes management plan. However, snacks *must* be included in your total meal plan. Don't overdo snacks just like you don't overdo eating your regular foods. One way to do this is to schedule your snacks. It is often helpful to have your snacks at the same time each day. What time of day do you get hungry—mid-morning, mid-afternoon, evening, all the time? Choosing healthy snacks may get you through the day without overeating. Healthy snacks do not have to be "fat free" either. If not eaten too much, fat is an important source of energy. Talk with your diabetes care team to help you plan for a tasty snack like a bagel pizza. The *Snack, Munch, Nibble Nosh Book* is available through the American Diabetes Association bookstore and has many healthy snack recipes.

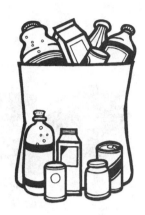

*W*hat foods should I keep on hand for quick
meal preparation and snacks?

TIP:

This depends on a lot of things. Every person has different tastes
and preferences. However, some foods are good to keep
available for last-minute meals or healthy snacks no matter what your
taste preference. These foods can be combined to make many
different items. They are healthy, low fat, and will not spoil quickly.
Be sure to check labels and don't eat out-dated foods. Below are
some foods that you may want to keep on hand.

vegetables (mixed
   and varieties)
fruits (water
   packed)
meats (water
   packed, low fat,
   low salt)
soups/broth (low
   fat, low sodium)
evaporated milk
tomato sauces
   (low fat)
macaroni

spaghetti
beans
rice
peanut butter
   (low fat)
pudding (low fat,
   low sugar)
gelatin (low sugar)
spices/Worcester-
   shire sauce
cooking spray oil
salad dressing
   (low fat)

mustard/mayon-
   naise (low fat)
salsa/relish
fruit spread
   (low sugar)
syrup (low sugar)
soda crackers
graham crackers
flour/biscuit mix/
   pancake mix
non-fat dry milk
   powder
spices

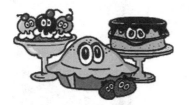

*C**an people with diabetes eat foods
that contain sugar?*

TIP:

In the past, sugar was strictly off limits for people who had
diabetes. It was believed that simple sugar (like table sugar) would
be more quickly absorbed and lead to a higher blood sugar than other
carbohydrates. Research has shown that this is not true. The
American Diabetes Association has relaxed its guidelines on sugar for
people with diabetes. Now you can eat foods containing sugar. Just be
sure to count the sugars as part of your total carbohydrates, just as
you would with starches. Many exchange lists exclude dessert foods.
Below is a chart giving approximate carbohydrate counts for some
sample dessert foods:

Dessert	Size: 1 exchange, which is 15 grams of carbohydrate or 1 bread or fruit exchange
Cake, unfrosted	1 1/2 inch square
Cake, with frosting	1 inch square
Ice cream, ice milk, sherbet, frozen yogurt	1/2 cup
Cookies, round sandwich type	1 cookie
Table sugar	1 tablespoon

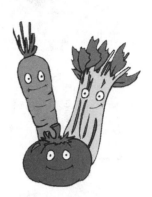

*H*ow do I get protein in my diet if I am
vegetarian?

TIP:

M any foods contain protein, but meat, eggs, and dairy foods
contain "complete proteins." Grains and legumes (beans, peas,
and lentils) contain "incomplete proteins." If your vegetarian diet
includes eggs and/or dairy products, then your diet likely provides
enough "complete proteins." If you do not eat eggs or dairy foods you
must combine two incomplete protein foods in a meal so that each
meal provides the complete proteins you need.

The following table shows some of the ways incomplete proteins
can be combined to make a complete protein:

Rice plus:	Wheat plus:	Legumes plus:
Wheat	Legumes	Corn
or	or	or
legumes	soybeans and nuts	rice
or	or	or
sesame seeds	soybeans and rice	wheat

The serving size is 1/3–1/2 cup.

Your diabetes care team and a dietitian can determine your protein
needs, as well as your likes and dislikes, to create a meal plan that
works for you.

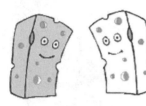

*I*s white cheese better for my diabetic diet than yellow cheese?

TIP:

No. All cheeses (hard, soft, and processed) have a high fat content. Color is added to cheese and is not related to how much fat is in the cheese. In most cheeses, about 75% of the calories come from fat! There are several "low-fat" cheeses on the market, but the taste and texture are usually different from regular cheese. Read the labels and experiment with different varieties to find the types you enjoy most. The chart below lists cheeses, the percent fat for a 1-ounce serving (about one slice), and exchange information for each cheese. More "cheesy" information can be found using the Internet. The key words to use are "cheese" or "diet and nutrition."

Cheese (1 ounce)	% fat	Diabetic exchanges
Cheddar	74	1 meat
Mozzarella	56	1 medium fat
Bleu	73	1 medium fat
Feta	59	1/2 medium fat
Parmesan	62	2 medium fats
Velveeta®	62	1 medium fat
Brie	75	2 fats
Swiss	66	1/2 fat plus 1 medium meat
Gouda	69	1/2 fat plus 1 medium meat
Cream Cheese	90	2 fats

D *o I need to pay attention to how much fiber I eat?*

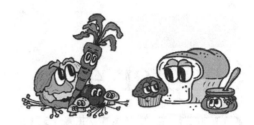

▼ TIP:

Fiber is the part of plant food that doesn't get digested. The ADA recommends eating 20 to 35 grams of fiber each day. Fiber is important in your diet because it can slow the absorption of sugar into your blood. Fiber helps your bowels stay regular, lowers the level of cholesterol in your blood, and helps you feel full and satisfied. Some studies have also shown high-fiber diets can improve A1C. Fiber is found in whole grains, breads, rice, pasta, dried beans and legumes, as well as fruits and vegetables. These foods may also reduce your risk for colon cancer and heart disease. If you eat a diet rich in these foods, you will not need a fiber supplement.

Food	Portion size	Fiber	Exchange rate
Rolled oat meal	1/2 cup dry	4 grams	2 bread exchanges
Whole-wheat bread	1 oz slice	2 grams	1 bread exchange
Green peas	2/3 cup	4 grams	1 bread exchange
Wax beans	2/3 cup	2 grams fiber	Not counted as an exchange
Apple	1 large	5 grams fiber	2 fruit exchanges

Chapter 4
GET MOVING!

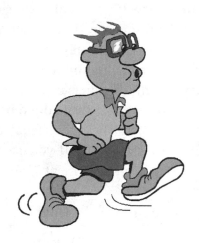

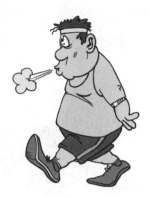

*H*ow do I know if my exercise program is "aerobic"?

TIP:

The term "aerobic" refers to exercise that increases your heart rate. You can check your heart rate (or pulse rate) with the help of a stopwatch or a watch with a second hand. Place your index and middle finger on your wrist, just below the base of your thumb, or on your neck on either side of your Adam's apple. Count the number of beats for 15 seconds and then multiply this number by 4 to determine your heart rate per minute. Your resting heart rate should be 60–100 beats per minute. To find if your exercise program is aerobic, determine your target heart rate range (see chart below) and count your heart rate during or after exercise. When any activity raises your heart rate to within your target heart rate range, you are "aerobic."

Age	Normal resting heart rate	Target heart rate range
30–39 yrs	60–100	95–133
40–49 yrs	60–100	90–126
50–59 yrs	60–100	85–119
60–69 yrs	60–100	80–112
70–79 yrs	60–100	75–105
80–89 yrs	60–100	70–98
90+ yrs	60–100	65–91

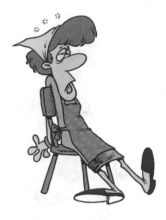

*C*an I consider household chores
  exercise?

▼
TIP:

Yes. Have you ever raced around the house to get the dusting and vacuuming done before guests arrive, and then found you're out of energy? Have you noticed your blood glucose level gets low whenever you mow the lawn? The U.S. Surgeon General suggests 30 minutes of moderate physical activity at least 5 days per week. Moderate intensity is anything that raises your heart rate. Thirty minutes sounds like a lot, but you don't have to do it all at once. If your chores increase your heart rate for 10 minutes or more, you can count it toward your exercise goal. Ten straight minutes of moderate-intensity activity 3 times per day would give you the recommended 30-minute workout. Mowing your lawn with a push mower, moving furniture when you vacuum, chopping wood, and washing the floor on your hands and knees are all good examples of moderate-intensity exercise. Light dusting, washing dishes, and ironing are considered to be light-intensity activities and would not count toward your daily activity minutes. So, go ahead . . . retire the housekeeper and the lawn crew—do these household chores yourself and build a healthier you!

*W*hy should I exercise?

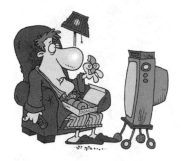

▼
TIP:

B ecause it might save your life! Exercise has been recommended for people with diabetes for many years and is one of the basic elements of diabetes treatment. However, it was not scientifically proven that exercise led to better health or a longer life span with diabetes until recently. In a new study, more than 1,200 men with type 2 diabetes were followed for an average period of 12 years. Death rates in these men were examined based on their level of physical fitness. Men who said that they were not physically active had a 70% higher death rate compared to men who were. In addition, men in the lowest fitness group had double the death rate of the men in the highest fitness group. Exercise continued to help even after other factors—such as glucose levels, cholesterol levels, body weight, smoking, and high blood pressure—were under control. So now we can say with certainty that exercise can help you live a longer, healthier life with type 2 diabetes. This is the best reason we can give you to get off the couch and start exercising!

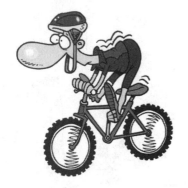

Does my diabetes make it harder for me to exercise?

TIP:

It's possible that if you are not in good shape, having diabetes might make exercise harder for you, especially at first. Researchers believe there is a possibility that diabetes may damage the cells that line the blood vessels, which would mean your blood vessels wouldn't dilate correctly during exercise. To get blood to your muscles while you exercise, your blood vessels need to dilate normally. If this doesn't happen, it may be harder for you to do the same exercise as another person your age or in the same shape as you. This can be frustrating, and may make it difficult for you to keep exercising. Even though it is hard, it's worth it to make the effort. Research has shown that exercise lowers blood sugar and cuts down on stress. Keep in mind that exercise will affect your blood sugar levels. If you're just starting out, you may need to adjust your medication to match these blood sugar changes. Remember— exercise gets easier the more you do it. Once you get in the swing of things, diabetes should not keep you from meeting your exercise goals.

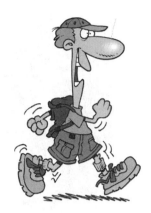

*H*ow can I measure the distance I walk
each day?

▼

TIP:

A pedometer is a little, watch-sized device that counts your steps
for you. Pedometers can be found at most sporting goods stores
and cost about $10.00. Pedometers need to be attached to your
clothing around your waist first thing in the morning and worn the
entire day. Begin the first few days recording your steps and log this
number on your calendar. If you walk fewer than 8,000–10,000 steps
per day, you need to increase your daily activity. Fewer than
8,000 steps per day is considered sedentary, which means you're
not getting enough exercise. Between 8,000 and 10,000 steps is
considered active. Increase your total daily steps by walking 100
extra steps every day. Set a higher goal each month until you are
walking 9,000–10,000 steps per day. Then try to build up to more
than 10,000 steps each day. Depending on the length of your stride,
these additional steps will add up to approximately 2 miles. This can
help you lose weight and feel better. So keep walking!

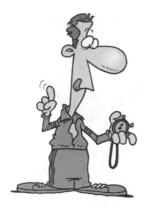

*D*o *I need a personal trainer to help me with my exercise program?*

▼

TIP:

A personal trainer is not necessary. However, if you no longer see results from your exercise, can't reach your weight goal, or are just bored with your routine, a personal trainer can help you get back on track. Just two or three sessions with a personal trainer can be helpful. Most gyms offer personal trainers free of charge if you're a member. When choosing a trainer, be careful. Many people who claim to be trainers are not professionally certified. It is important that you know how to choose a certified personal trainer. Listed below are three organizations that certify trainers.

■ American College of Sports Medicine (ACSM)
■ American College of Exercise (ACE)
■ National Strength and Conditioning Association (NSCA)

If your trainer is certified by any of these organizations you can be sure that he or she is a professional. For more information, you may contact your gym manager or use the web site *www.acefitness.org* for help.

Chapter 5
WHAT TO DO WITH
HEALTH CARE

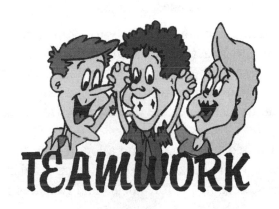

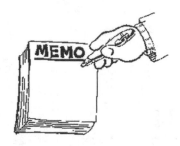

How can I make the most out of my appointments with my diabetes care team?

▼

TIP:

There are several ways you can get the most from your appointment. For instance:

Be prepared and come a little early to allow time for check-in.

If you were told to get lab tests, get them done several days before your appointment. If they were done somewhere else, call to make sure your results were sent to your doctor's office. It might be up to you to get the results and bring them with you to the visit.

Bring your blood sugar meter and a log of your blood sugar readings. If you do not check your blood sugars regularly, take several blood glucose readings before meals and two hours after meals during the week before your appointment.

Bring your prescription bottles with you. If you are taking vitamins, supplements, or herbal remedies, bring them with you, too.

Jot down questions you want to ask your diabetes care team.

If you need a referral, make sure you have it with you when you go to your appointment.

Bring a pen and paper to write down instructions and other information.

Take off your shoes and socks as soon as you get into the room so that your provider can examine your feet.

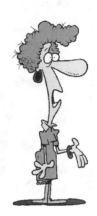

*W*hat should I do if my diabetes treatment plan isn't working?

▼
TIP:

If you are not meeting your diabetes treatment goals, one of two things could be happening:

1. You are not completely following your treatment plan.
2. Your treatment plan is not right for you.

Meet with a certified diabetes educator or a registered dietitian to talk about your diet if you have not yet done so or if it has been longer than two years since you've had any dietary counseling. You may also need to meet with an exercise trainer if there's something keeping you from regular exercise. An exercise trainer can design an exercise plan that fits your abilities. Finally, discuss your medications with your doctor. Are you taking them in the right amount and at the right time of day? The American Diabetes Association states that an A1C level of less than 7.0% is what you're shooting for with therapy. If your doctor's care does not give you an A1C of less than 8.0%, it's time to talk with your diabetes care team. You can request a meeting with a diabetologist or a certified diabetes educator. He or she will work with your diabetes care team to help you meet the goals of your diabetes treatment plan.

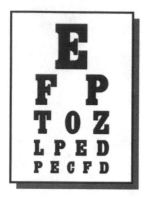

How often should I get my eyes examined?

TIP:

Currently, the American Diabetes Association recommends that if you have diabetes you should have your eyes checked by an ophthalmologist once a year. However, this is not a rigid recommendation. Doctors have suggested that in some patients, an eye exam every two to three years is enough. You probably do not need an eye exam every year if

- You have had a recent normal eye exam
- You have had type 1 diabetes for less than 10 years
- You have excellent glucose control
- You do not also have diseases that lead to a high rate of retinopathy, such as high blood pressure or kidney disease

If you have background retinopathy (changes in the back of your eye that indicate your diabetes is affecting your eye but not threatening your vision at the moment), you should continue to have yearly eye exams. The best person to recommend how often you should get an eye exam is your own eye doctor. Be sure to ask him at your next visit how often you should get an eye exam.

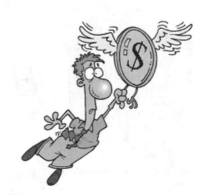

How can my social security check cover the cost of a healthy meal plan?

▼

TIP:

When your personal income only covers the bare essentials, it's difficult to afford healthy foods like cherries, bell peppers, and whole-wheat bread. If you want to make healthier food choices, how can you fit it into your budget? Your community may be the answer. The government and your community offer many programs to help people eat healthy. These programs are not charity. They're a public service to the entire community. Look through the city and government pages of your telephone book for the following:

- ■ Health Department
- ■ Families First Program
- ■ Women, Infant, and Children Program
- ■ Human Services Department
- ■ Senior Services
- ■ Senior Companion Program
- ■ Family and Community Services

These resources can help you get the healthy meals you need. And remember, unhealthy food such as fast food and processed food can be even more expensive than healthy food. Try to get the food your body needs. It's worth the effort.

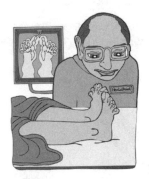

*H*ow can I keep my feet healthy?

TIP:

First of all, it's good that you're concerned about your feet. People with diabetes often develop foot problems, but some simple care can prevent complications. Try the following:

☐ Keep your feet clean and don't forget to check them every day. Better yet, have someone check your feet for you.

☐ Make sure someone trims your nails on a regular schedule.

☐ If you have toenail problems, poor circulation, and/or nerve damage, you should see a podiatrist.

☐ Be sure to wear socks or shoe inserts that absorb sweat.

☐ Always check your shoes for foreign objects.

☐ Make sure that new shoes fit properly and take the time to break them in slowly.

☐ When you find shoes that are particularly comfortable, buy two pairs.

☐ Try wearing two different pairs of shoes every day. Wear one pair to work in the morning, and then change into the other pair half way through the day. If you alternate shoes each day, it's better for your feet and for your shoes.

For additional tips on foot care, see the section *101 Foot Care Tips for People with Diabetes.*

*H*ow can I get my HMO to provide
better care for my diabetes?

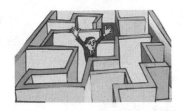

▼
TIP:

G etting proper medical care can be tricky with managed health
care, but you'll probably find that you can get excellent care
once you have learned how to work the system. Your primary care
provider is the key to getting good care in a health maintenance
organization (HMO). He or she is the person who can help you find
resources in your health care organization, including specialists,
diabetes educators, and dietitians. You must also know the current
standards of care for diabetes. Make it clear to your primary care
provider that you expect these standards to be met. This means
providing the supplies you need for home blood glucose monitoring,
testing of your A1C level every three months, prescribing
medications, and yearly checkups of your eyes, kidneys, and
cholesterol levels. Finally, many HMOs have special programs for
people with chronic diseases like diabetes. Ask your primary care
provider about Case Management services in your HMO. Case
managers include nurses, social workers, and diabetes educators.
Case managers can be helpful because they know the ropes and can
help you get through the red tape of your HMO.

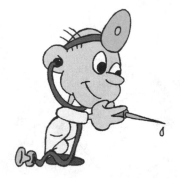

*W*hat vaccinations should I receive if I
have diabetes?

TIP:

V accinations are very important for everyone, but even more so if
you have diabetes. This is because high blood sugar may lower
your body's ability to fight infections. Below is a list of the
vaccinations you should get if you have diabetes.

■ Flu (influenza)—Including pregnant women who are in their second or third trimester during the flu season.
■ Pneumonia—Especially if you've had your spleen removed.
■ Hepatitis A—Especially if you're traveling to a foreign country
that may not have clean water and good sewage disposal. Also, if
you have liver or kidney disease or blood clotting disorders.
■ Hepatitis B—Especially health care workers, travelers to certain
countries, people on dialysis, and people who must receive donor
blood products.
■ Measles, mumps, rubella—If you were born in 1957 or later.
■ Chicken pox—If you are 13 years or older and have not already
had chicken pox.

Vaccinations may not be safe for everyone, so be sure and talk to
your diabetes care team about which vaccinations are right for you.

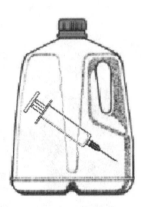

*H*ow can I throw away my insulin syringes
safely?

▼
TIP:

W hile it's true that insulin syringes in your trash can be a health
risk to the people who handle your trash, there are no laws that
require you to throw away your used syringes any special way. On the
other hand, hospitals and medical clinics are required to dispose of
sharp medical waste in puncture-resistant containers. The companies
that make insulin syringes also make containers that allow you to
dispose of syringes safely. However, these containers are often
expensive and hard to find. If you use insulin syringes, you can safely
throw them away by putting them in a strong plastic container with a
lid, such as a used milk bottle or an empty dishwashing or laundry
detergent bottle. Make sure the lid is tight and won't come off. People
with blood-borne diseases such as hepatitis or HIV should be very
careful of how they get rid of their insulin syringes and should
discuss what they can do to be safe with their diabetes care team.

*W*ill my mother receive good care for her diabetes in a nursing home?

TIP:

It's possible, but not certain. Diabetes is common among the elderly. Unfortunately, since some patients in nursing homes suffer from other serious and chronic conditions, day-to-day diabetes care may be overlooked. It is important to find out if your mother's nursing home follows the ADA guidelines for standard care. You or another family member may want to meet with the nursing home staff and see how they handle diabetes. Questions you might ask:

How many times a day is blood sugar monitored?
When are diabetes medicines given during the day?
What are the diabetes treatment goals?
How often will her feet be checked?
How quickly is hypoglycemia recognized and treated?
Is blood pressure normally monitored?

You should also see if they evaluate for diabetic complications of the eye, kidney, and heart at least once a year. Schedule a periodic review of her status with the charge nurse or administrator. By making it clear that you expect excellent diabetes care for your mother, you can help make your mother's stay at the nursing home a positive experience.

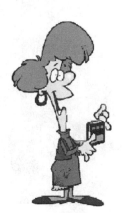

*W**hat is involved in starting insulin pump therapy?*

TIP:

Starting pump therapy takes time and money. However, most insurance plans will cover insulin pumps (which cost about $5,000) for patients with type 1 diabetes. Supplies (tubing, insulin reservoir, adhesive tape, IV prep, etc.) add another $100 to $200 a month. It then takes several hours of training to learn to use a pump. This training includes

■ Checking your blood glucose after food, activity, and medicine
■ Reviewing the factors that are affecting your highs and lows
■ Adjusting the doses to find what works for you
■ Reviewing your meal plan strategy with a registered dietitian
■ More structure in your daily routine until your insulin needs have been determined

Once your training period is complete, you will probably have better diabetes control and fewer episodes of low blood sugar. Ask your diabetes care team to refer you to someone who uses a pump and is willing to discuss his or her experiences. It is important to take the time to learn about insulin pumps before making a decision to buy one.

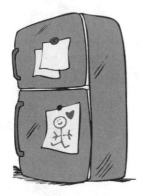

*S*hould I refrigerate my insulin?

▼
TIP:

The vials of insulin that you are using right now should be left at room temperature and away from heat sources and light. Don't leave insulin in your car where it can become hot or cold very quickly. If you take insulin with your food, you need to keep that insulin with you. You probably don't need to carry an insulin cooler. Your pocket or purse will work just fine (just don't leave it some place that's very warm or cold), since modern insulin is stable for at least one month at room temperature.

You should keep unopened vials of insulin in the refrigerator but never in the freezer. However, don't put the vials in the refrigerator door, because the jarring movements of the door may lower the activity of the insulin. Try to keep your insulin on a low shelf in the refrigerator so it doesn't run the risk of freezing. Always examine your insulin before injecting it. Do not use insulin that is past the expiration date on the label and do not use insulin that is discolored or has clumps in it.

C^{*an I reuse my syringes?*}

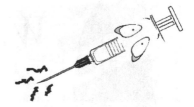

▼
TIP:

M any people reuse their syringes until the needles become dull. For most, this is safe and practical. However, the makers of disposable syringes recommend that syringes be thrown away after only one use. This is because after a syringe is used, there's no guarantee that it's sterile. If you plan on reusing a syringe, keep these things in mind:

■ Recap the syringe after each use.
■ Throw away a syringe if the needle bends or becomes dull, or if you can't read the numbers on the side.
■ Do not clean the needle with alcohol because this may remove the lubricant and make the next injection uncomfortable.
■ Never use a syringe that has been used by someone else. You could possibly be infected with very dangerous illnesses (such as AIDS and hepatitis).

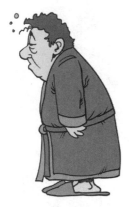

*W*hy do I feel tired all the time?

▼

TIP:

There could be lots of reasons. It could be a sign that your blood sugars are too high, or you're not getting enough exercise. Your heart may not be getting oxygen to your body correctly. It could also be a sign of depression. High blood sugars can make you feel very tired, and people with diabetes who are depressed are more likely to have high blood sugars. The more tired you are, the harder it is to take care of your diabetes. The combination of depression and poorly controlled diabetes can lead to a powerful sense of fatigue and loss of control. To break this cycle, work with your diabetes care team to get your blood sugars under control. Be patient. It may take several weeks for the effects of lowered blood sugar levels to provide you with more energy. Tell your diabetes care team your thoughts and feelings about being tired. If you improve your glucose control but still feel like you are failing and that nothing helps, you may be clinically depressed. Negative thinking makes you feel helpless. Counseling may help you learn how to change your thoughts, which may help your depression.

W *hy do I keep having bladder infections?*

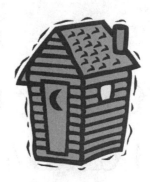

TIP:

B ladder infections are common in women with diabetes. Unlike regular bladder infections, however, women with diabetes may not have pain or burning with urination, or bloody urine. These are called "asymptomatic" bladder infections (meaning there are no symptoms) and a recent study showed that 26% of women with diabetes had this type of bladder infection. Because there are no symptoms, only a urine test can tell you if you have an asymptomatic bladder infection.

These bladder infections probably occur because glucose in your urine provides a good place for bacteria to grow and your body's normal response to infection may be impaired because of your diabetes. Asymptomatic bladder infections are more common if you are older, have long-standing diabetes, spill large amounts of protein in your urine, or have had a bladder infection during the previous year. If your doctor prescribes medicine, be sure to follow the full course of treatment. If you notice a change in the color, concentration, or smell of your urine, you should talk to your diabetes care team.

Chapter 6
I CARE ABOUT NUTRITION

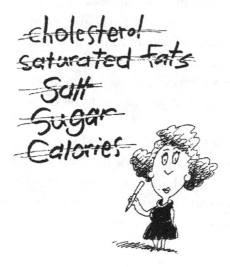

Is there a good way to figure out how much carbohydrate is in a casserole?

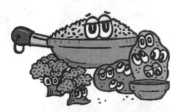

▼
TIP:

If you are making a casserole at home, you can get a very good carb count by adding up the carbohydrates in the ingredients and then dividing the total carbohydrates by the number of servings. However, this isn't going to work if you are eating at someone else's home or in a restaurant. If you are eating a typical casserole (one with potatoes, rice or noodles, meat, vegetables, and sauce), you can figure that each 1/2 cup of casserole has about 15 grams of carbohydrate (equal to one fruit or bread exchange). This may not be exactly right, but it is a close guess. Check your blood sugar two hours after eating the casserole. If your blood sugar is higher than you expect, your casserole probably had more carbohydrate calories than you guessed. Either take more insulin or eat less casserole the next time.

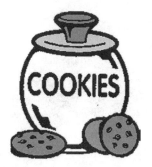

*I*s there a simple way to know how much
carbohydrate is in a homemade cookie?

TIP:

If you make the cookie yourself, you can add up the carbohydrates in the
ingredients and divide that number by the number of cookies in the batch.
Another way is to estimate based on the size of the cookie. On this page is a
cookie meter. Place the cookie in the center of the ring and estimate its size.

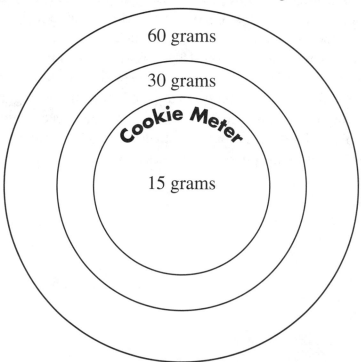

60 grams

30 grams

Cookie Meter

15 grams

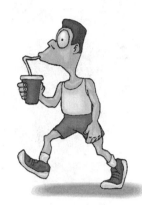

*A*re sports drinks such as Gatorade okay for
people with diabetes?

TIP:

Yes, but be careful. Some sports drinks have a lot of sugar and
could affect your blood glucose in nasty ways. Not having
enough fluid during or after exercise can lead to serious problems. So,
drinking plenty of fluids is very important. You should drink at least
2 quarts of fluid a day to avoid dehydration. Drinking an extra 4–8 oz
of fluid for each 30 minutes of intense exercise will help your body
achieve peak performance and recovery. Drinking something
other than water can add variety, but sports drinks contain about
15–20 grams of sugar and 50–70 calories per 8 oz, and the sugar is
often in the form of fructose corn syrup. Take the time to read labels
and compare ingredients, sugar, and carbohydrate amounts before
drinking these products. Always check blood sugar levels before and
after exercise. Listed below are some sports drinks and the grams of
sugar and calories for each.

Sport drink	Calories	Sugar
Allsport 8 oz	70	19 g
Gatorade 8 oz	50	14 g
Powerade 8 oz	70	15 g

*H*ow can I learn the carbohydrate and fat content of fast food?

▼

TIP:

ast food tends to be high in both fat and carbohydrate. However, fast food can be included occasionally in a healthy diet. Most national fast food chains have nutrition information available. All you have to do is ask the manager. Sometimes this information is in the form of exchanges, and sometimes it is given as grams per serving.

The ADA has an excellent book called *Guide to Healthy Restaurant Eating*, which lists information about food at popular fast food chains in the U.S. You can buy it at *http://store.diabetes.org* or call (800) 232-6733 to get a free catalog of ADA books.

H *ow can I add fiber to my diet and why should I?*

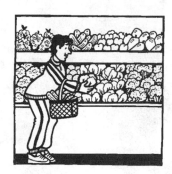

TIP:

When you eat a high-carbohydrate meal with very little fiber, your blood sugars may rise and then fall rapidly. Think of fiber as a sponge, absorbing and then releasing sugar. A high-fiber meal will slow down the rapid changes of blood sugar, preventing the "highs and lows" you get with a high-carbohydrate meal. The National Institutes of Health recommends that adults eat 20–35 grams of fiber per day.

Fiber can be found in many different types of plant foods, including whole-grain breads and cereals, fruits and vegetables, and many types of beans. The best way to add fiber to your diet is to slowly slip in more high-fiber foods. Add grated carrots, zucchini, or celery to your usual meals. Use a handful of rolled oats to top casseroles such as macaroni and cheese. Add garbanzo beans or kidney beans to rice dishes. When baking cakes or cookies, use oat flour for half the flour in the recipe and oat bran or oatmeal for the other half to provide extra flavor and crunch. High-fiber foods are low in fat and provide essential nutrients, such as vitamins C, B6, A, E, folate, and carotenoids.

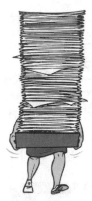

W *here can I find current dietary guidelines for healthy living?*

TIP:

I n 1980, the Department of Agriculture and the Department of Health and Human Services printed the first edition of *Dietary Guidelines for Americans*. These guidelines are revised every 5 years to keep up to date with advances in nutritional research. The 2000 edition gives 3 areas of specific recommendations for healthy living.

1. **Aim for fitness:** Your goals should be to be physically active each day and maintain a healthy weight.
2. **Build a healthy base:** Let the Food Pyramid guide your food choices. Choose a variety of whole grains, fruits, and vegetables daily. Store foods properly to keep them fresh and safe to eat.
3. **Choose food sensibly:** Eat a diet low in saturated fat and choles-terol, and moderate in total fat. Drink low-calorie beverages. Prepare foods with less salt. If you drink alcoholic beverages, do so in moderation.

To get a full copy of the *Dietary Guidelines*, go to *www.health.gov/dietaryguidelines*.

*W*hat are omega-3 fatty acids and
should I include them in my diet?

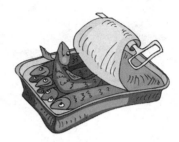

▼

TIP:

R esearch has indicated that omega-3 fatty acids play a role in
healthier diets. These fats have a different chemical structure
then other fats. They improve "good" cholesterol (HDL) and improve
blood flow by making your blood cells less "sticky." Boosting
omega-3 fatty acids in your diet appears to cut the death rate if you
have had a heart attack, lowers the risk of various other heart
problems, lowers the risk of strokes, lowers triglyceride levels, and
slightly reduces blood pressure if you have high blood pressure.
Because foods high in omega-3 fatty acids tend to be high in fat, they
should replace other fatty foods in your diet. Omega-3 fatty acids can
be found in fish such as mackerel, herring, sardines, salmon, and
trout. The best plant sources for omega-3 fatty acids are ground flax
seed, flax seed oil, tofu, soybean oil, canola oil, and nuts. Fish oil
supplements containing omega-3 fatty acids are also available, but it
is better to eat a healthy diet than to add supplements.

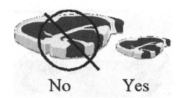

No   Yes

*I*s protein good for me?

▼
TIP:

It is a popular belief that protein is good for your health. However, most Americans get more protein than they need. If 10% of your diet is protein, this is usually enough for your body's needs. Too much protein can damage your kidneys and add to kidney failure down the road. The best way to prevent kidney damage is to keep your sugar values as close to normal as you can, keep your blood pressure low, and eat a low-protein diet.

Protein is found in many foods but is particularly high in meat, dairy products, chicken, and eggs. Cutting down on protein has been shown to slow damage to kidney function in both type 1 and type 2 diabetes. Discuss with your diabetes care team what your kidney filtration rate is and whether a low-protein diet would be good for your kidney's health.

W*hat is a diabetic recipe?*

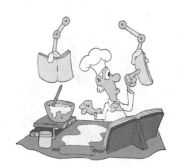

TIP:

G enerally speaking, there are no strict guidelines for a diabetic recipe. Most "diabetic" recipes just follow the American Diabetes Association nutrition guidelines and include diabetic exchanges. Also included is information on calories and the amount of carbohydrate in a serving. Many recipes use artificial sweeteners such as saccharin, aspartame, and acesulfame-K in place of part or all of the sugar. This helps keep the sugar levels down. However, even though less sugar is used, the final product may still have quite a bit of carbohydrate, especially if the recipe includes flour, milk, or fruit. When it comes to cooking, your main focus should be cutting down the carbohydrate, not just the sugar. Foods that used to be frowned upon because of sugar can now be worked into your meal plan. Remember, if you eat too much carbohydrate, you may cause a rise in your blood glucose. Always account for all of the carbohydrate you eat. Numerous books provide diabetic recipes. The bookstore on the ADA web site (*store.diabetes.org*) has available recipe books published by the American Diabetes Association.

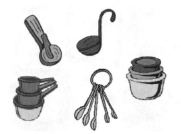

*I*s there a simple way to estimate how much I'm actually eating?

TIP:

O ne good idea is to use measuring cups as serving cups at home. If you regularly use 1 cup, 1/2 cup, and 1/3 cup measuring cups to serve your food, you can get very good at "eyeballing" the size of your portions. The portions restaurants serve are often much larger than you need. For example, a 1/3 cup of cooked rice has 15 grams of carbohydrate and is equal to 1 bread exchange. However, you usually get 2 full cups of rice in a restaurant, which is equal to 6 bread exchanges. If you normally measure your rice portions using a measuring cup at home, you can better judge a good amount of rice to eat in a restaurant. Request a doggy bag at the beginning of your meal. Take the extra food off your plate and you will be less tempted to eat more than you need. The table below gives some examples of how much food gives you 15 grams of carbohydrate for different foods.

Food	Amount	Carbohydrate grams	Servings/ exchanges
Popcorn	3 cups	15	1 bread
Mashed potatoes	1/2 cup	15	1 bread
Pinto beans	1/3 cup	15	1 bread
Strawberries, raw	1 1/4 cup	15	1 fruit
Cantaloupe, cubed	1 cup	15	1 fruit

*H*ow can I estimate how much salt is in my food?

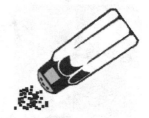

▼

TIP:

R ecommended salt intake for people with diabetes is the same as for the rest of the population. To stay healthy, you should get about 4 grams of salt per day (4,000 mg). Most food labels do not give any information on salt content but do list "sodium" as one of the ingredients (salt is made of sodium and chlorine). Sodium is the part of salt that can be bad for your health, especially if you have high blood pressure or heart problems. Four grams of salt contain 1,407 milligrams of sodium, which is equal to about one teaspoon. Therefore, all you need is about one teaspoon of salt per day. This sounds easy, but remember, many foods are soaked with sodium. You should carefully read the sodium content on food labels (they'll be in milligrams) and then convert it back into teaspoons of salt. What is listed on the food label as sodium is less than half of the amount of salt in that food. For example, if a can of soup contains 1,200 milligrams of sodium, then that equals approximately one-half teaspoon of salt (2 grams). Four grams of salt a day is usually included in a regular diet without adding table salt to any food.

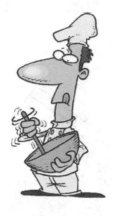

*H*ow big is a serving?

TIP:

This is a tricky question to answer. Good nutrition comes in many different shapes and sizes, and suggested servings of foods and liquids may be difficult to figure out. The USDA Food Guide Pyramid gives a wide range of servings from each of the six major food groups. However, serving sizes are different within each group, and from group to group. Serving sizes are used to keep the level of calories, carbohydrates, protein, and fat the same within each group. When calories and carbohydrates are the same in your daily meal plan, then it's easier to keep your blood glucose stable. Following is a list of some serving sizes.

1 slice bread
1/2 cup cooked cereal
1/2 cup rice or pasta
1/3 cup cooked beans
1 cup milk or yogurt
1 oz cheese
1 cup raw vegetables
1/2 cup cooked vegetables
1/2 cup vegetable juice

1 medium apple, banana, orange
1/2 cup fruit chopped, cooked, or canned in water
1/2–3/4 cup fruit juice
3 oz cooked beef, poultry, or fish
1 egg

A re soybeans good for me?

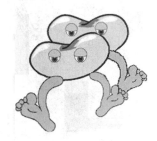

▼
TIP:

S ome studies have shown that soy may be good for you. Soybeans contain compounds called isoflavones, which are plant hormones that may be helpful in fighting problems like osteoporosis, certain cancers, and hot flashes during menopause. But soy's biggest strong point might be in how well it can lower cholesterol. At least 38 studies have found that people with high cholesterol levels who ate soy protein instead of animal protein lowered their total cholesterol, triglycerides, and LDL. The HDL ("good") cholesterol remained the same.

There are several ways to add soy to your diet. You can eat tofu, which is made from curdled soy milk. Tempeh is a formed cake made from fermented soybeans and has a firmer texture than tofu. Canned soybeans can be added to soups, stews, salads, etc. Soy milk makes great "smoothies." Now that soy is becoming accepted as a healthy food, soy products can be found just about everywhere. A good way to try some soy products is to go to the deli section of a health food store and ask for samples. You can also learn more about soy foods and how to prepare them by getting a good vegetarian cookbook.

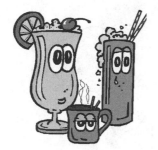

Do sugar alcohols raise my blood glucose?

▼

TIP:

Yes, sugar alcohols can raise your blood sugar. Sugar alcohol is not the same as the alcohol found in alcoholic beverages. Many fruits and vegetables naturally contain sugar alcohols. Artificial sugar alcohols such as sorbitol, mannitol, and xylitol are often used as sweeteners and are classified as nutritive sweeteners. Nutritive sweeteners contain about 2 to 3 calories per gram instead of the 4 calories per gram you get from other carbohydrates. Because they still contain calories, sugar alcohols may affect your blood glucose levels and must be included in your meal plan. Other sweeteners (saccharin and aspartame) are not sugar alcohols and do not raise your blood sugar (they are calorie free). You should eat foods with sugar alcohols in moderation, since some sugar alcohols (sorbitol and mannitol) can have a laxative effect if you eat large amounts. Take time to read product labels, and become familiar with the food items in your grocery store that contain sugar alcohols.

*W*hy should I use a sugar substitute?

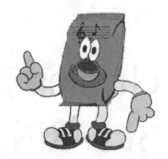

▼
TIP:

I n the past, people with diabetes used sugar substitutes because it was believed that eating sugar caused high blood glucose levels. Today, we know that sugars are just like any other carbohydrate and must be treated in the same way. However, by cutting down on sugar, you can seriously cut down on your total carbohydrates. Sodas, gelatin desserts, and chewing gums that are sugar free will all contain less carbohydrate. All of the sweeteners listed here are caloric free.

Generic name	Brand name	How available	Notes
Aspartame	Nutrasweet	Many prepared foods	Loses flavor if heated
Saccharin	Sweet 'N Low	Many prepared foods— individual serving packets	Fine for cooking
Stevia	several	Pellets, at health food stores	Sold as a supplement, not approved as a food additive
Acesulfame K	Sunett	Many prepared foods	Fine for cooking

Chapter 7
BREAKING NEW GROUND:
DIABETES RESEARCH

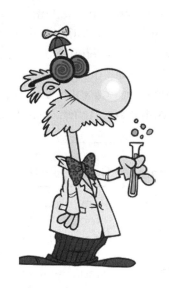

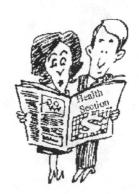

*W*ill being in a clinical trial help my
diabetes?

▼
TIP:

Probably. No matter what, being in a clinical trial means you will
be examined more often than usual, which could lead to
problems being found earlier than they might have been. You may
also have the chance to test new therapies for diabetes. You should be
aware that if you take part, you might be given a placebo, or a
dummy pill with no real medication. It may surprise you, but many
patients actually get better even when they receive a dummy pill. This
is called a placebo effect. You may also receive the active treatment,
usually made up of a new medication of some type. Be aware that
new medications may have unknown side effects that are not
discovered until patients try the medications. But one thing is certain.
Before you participate in any clinical trial, you should read the
consent form very carefully and ask questions. If you are still
confused, bring the consent form home and go over it with a relative
or friend. Understand the consent form before you sign it.

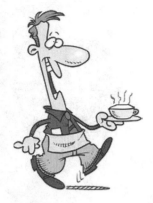

*I*s there any way to improve my awareness of low blood sugars?

TIP:

Most people with a blood sugar level less than 50 mg/dl suffer from nervousness, shaking, sweating, hunger, difficulty concentrating, and a rapid heart beat. Although these symptoms sound terrible, having them tells you that you have low blood sugars and allows you to correct them before something bad happens. Unfortunately, not being able to notice your low blood sugars (hypoglycemia unawareness) is common if you have long-standing diabetes, especially in people with type 1 diabetes. This unawareness is also common in people with very well-controlled blood sugars.

Usually, your health care providers will relax target blood glucose goals slightly if you lose your ability to notice your low blood sugars. Avoiding hypoglycemia for a week or two will probably improve your ability to sense a low blood sugar. Interestingly, a recent study showed that people who took caffeine (equal to about 2 cups of coffee) had more frequent and more intense low blood sugar symptoms than those who didn't. Thus, drinking 2 cups of coffee every day may improve your ability to feel when your blood sugar is getting low.

W hat do I need to know about C-peptide?

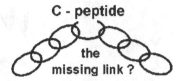

▼
TIP:

W hen cells in the pancreas produce insulin, they also produce a protein called C-peptide. C-peptide stands for "connecting peptide." If you don't have diabetes, C-peptide is secreted with insulin in equal amounts. Until recently, it was thought that C-peptide didn't serve much of a purpose. However, recent studies seem to suggest that daily injections of C-peptide may prevent kidney, bowel, sexual, and circulatory complications in type 1 diabetes. People with type 1 diabetes do not receive any C-peptide when they inject their insulin because C-peptide is not included in their bottle of insulin. If C-peptide proves to be helpful, it may be added to every insulin bottle. Since C-peptide can be made commercially, this should give us an additional tool for managing diabetes.

Because of the interest sparked by these first studies, new research on C-peptide being added to insulin has been started in both Europe and the United States. You will likely hear more about this exciting development over the next several years.

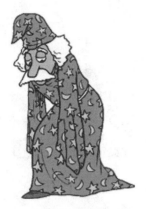

*W*hen will there be a cure
for diabetes?

TIP:

No one knows the answer to your question because diabetes isn't just one disease. A more realistic question would be: "When will we have effective and safe treatments for diabetes?" Many effective treatments for chronic diseases are not cures at all. A good example is the treatment of hypothyroidism (low thyroid). There is no "cure" for hypothyroidism. However, the treatment (one thyroid pill per day) is simple, safe, effective, inexpensive, and completely erases the effects of the disease. If something like this were available for diabetes, the need for a "cure" could wait awhile.

The good news is that many new treatments for diabetes are becoming available each year. In just the last 5 years, diabetes treatment has come a long way. Unfortunately, many of these new treatments are expensive and have some pretty bad side effects. Right now, at least 35 new therapies for diabetes are being developed. The successful ones will not only be better than the treatments already available, but they'll probably lower the cost for all treatments due to competition in the marketplace.

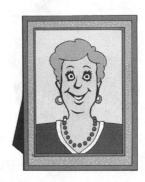

S hould I take estrogen after menopause?

▼

TIP:

This issue is still being debated. Taking estrogen prevents osteoporosis (when bones become weaker from aging) in women who take it regularly after menopause. It was also thought that estrogen prevented heart disease. Because women with diabetes are at a higher risk for heart disease, it seemed to make sense that women with diabetes should take estrogen after menopause. Recent studies, however, suggest something different. The Heart and Estrogen/ Progestin Replacement study showed that taking estrogen did not prevent the advancement of heart disease in women who already had heart disease when they started taking it. In addition, the Women's Health Initiative demonstrated that estrogen does not prevent heart disease in healthy postmenopausal women and may increase the risk of breast cancer. Every woman with diabetes who has been through menopause should discuss the risks and benefits of estrogen therapy with her diabetes care team before making this important decision.

W^{hat} *is the HOPE Study?*

TIP:

The major cause of death in people with diabetes is heart disease. It is 5 times more common in men with diabetes than in men without diabetes, and 10 times more common in women with diabetes than women without diabetes. Because of this, any treatment that will reduce the risk of heart disease in people with diabetes will save many lives. The Heart Outcomes Prevention Evaluation (HOPE) study was a very large study examining the effects of ACE inhibitors (or rampril, an ACE inhibitor medication) on lowering the death rate from heart attacks and strokes in high-risk patients. In the large group of 9,297 volunteers who were being studied, 3,577 had diabetes. Patients were randomly given either an ACE inhibitor or a placebo (a dummy pill) and then studied for 5 years. Because the ACE inhibitor worked so well in lowering heart attacks, stroke, and death from heart-related events, the study was stopped early. If you have any signs of kidney disease, ACE inhibitors can help because they slow the progression of this complication of diabetes. If you are not taking an ACE inhibitor, you should talk to your doctor about whether you should start.

*W*hat are impaired fasting glucose and
impaired glucose tolerance?

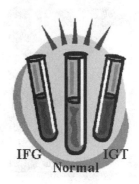

IFG   IGT
Normal

▼
TIP:

Impaired fasting glucose and impaired glucose tolerance are blood
sugar levels that are higher than normal but not high enough to be
diabetes. In the past, these conditions would have been called
borderline diabetes.

If you have impaired fasting glucose and impaired glucose tolerance you're at a higher risk for type 2 diabetes. If you have impaired
glucose tolerance you're also at a greater risk for heart disease. The
treatment for either of these conditions is aerobic exercise and
weight loss through meal planning. Resistance training (lifting
weights) may also help by building your muscle mass. You and
your doctor can decide on the best course of treatment. Below is
a comparison between normal glucose values and the values of
impaired fasting glucose or impaired glucose tolerance.

Normal	Impaired fasting glucose or impaired glucose tolerance
Fasting plasma glucose <100 mg/dl	Fasting plasma glucose ≥100 and <126 mg/dl (impaired fasting glucose)
Plasma glucose <140 mg/dl two hours after drinking 75 g of glucose	Plasma glucose ≥140 mg/dl two hours after drinking 75 g of glucose and <200 mg/dl (impaired glucose tolerance)

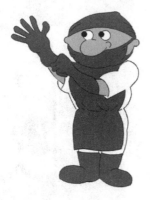

W̶ill an islet cell transplantation cure my diabetes?

▼
TIP:

Y̶ou're not alone in looking toward islet cell transplantation for hope. A recent study successfully transplanted islet cells in 7 patients with diabetes. After the transplantation, the diabetes disappeared for at least 1 year. If longer-term trials go well, then islet cell transplantation will be a major medical breakthrough. Before this happens, however, several questions need to be answered, including:

- How long will the transplant last?
- Will a second transplant (if needed) be as successful as the first transplant?
- Will the medications that prevent transplant rejection (when your body won't accept the new tissue) have any long-term side effects, such as cancer or kidney failure?
- Where will all the islets cells come from?
- How much will transplantation cost and who will pay for it?

As you can see, there's still a lot of research that needs to be done before we can properly answer your question.

*W*hat are the advantages of the new
    blood glucose meters?

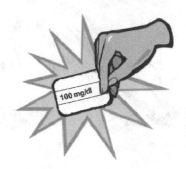

▼
TIP:

Several new blood glucose meters are on the market, including the
Lifescan Ultra (LifeScan), the FreeStyle (Therasense), and AtLast
(Amira). These meters use less blood, are smaller and lighter (usually
the size of a credit card or shaped like a pen), give a reading within
15 seconds, and can draw blood from a variety of places, including
your forearm and thigh. If your life is hectic, a quicker meter may
make it easier to check your blood sugars more often, and a smaller
meter is easier to carry with you. Not having to prick your finger also
makes it a lot less painful. However, your insurance company may
not see the need for a different meter. Many insurance plans cover
only one brand of meter and strips. To get the strips for another meter,
your doctor or diabetes educator may need to write "a letter of
medical necessity" explaining why you need the new meter. Since the
new meters require a smaller blood sample, many insurance plans
will pay for your switch to another meter if you have calluses on your
fingers, which makes it hard to get a drop of blood.

How can I reduce hypoglycemia by changing my pen injector technique?

TIP:

A recent study looked at 109 patients with diabetes who used pen injectors to see how well the NPH insulin in the pen was mixed before injection. The study found that the NPH insulin in the insulin cartridge had an unacceptable degree of variability in more than 70% of the patients. The study also found that by turning the pen upside down and then rightside up at least 20 times before you inject it could help this. This method works much better than just shaking the pen up and down. Low blood sugar was reduced among the patients who used this new method. This suggests that poorly mixed NPH insulin in injector pens can cause some attacks of unexpected low blood sugar. If you have not been mixing your cartridge insulin well enough, you may have fewer episodes of hypoglycemia when you mix your insulin this way.

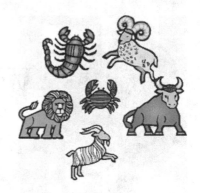

*H*ow does my personality affect my
blood sugar control?

▼

TIP:

It is likely that personality may play a part in how well you care for
your diabetes. But which types of personalities will help and which
won't? One recent study tried to answer this question. Detailed
personality tests were given to 105 people with type 2 diabetes. The
results of these tests were studied to see how well the personality of a
person predicted his or her average blood sugar levels. Surprisingly,
they found that people with personality traits such as anxiety,
hostility, vulnerability, and self-consciousness usually had good
diabetes control. On the other hand, people who had fewer negative
emotions and a general focus on the needs of others were more likely
to have poor diabetes control. These data suggest that people who are
more focused on themselves are more likely to have good diabetes
control than people who are not.

However, medical science is only starting to understand the relationship between personality and disease. More research is necessary before this information will become useful in your diabetes
care.

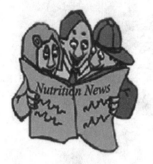

Why does diabetes nutrition news change?

TIP:

It can be frustrating, but nutrition news changes as new information becomes available. Nutrition news is often based on research, which is usually based on one scientist's idea or theory. If it makes it through testing, the scientist's idea is thought to be well-founded—until another study is published with information saying something different. For example, early research suggested low-carb diets were best if you had diabetes. Now, it's recommended that carbohydrates be included in meal plans for a more balanced diet.

The problem is that separate studies are needed to answer a single question. Over time, all of the test results build a more complete picture of the truth. Unfortunately, the research results of one study are often presented to the public as the whole picture instead of just one piece of a larger picture. You might want to think of it as just one piece of a jigsaw puzzle. The next time you hear about "good" or "bad" diabetes nutrition news, remember that the information may be only a piece of the puzzle.

*W*hy did I gain weight after I started
my new insulin sensitizer?

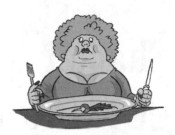

TIP:

Insulin sensitizers are a powerful new class of type 2 diabetes drugs
that work by lowering your insulin resistance. This category of
diabetes medicines includes rosiglitazone (Avandia) and pioglitazone
(Actos). Metformin also increases sensitivity to insulin but is not
usually thought of as an "insulin sensitizer."

Insulin sensitizers have worked wonders for many people with
type 2 diabetes. Unfortunately, you're probably also going to gain
about 2 to 10 pounds when you use them. Part of this weight gain is
from retained water, which may cause your shoes to be tight, make
it difficult to get your rings on and off, and give you a feeling of
tightness in your hands. This can usually be helped with a low dose
of a diuretic medication. If you have a heart condition, be careful,
because water retention can bring on congestive heart failure.

Studies have also shown that insulin sensitizers can increase
your subcutaneous fat (the fat under your skin) and may result in a
decrease in visceral fat (the fat around your midsection). Therefore,
it is possible that these drugs move the fat from your stomach to the
fat under your skin and that there is no real rise in total body fat.

Chapter 8
CUTTING THE RISKS

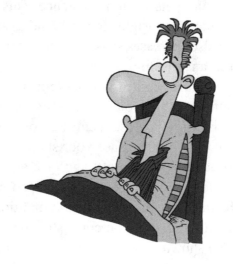

*W*ill *drinking a little alcohol lower my risk of heart disease?*

▼ TIP:

Recent newspaper and magazine articles have suggested that one alcoholic drink a day can help people without diabetes lower their risk for heart disease. Whether or not this applies to people with diabetes is still unclear. Recently, a study was conducted of 983 people with type 2 diabetes, including people who did not drink at all and people who drank one or more drinks per day. This test group was followed for 12 years, and it turned out that previous drinkers and people who did not drink at all had the highest death rate from heart disease. People who had at least one drink a day had the lowest death rate. Therefore, the answer is "Yes, alcohol does appear to reduce the risk of heart disease in people with diabetes." However, as you are probably aware, alcohol can have a lot of side effects, including hypoglycemia, alcohol addiction, and a worsening of blood fat levels. With this in mind, one drink per day with dinner is probably okay, but any more than that may be bad for your health.

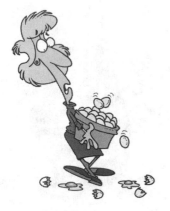

*W*ill eggs increase my risk for
heart attack?

TIP:

Egg yolks are very high in cholesterol, and many experts suggest
lowering how much cholesterol you eat to reduce your risk of
heart disease. A recent study of more than 117,000 men and women
showed that eating up to one egg a day did not increase your risk for
a heart attack or stroke—unless you have diabetes. For people with
diabetes, eating one egg a day doubled the risk for a heart attack in
men and raised the risk of heart attack in women by 50%. Instead of
eating an egg, try eating an egg substitute, such as Egg Beaters. Or,
simply separate the white from the yolk and eat only the whites of
your eggs. Although scrambled whites taste a little different than
regular scrambled eggs, if you scramble 2 whites with 1 yolk every
now and then, you probably won't be able to taste the difference.
There is no cholesterol in egg whites, and by removing the yolks, you
can halve your eggs and eat them, too!

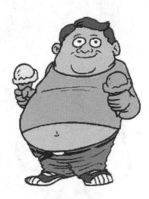

*H*ow can I help my child lose weight?

TIP:

R ight now, there is an epidemic of obesity in children and
teenagers in this country. Because of this, there has also been a
rise in type 2 diabetes at younger ages. Many studies show a high
level of impaired glucose tolerance (pre-diabetes) and high fat levels
in the blood of obese children. Since impaired glucose tolerance is a
condition that leads to type 2 diabetes, you should have your child
tested. This is especially important if you or others in your family
already have type 2 diabetes.

The best way to help your child lose weight is to set an example
of healthy eating and exercise. Include your child in family activities
such as riding bicycles, hiking, or swimming. That way your child
will not feel singled out and ashamed. If the whole family is living a
healthy lifestyle, it is easier for the child to do it, too. The family
can have fun setting goals, awarding prizes for accomplishing goals,
and simply working together to prevent obesity and the risk of diabetes. If you make these changes and your child still fails to lose
weight, you might consider seeing a specialist for help.

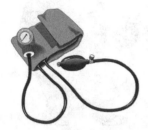

*H*ow low should my blood pressure be to prevent complications?

TIP:

The benefits you get from low blood pressure get better the lower your blood pressure goes. This is based on the recently completed, long-term United Kingdom Prospective Diabetes Study. This study, which lasted over 15 years, followed about 4,000 patients with type 2 diabetes and monitored how often they had diabetic complications. Besides showing that blood sugar control is important in stopping complications before they start, the results also showed the importance of blood pressure control. Almost every diabetic complication was linked with systolic high blood pressure (the top number of your blood pressure reading). In fact, for each 10 mmHg of lowered blood pressure, the risk of having any complication was reduced by at least 12%. Just like with blood glucose levels, the lower the blood pressure, the lower the risk of complications. With this in mind, your blood pressure should be as low as possible without causing you problems. Your target should be a blood pressure below 130/80. The bottom line—controlling your blood pressure is just as important as controlling your blood sugar.

A re high blood sugars after
  meals dangerous?

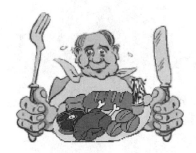

▼
TIP:

Y es, they are. As you know, high blood sugars can cause
  problems with your eyes, nerves, and kidneys. They may even
put you at a higher risk for a heart attack. It is normal for your blood
sugars to go up after a meal, but this can raise your average daily
blood sugar. The perfect blood sugar after meals should be less than
150 mg/dl. There is a stronger relationship between your A1C and
after-meal blood sugars than between A1C and your overnight fasting
sugars. Since A1C is the measure of your long-term exposure to
blood glucose, your blood sugars after meals may be the most
important factor in your risk for diabetic complications. If you are
interested in learning your blood sugar level after a meal, check your
blood sugar level 2 hours after eating (when it is usually at its
highest). Talk to your diabetes care team and develop treatment
strategies to keep your meal-related sugars as normal as possible.

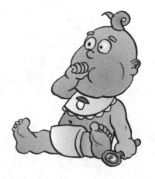

*W*hat is preconception counseling and why
is it important?

TIP:

I f you have diabetes, your chances of giving birth to a deformed
baby are almost 5 times higher than if you didn't have diabetes.
Preconception counseling can drop this risk down to normal levels.
Preconception counseling is therapy for women who wish to become
pregnant, and it can lower the risk of something going wrong with
your pregnancy. There are 3 goals for preconception counseling:

■ To achieve and maintain excellent glucose control before and
during the pregnancy.
■ To identify, evaluate, and treat complications of diabetes and risk
factors that can have negative effects on you or your baby.
■ To delay pregnancy until it is safe and wanted.

Unfortunately, preconception pregnancy counseling is not common
in the United States. Many studies show that less than 25% of pregnant women with diabetes seek preconception counseling. If you are
pregnant, or wish to become pregnant, and you have diabetes, do
yourself and your baby a favor—cut the risk of something going
wrong and seek preconception counseling.

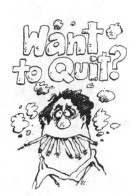

*H*ow can I stop smoking?

▼
TIP:

The first step to a smoke-free lifestyle is realizing how horrible smoking is to your health. In fact, if you have diabetes, smoking is just about the worst thing you could do to your body. The thing is, you probably already know that smoking is bad for you, and you've probably already tried to quit more than once. By now you may think that your addiction to nicotine is so strong that you'll never be able to quit. But keep the following in mind:

■ First, realize that many people have quit smoking who were just as addicted to nicotine as you are.
■ Second, most people who quit smoking have tried to quit several times before they finally succeed.
■ Third, trying to quit by yourself is very hard. Most people need help from outside support groups.
■ Fourth, you'll probably get the best results by joining a behavioral modification program, combined with a nicotine patch and/or medications that lower you withdrawal symptoms.

Almost all communities have programs to help you quit smoking. Ask your diabetes care team what's available in your area. Quitting smoking is a long-term commitment. It is not easy to quit, but your health is worth the effort.

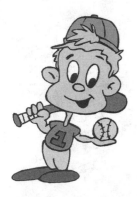

*W*hat can I do to prevent my child from getting type 2 diabetes?

TIP:

D iabetes is a growing health problem among American children. Until recently, almost all of the diabetes that occurred in children was type 1 diabetes. Type 2 diabetes in children was rare. Now, things are different. But why? More than likely it's because kids are getting less exercise and suffering from high rates of obesity. In order to prevent type 2 diabetes in your child:

■ Do whatever possible to keep him or her thin.
■ Limit how much time your child spends doing sedentary activities (like watching television or playing on the computer).
■ Be aware of what and how much your child eats.
■ Encourage your child to take part in lively, outdoor activities.
■ Check age, height, and weight charts so you know how much your child should weigh compared to others of his or her age and height.
■ Ask your diabetes care team to help you evaluate your child.

Remember, if you or other members of your family have type 2 diabetes, your child is at an even higher risk.

Chapter 9
MORE QUESTIONS, MORE ANSWERS

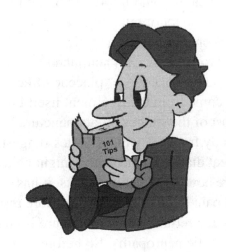

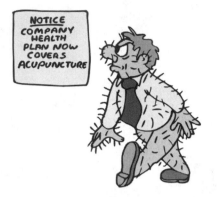

*W*ill acupuncture help the pain I
have from neuropathy?

▼ TIP:

A lot of therapies can help you with the pain from neuropathy,
including medications and improved blood glucose control.
Recently, there's been a lot of talk about acupuncture, mostly from
popular magazines on alternative therapies. As with all alternative
therapies, it's hard to tell how well acupuncture really works. Many
of the benefits could be linked to a "placebo effect," or benefits that
don't necessarily come from the treatment itself but from the idea of
being treated. Most of the studies on acupuncture have been done in
China, but one study from the United States suggested that using
acupuncture to treat diabetic neuropathy might be useful. Although
we're still not sure how acupuncture works, it has been used to
successfully treat pain in other conditions. More research is needed
before we can say for certain that acupuncture is an effective way to
treat pain from diabetic neuropathy. So before you start acupuncture
therapy, talk with your diabetes care team about whether they think
it's okay for you. If you decide to try acupuncture, don't stop using
your regular medications. Remember that all treatments do not work
the same for everyone, and acupuncture may help some people more
than others.

*W*hy should I educate my friends
 about diabetes?

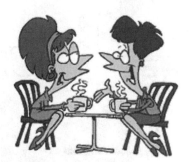

TIP:

W hen people don't understand something, they often feel
 uncomfortable or frightened. The best way to deal with this is
to educate them. Tell them about diabetes—what is true and what is
not true. For example, many people believe that you get diabetes from
eating too much sugar, or that you can catch it from someone else.
This, of course, is not true. Unfortunately, some people also think that
type 2 diabetes is not a serious disease. Type 2 diabetes has many
serious complications if you don't treat it right.

   If you want to help, try lending your friends some books to read
or show them *Diabetes Forecast.* If you are on insulin, explain
hypoglycemia to them and show them exactly what they can do if
you ever need help. Including others in your fight against diabetes
can give you a valuable support group. Diabetes is much easier if
you don't approach it alone. Most of all, show your friends by
example that you can have diabetes and live a very normal life.

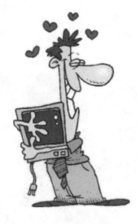

Can my computer help me with my diabetes?

TIP:

The computer can be a big help in managing your diabetes. You can use it to track the food you eat, how much activity you get, and what your blood sugars are. Then you can use this information to get a better understanding of your diabetes data and make good management decisions. For example, you could compare how many calories you eat, how many calories you burn, and blood sugars over a six-month period. Using this information, you could make changes in your diet or activity plan to better meet your goals. Share your information with your diabetes care team so they can use your computer information to help you.

Several programs are available for people with diabetes. For example, *Lifeform* allows you to track calories, food composition, exercise, body weight, lab results, and how you feel each day. You can download a 21-day free trial from the web site: *www.lifeform.com.* If you do not have your own computer, you can go to the public library and use their computers. Always keep in mind that computers are only as reliable as the information you give them. It's still up to you to review, adjust, and improve.

M y diabetes is making me depressed.
   Will counseling help this?

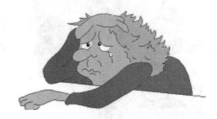

▼
TIP:

If your doctor has suggested you get counseling for your depression, he may be worried about how you are feeling and what effect that might have on your diabetes. People get tired of dealing with a long-term illness like diabetes. They may begin to feel that there is no point in caring for their diabetes. It is important to find out what is causing or adding to your depression. Both professional counseling and medication can be helpful. People are often slow to ask for help because they think that they should be able to handle everything by themselves. However, at your first counseling visit, you will find that a good counselor is supportive and helpful. Counseling and/or medication for depression can be helpful tools for your diabetes management.

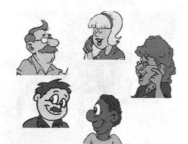

W<i>ho should I have on my diabetes care team?</i>

TIP:

A diabetes care team is a group of health care professionals, friends, and family who focus on improving your health.

Primary group	Function
Primary care physician	Primary medical care
Dietitian	Healthy diet advice
Certified diabetes educator	Diabetes education and advice
Friends and family	Support and motivation
Dentist	Dental health
Pharmacist	Medication supply and advice
Secondary group	
Diabetologist	Endocrinologist specializing in in diabetes
Nephrologist	Kidney specialist
Neurologist	Nerve specialist
Ophthalmologist	Eye care and laser therapy
Podiatrist	Toe and foot care
Social worker	Financial advice
Mental health care professional	Psychological support
Exercise physiologist	Healthy exercise program

*H*ow can I contact other people with diabetes?

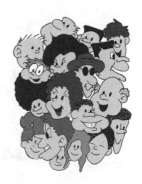

▼
TIP:

It's always a good idea to talk to other people who are dealing with the same health problems that you are. Ask a diabetes educator if there are any support groups or classes in your area that you could attend. You might also ask friends and family if they know someone who has diabetes. Another good way to contact people is the "Making Friends" section of the ADA's *Diabetes Forecast* magazine. This is a great way to get in touch with other people with similar problems. To meet others through the magazine, write to:

Making Friends, ADA
1701 N. Beauregard Street
Alexandria, VA 22311

Diabetes summer camp is also a great way for children to meet each other.

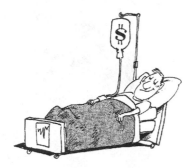

W hy won't my insurance company pay for the diabetes supplies I need?

TIP:

S tudies have shown that preventing the complications from diabetes is cheaper in the long run than getting the medical care to treat them right. In fact, the two largest prospective studies for type 1 and type 2 diabetes (the Diabetes Control and Complications Trial and the United Kingdom Prospective Diabetes Study) clearly showed the money you can save with intensive diabetes management. Unfortunately, the health care industry sees these savings as "future savings," and not a way to save money in the here and now. When health care plans are trying to save money in the short term, they reduce how much they'll provide for diabetes expenses, and you suffer. Even though this attitude is shortsighted, it is typical of most insurance providers, especially Medicare and Medicaid, which are run by the United States government. This is why it is very important that you support the efforts of organizations such as the American Diabetes Association. They are working hard to increase your health care benefits. A reasonable health care policy that gives people with diabetes proper medical supplies is urgently needed.

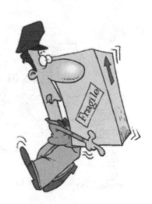

*S*hould I order my diabetes medication
through the mail?

▼
TIP:

If your medications and supplies stay about the same from month to
month, mail order is a great way to go. For instance:

Mail-order pharmacies can deliver 2 to 3 months' worth of medication and supplies at a time.

Prescriptions can be written for refills so that you automatically
receive shipments every 30, 60, or 90 days.

■ The items come directly to your door.

Some mail-order pharmacies can bill your insurance company
directly.

However:

If you need a drug quickly, mail order does not work well.

If you prefer the personal attention you get at a local pharmacy,
it's also not a good idea.

Your order could get lost or delayed in the mail.

If you are starting a new medication, you should buy it in person
so you can ask your pharmacist questions. If you find that this
new drug works for you and you will be on it for a while, mail-
order may be a good option.

Call your HMO or insurance company and ask if they have a mail
order option.

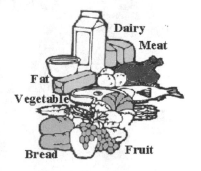

What is a meal plan?

TIP:

B asically, a meal plan is when you take time to think about a meal before you eat it. Sometimes meal planning happens 10 minutes before your next meal. Other times you can plan an entire week. No matter when it happens, an eating plan is an important part of diabetes therapy and can help you keep your blood sugars under control. A meal plan helps you manage the amount of carbohydrates and calories you take in on a daily basis. Meal planning is good if you have type 1 diabetes because you can match your insulin dose to the amount of carbohydrates you plan to eat. For type 2 diabetes, controlling the carbohydrates you take in can help keep your blood glucose in your target range. Meal plans can be developed to fit your tastes and your schedule, as well as your lifestyle. The USDA Food Guide Pyramid is a useful tool to develop a balanced meal plan. To make sure you and your family get the nutrients and fiber you need to stay healthy, choose foods from the 5 major food groups (bread, fruit, meat, dairy, and vegetable). Use as little as possible from the "fat" section. Take the time to develop a meal plan using the Food Guide Pyramid that will fit your lifestyle and that of your family.

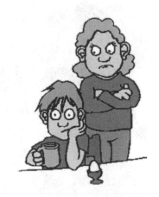

*W*hy do I resist when my family tells me what to eat?

▼

TIP:

Your family is probably worried about you and wants you to stay healthy. Unfortunately, telling you what to cat is probably the wrong way to approach the situation. It is a natural human response to get defensive, especially if you feel you're being judged or criticized. You may also feel guilt and shame from not sticking to your meal plan, and this can cause you to resist as well. All of this is normal. There is no evidence that having a family member hound you all the time helps you improve your diabetes care. Only you can make the decision to improve your dietary habits. However, your family can encourage you. Think about what you would like your family to say to you and tell them exactly what might help. Perhaps you don't want to hear comments on what you eat. Ask them to stop bugging you when you are not following your diet because that makes you resentful. If you have a hard time talking to your family, talk to your diabetes care team and see if they can help. A meeting between your family and your diabetes care team may help them understand that you are the one responsible for your diet.

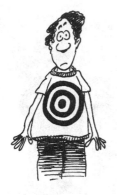

I'm always afraid my diabetes care team is going to be upset with me if I don't meet my goals. Am I being silly?

TIP:

Your diabetes care team is not there to judge. They are there to help you get better control over your diabetes. Use them. The only way they can help is if you communicate. Still, it's common to worry about what your doctor might say. It can be very hard to change your lifestyle, especially if you need to lose weight and exercise. Many people struggle with lifestyle changes, and your diabetes care team knows that. It's easy to feel like there is something wrong with you when you can't "just do it." Unfortunately, this can cause you to avoid talking to the very people who can help you. Go to your appointment. Tell your doctor or another diabetes care team member what you're having trouble with. You may just need some help setting realistic goals. If members of your care team do get mad, you have the right to ask why. If it remains a problem, try and find professionals who won't judge or shame you. It's your life—you're the one in control.

*I*s it okay if my 11-year-old daughter with diabetes attends a friend's slumber party?

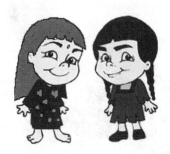

TIP:

C hildren with diabetes, and especially young teenagers, are often worried about being accepted by their friends. They want to be just like everyone else. By the time she's 11, your daughter may be taking on some of the responsibility for her diabetes care. If she hasn't started, now is a good time. Help your daughter take responsibility by making sure she understands what is needed and why. To best prepare her for her slumber party, make sure

- She can take insulin without supervision
- She can check her blood glucose
- She can tell when she's having low blood sugar
- She has the snack she needs
- She parents of the child having the party are willing to help if she needs it
- You can be contacted if she needs anything

It is important for her to know that the better she manages her diabetes, the more like everyone else she will be. When both of you are comfortable about her diabetes management, you will feel better about letting her out into the world.

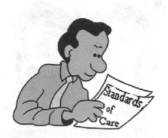

Why are the Standards of Medical Care for Patients with Diabetes Mellitus *important to me?*

▼
TIP:

The *Standards*, published by the American Diabetes Association, are very important to your health and to other people with diabetes. These standards, or treatment guidelines, need to be followed by doctors, nurses, dietitians, and other health professionals who treat people with diabetes. They are often revised to stay up to date with the most current research in diabetes care. They are available on the web at *http://care.diabetesjournals.org/cgi/content/full/27/suppl_1/s15* and in medical journals such as *Diabetes Care*. These guidelines describe the basics of acceptable medical therapy for patients with diabetes and include the tests that should be done during your annual physical, as well as other tests you should have. If you have a problem related to your diabetes, such as high blood fats, you should examine these standards to be sure that your health care team is doing what it should to get your levels in the healthy range. It is important that you understand what the goals of treatment are. By doing so, you can be sure you're getting good medical care. If your physician does not follow the *Standards*, we suggest changing to a physician who follows the *Standards of Medical Care for Patients with Diabetes Mellitus.*

101 TIPS FOR COPING WITH DIABETES

▲

A project of the
American Diabetes Association

▼

Written By

Richard R. Rubin, PhD, CDE
Gary M. Arsham, MD, PhD
Catherine Feste, BA
David G. Marrero, PhD
Stefan H. Rubin

101 TIPS FOR COPING WITH DIABETES

▼

TABLE OF CONTENTS

Chapter 1
MANAGING STRESS AND NOURISHING YOUR SOUL

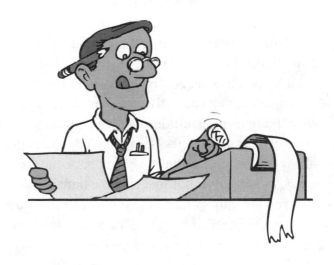

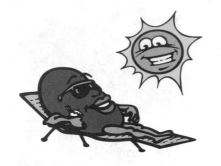

*I*s it okay to take a vacation *from diabetes when I take my summer vacation at the beach?*

▼

TIP:

Everyone needs vacations—even from diabetes. Trouble is, it's hard to take one. When you're on vacation you want to enjoy yourself as much as possible. To do that you have to feel good, and to feel good you can't take a complete vacation from your diabetes. However, you can probably take a more relaxed approach to at least some parts of your normal routine.

Think about one or two things you do to manage your diabetes from which you would most like a vacation. Things like monitoring your blood glucose, getting up early in the morning to take your insulin, or eating carefully. Are there ways you could take a vacation from these responsibilities—at least once in a while—without losing control of your diabetes? Are there adjustments you could make that allow you to miss a glucose check here and there, sleep in a little extra, or work in foods that aren't a normal part of your diet?

You are only human, and it is vacation. You need it and deserve it. There's plenty of time to get back on track later. Talk to your diabetes care team about changes you can make to your routine that can help vacation be a little more relaxing.

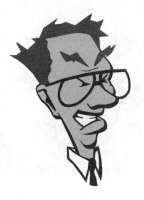

*C*an stress affect my blood glucose
levels?

▼
TIP:

It sure can. Stress can affect your blood glucose in 2 ways. First,
some people find that stress has an immediate effect on their blood
sugars. Most people who notice an effect say that stress pushes their
blood sugars up, but a few say that stress has the opposite effect.

Second, stress can also have a long-term "wear and tear" effect on
blood glucose. Most people who have diabetes experience this effect,
at least from time to time. When people feel stressed they often stop
taking good care of themselves, because they are overwhelmed and
don't have the energy. Ultimately, stress can trigger a negative spiral
of feeling overwhelmed, doing less to manage diabetes, and having
higher blood glucose levels.

Finding ways to cope with stress can help your body and your
soul.

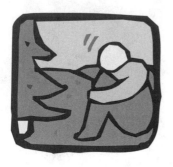

How can I keep going when nothing I do to control my diabetes seems to work?

▼ TIP:

First, make sure your goals are realistic. Perfect diabetes control is impossible, so if this is your goal, you'll probably be disappointed. You'll also be disappointed if you set goals that are personally unrealistic. Some people can run 6 miles every day, but you may not be one of them. If not, don't make that level of activity part of your diabetes management plan.

Naturally, there are times when even the most realistic goals aren't met. That's the time to remind yourself why you set the goal in the first place. If that reason still holds, it could help you get back on track. You can also think of one step, no matter how small, you could take to get you immediately on the path toward your goal. Sometimes just realizing it's possible to take a positive step can really help. And remember; if all else fails to rally your spirits, call on a family member, friend, or health care provider for the support you need.

Talk "sense" to yourself. Give yourself affirming messages for all that you're doing to manage your diabetes. Then, focus on healthy living and enjoying life. Let life be your focus, not diabetes. Remember what former American Diabetes Association (ADA) president Dr. Fred Whitehouse so wisely said, "Manage your diabetes to live; don't live to manage your diabetes."

*C*an stress management help my diabetes?

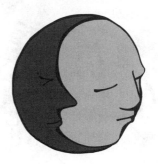

▼
TIP:

It could. Everybody's life is stressful, so doing things that help you relax is always good. Relaxing and managing your stress can also help you control your blood glucose, since uncontrolled stress can throw glucose levels out of whack.

There are lots of ways to relax. Think about what works for you. How about a nice soak in a warm tub? Or a quiet time reading your favorite magazine? Or talking on the phone to a good friend? How about gardening or attending religious services? Some people do formal meditation exercises or yoga or other physical activities to relax. All of these are wonderful ways to control stress.

Diabetes adds stress to your life. Finding ways to relieve stress can help you feel better and more able to manage your diabetes.

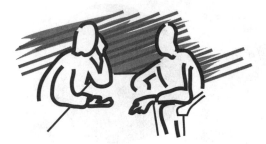

Where can I find people to talk to about living with diabetes? My family doesn't seem to get it.

▼
TIP:

Some hospitals offer educational programs and support groups for people who have diabetes. You could ask a family member to join you at a class or meeting, if you think that would be helpful. In some areas, the American Diabetes Association sponsors similar activities. Dial (800) DIABETES (342-2383) and ask them what they offer and where programs are held. Your health care provider may also be able to put you in touch with other people who have diabetes.

You might also try the Internet for a "virtual" support group. The ADA web site, *www.diabetes.org*, is a good place to start. Be aware that what other people say on the Internet ranges from brilliant to bunk, so be sure to check out anything you see online with someone you trust before giving it a shot yourself. The ADA also publishes a wide variety of materials to help you, including *Diabetes Forecast*, and books like this one with tips for living better with diabetes.

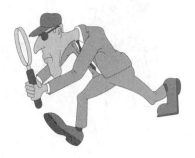

*H*ow can I deal with the
discouragement I feel when
I don't get the results I want?

▼
TIP:

*F*irst, be sure your expectations are realistic; unrealistic expectations almost guarantee disappointment. If your goals are realistic,
problem solving can boost your self-confidence and, thus, lift you out
of discouragement.

The basic, time-honored process of problem solving has four
steps:

1. Identify and define your problem.
2. List possible solutions.
3. Select and act on the most promising option.
4. Evaluate the outcome and keep going on your list of solutions until
   you feel the problem is solved.

Keep in mind the resources you have to help you problem solve.
Your health care team is a good source of practical suggestions,
having worked with many people who live with diabetes. Finally, by
talking positively to yourself you can alleviate the stressful feelings of
discouragement. Thomas Edison considered every failed experiment
not as a failure, but as a lesson in what didn't work.

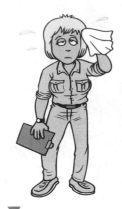

Can stress cause type 2 diabetes?

▼
TIP:

After lots of studies and research, the best we can say is maybe. Stress can elevate blood glucose levels. Sometimes this is the direct effect of stress hormones. Other times, it's because stress leads people to eat more and be less active, which can also raise blood glucose levels. We know this is true for people who already have diabetes. So, it seems likely that if your blood glucose levels are already higher than normal (but not yet high enough to call it diabetes), stress could push your levels into the diabetes range.

So the stress of a serious life event, such as the death of a loved one or the loss of a job, could play a part in developing diabetes. However, it is likely you would have eventually developed diabetes anyway as insulin resistance increased or insulin production decreased.

*H*ow can I tell if I am depressed?

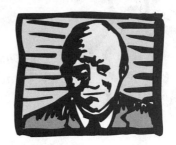

▼
TIP:

Being sad is normal. Just because you're sad, doesn't mean you're "depressed." Generally, if for at least two weeks you have been feeling really sad almost all day long, or you have lost interest in most things you used to enjoy, you could be suffering from depression.

Other signs of depression include:

- Feeling bad about yourself
- Trouble concentrating and making decisions
- Feeling hopeless
- Thoughts of dying
- Trouble sleeping
- Big changes in appetite and weight

People with diabetes are much more likely to be depressed, and the consequences of this can be especially severe—depression can make it much harder to manage your diabetes. So talk to your health care provider. There are treatments for depression that work for people with diabetes.

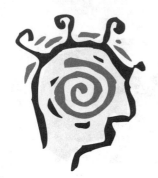

What should I do if I think I am depressed?

▼
TIP:

First, talk to your health care provider. Tell your provider that you think you might be depressed. Your health care provider can help determine whether or not this is true, or refer you to a mental health professional for diagnosis and treatment.

The good news is that there is effective treatment. Research shows that both counseling, especially a form of counseling called cognitive behavioral therapy, and antidepressant pills work to relieve depression in most people who have diabetes. Not only that, people in these studies whose depression was resolved also had closer-to-normal blood glucose levels.

So if you think you are depressed, trust your feelings and seek some assistance. Treatment can make your life happier, and healthier as well.

Could the fact that I was diagnosed
with diabetes a few months ago be
the reason I feel angry all the time?

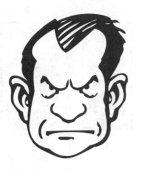

▼

TIP:

Maybe. Your life has changed a lot over the past few months, and it has changed in ways you didn't choose. It is normal and natural to feel angry about that. Your anger is even more understandable if your life was already pretty stressful before you developed diabetes.

Unfortunately, understandable as your anger may be, it can hurt you. Anger can burn you up and it can burn you out. Anger can push people away and cost you important support at a time when you really need it. Anger can increase your risk of having a heart attack or stroke, the leading causes of death for people with diabetes. And anger can sap your motivation for diabetes self-care. Some people even say that their blood glucose levels shoot up right away when they get angry.

So finding ways to deal with your normal, natural anger could really help.

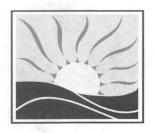

How can I find a positive way to look at diabetes management?

The real goal in diabetes management is quality of life. While diabetes management is measured by the amount of sugar in your blood, quality of life is measured by spiritual qualities like joy, peace, and love.

Inspiring stories are a source of nourishment. Stories like the poor shepherd boy, David, taking on a foe like Goliath, the giant, can inspire people to believe that they can "take on" the challenge of diabetes with the same faith as David.

Metaphor is a great way to see an old or negative situation with a new and more positive viewpoint. The author Louisa May Alcott said: "I am not afraid of storms, for I am learning how to sail my ship." Like sailing, diabetes management requires specific skills. To sail our ships successfully we need to know how to manage the physical aspects of diabetes. Equally important is the psychological, social, and spiritual stamina that helps us to cope with diabetes and any other storm that life presents. As captain of your ship, you need to make sure that you have access to resources that can provide physical, mental, and spiritual ballast.

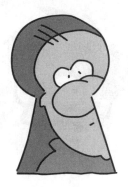

*W*hy do I feel anxious all the time?

▼

TIP:

*L*ots of people feel anxious, whether they have diabetes or not, especially these days. Having diabetes only adds to the burden of worry. It can be hard to tell the difference between normal, and even useful, worrying and the kind that indicates a problem.

If you feel anxious all or almost all the time, it is probably a problem. Try to picture as clearly and specifically as you can what worries you. Picture it and describe it to yourself in detail. Does anything help you manage your worry? If so, how can you more often do what helps? If nothing helps and you can't think of anything that would help, talk to your health care provider for suggestions.

Low blood glucose levels can also contribute to anxiety. When people are low, they often say they feel shaky and agitated, and since low blood glucose can be embarrassing and even dangerous, many people worry a lot about getting low. In a sense, you can get anxious about low glucose anxieties. Preventing lows is important, but so is preventing highs, so you want to deal realistically with your anxiety about low blood glucose.

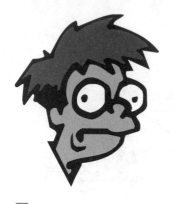

I've just been diagnosed with type 2 diabetes and it all seems very overwhelming. How can I make all the changes I'm supposed to make?

▼
TIP:

First, remember that you do not have to do everything at once. There are lots of changes to make, but they don't need to be made overnight. Also keep in mind that you are not alone in this. People who want to help you, including your health care team, family, and friends, are all around you. Make sure you draw on these resources to help you make needed changes. In addition to the support, you need the following three things to make changes:

■ Knowledge (about your diabetes)
■ Motivation (a reason to change that means a lot to you)
■ Resources (health care providers, family, personal strengths)

You can learn more about your diabetes by talking to your health care provider or participating in a diabetes education program at the local hospital. Call the American Diabetes Association at (800) DIABETES or visit *www.diabetes.org*. Having a reason to change is so important. Take time to be clear in your own mind and heart why you want to make changes. Then you can remind yourself later, when your commitment may be wavering. Resources to help you change are everywhere, and they can be very helpful once you are committed to making a change.

*M*aking changes to manage my diabetes is so hard. How can I make it easier?

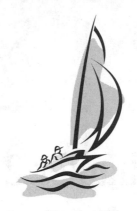

▼
TIP:

By making your changes more tangible. Consider a change you've been thinking of making. Pick a specific thing you want to do differently. Ask yourself, on a scale of 1 to 5, how important that change is to you. Next, ask yourself, on a scale of 1 to 5, how confident you are that you can make this change. Reflect on the barriers you may encounter as you attempt to reach your goal, and how you would overcome those barriers. Have you ever failed at an attempt to overcome this behavior? What's different about this time? Why are you confident that you will succeed?

As you list your reasons for success, list the rewards—both internal (like the pleasure of knowing you have succeeded) and concrete (like buying yourself a new article of clothing, a book, tickets to an event). Continue asking yourself the questions:

■ How important is this to me?
■ How confident am I that I can do it?

And, never give up. A German proverb says, "Patience is a bitter plant, but it has sweet fruit."

Chapter 2
EATING HEALTHIER AND CONTROLLING YOUR WEIGHT

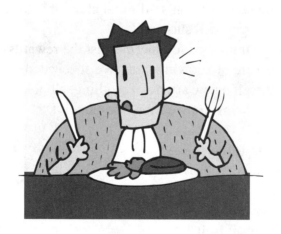

I *know I need to eat healthier* *because I have diabetes. How* *can I get my family to stop* *insisting I cook meals with lots of* *fat and sugar?*

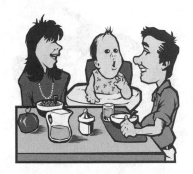

▼

TIP:

Try to strike a compromise with your family. For every time you cook a "rich" meal, they have to eat a meal low in fat and sugar. You can work out the most agreeable trade-off.

Also, you can probably make switches to cut "hidden" fat and sugar, like salsa on your potato, and skim milk instead of whole. Check out the many wonderful cookbooks that the American Diabetes Association has published. There are lots of great tips for cooking low fat and keeping carbs under control.

If you and your family have been accustomed to meals that are high in fat and sugar, you may want to make changes as slowly as possible. Instead of a high-fat salad, high-fat entrée, and a high-fat, high-sugar dessert, substitute a healthier item for one of the high-fat dishes. At another meal make a similar change with another dish. Slow changes will be more acceptable to your family and are more likely to stick. You can even avoid telling your family you've made the switch to healthier fare. They may not notice!

As you know, a diet that's good for people with diabetes is good for everyone. You're not helping just yourself, you're helping your whole family.

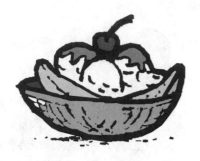

How do I deal with the temptation of desserts when I eat at other people's houses?

▼
TIP:

Offer to bring the dessert. Make something you really like that your family and friends enjoy as well. Most people are happy to have a guest to bring some part of the meal.

And remember, you can work in dessert. Tips for successfully "working in" dessert include:

■ Skipping another part of the meal, like bread or potato
■ Having a small portion. Sometimes a few mouthfuls will satisfy your craving
■ Extending enjoyment by eating slowly, savoring the flavor
■ Doing some activity after eating
■ Monitoring blood glucose an hour or two after eating to see what adjustments are called for

*H*ow can I stick to a meal plan when my schedule at work is so unpredictable?

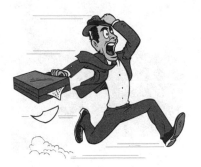

▼
TIP:

E ating something as close to your normal eating times as possible can help. Try carrying easy-to-eat foods with you, such as trail mix or carrots. That way you can satisfy your hunger without pushing your blood sugars too high. You can also check your blood glucose before you eat a snack or meal. If your blood sugar is on the high side, you don't need to eat unless you're hungry.

If you eat a snack to tide you over, try to eat a little less at your next meal. Focus on eating reasonable servings and avoiding large amounts of sweets. Finally, if you find yourself eating at an odd time, try to work in some exercise after your meal to help burn off a few of the calories and keep your blood glucose level closer to normal.

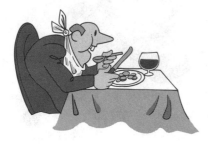

I find it hard to stay on my diet, and whenever I splurge I feel so guilty that I just keep on splurging for days. What can I do?

▼

TIP:

It was once said that the best way to deal with a temptation is to yield to it! Staying on a diet forever is extremely hard. So the first step is to recognize that *everyone* splurges. It's natural, normal, and even inevitable. If you accept this and it helps you feel less guilty, you might be able to splurge in a more controlled way.

You can also try the "3-to-1 rule." The 3-to-1 rule is as follows: Each time you indulge in a food splurge, follow it with 3 equal units of time in which you eat a more sensible, predictable diet. The time period in question can vary. It could be a single meal, a day, even a weekend. For example, if you eat voraciously for a day, eat conservatively for the following three days. Remember, good diabetes control is a game of averages, not a game of perfection!

I cannot control my eating in the evening between dinner and bedtime. What should I do?

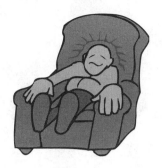

▼
TIP:

Get busy! Distract yourself from thinking about food by getting involved in an activity that so absorbs you, food doesn't even make it to your radar screen. Some people report that leaving the house is helpful. You could take a walk, do an errand, or visit a friend (and let your friend know what you're doing so that you're not offered snacks). If you are at home, clean a closet, do woodworking, play the piano, or read a book that you know will completely absorb you. Make a list of a few projects, so if you finish one you have another to start.

Make a decision (even a formal contract with yourself) about the times you absolutely will not eat, like when you're reading or watching television. Tell yourself that you will eat only while sitting at the kitchen or dining room table and only during mealtimes or scheduled snack times.

Another winning technique is to avoid overstocking the refrigerator and pantry. If there is not much food available, it is much easier to avoid eating between meals.

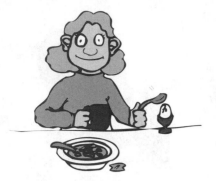

I'm shocked by how high my blood sugar is after a meal. Would eating smaller meals more frequently help?

▼
TIP:

It could help. Though this approach is not for everyone, it does have advantages for many people with diabetes, including

- Lower blood glucose levels after eating (because less food is eaten)
- Lower total insulin needs for those who take insulin
- Lower cholesterol levels
- Less hunger, so fewer calories are consumed throughout the day

There are some diabetes pills, such as acarbose (Precose) and miglitol (Glyset), that slow the absorption of food and have similar effects to eating smaller meals.

For more, talk to your health care provider about this approach to keeping your blood glucose level closer to normal throughout the day.

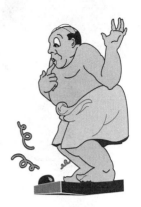

I'm struggling to control my weight. Should I see a dietitian?

▼
TIP:

EVERYONE who has diabetes should see a registered dietitian (RD). There are three very important reasons for this:

1. **Diabetes management** is greatly dependent upon the type of food you eat and the amount of food you eat.
2. **Good nutrition** is a basic and important part of a healthy life. A dietitian will recommend a meal plan that contains nutritionally well-balanced food and good taste.
3. A dietitian can help you with **weight management**, an important goal for most people with diabetes.

Weight management means taking in less energy (calories) than you put out (activity). That's a good way to remember that activity is an important part of weight control.

Both the American Dietetic Association—(800) 877-1600 ext. 5000, or *www.eatright.org*—and the American Association of Diabetes Educators—(800) TEAM-UP-4, or *www.aadenet.org*—have hotlines and web sites that can give you the names of dietitians in your area.

I almost always feel stuffed (and guilty) after eating at a restaurant. What can I do?

TIP:

This can be very difficult. Restaurants today serve almost criminal amounts of food as a single meal. Cleaning your plate usually means you've eaten enough food for three people. Therefore, portion control is very important. The following tips should help you keep your food intake at a reasonable level.

- First, become a taster. If you're dining with friends who like to share, trading tastes can add variety, and variety can help make up for quantity.
- Second, when you are served your main course, divide the portions (meat, vegetables, starch) in half, and ask the server to put your "leftovers" in a bag to take home for later. This will leave you feeling comfortably full rather than stuffed, and it means you'll have another delicious meal the next night.
- Finally, tune in to your body. Pay attention to how you feel when you are getting full. Learn to stop eating when you feel this way, even if your plate is not empty.

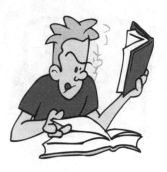

I *know I should be counting carbs*
to improve my blood sugar control,
but I'm having trouble learning how.
Where should I turn for help?

▼
TIP:

Talk with a registered dietitian who can help you figure it out. There is usually one associated with your local hospital. If this is not a good solution for you, look for an Internet site with carb counting help. For example, you could try using the carb counting flash card deck made by Carb Cards (*www.carbcards.com*). Each card has an image and the name of a type of food on it, along with the carbohydrate count for each item. You can combine the cards to build a food pyramid and create daily menus. Sometimes a picture is worth a thousand words!

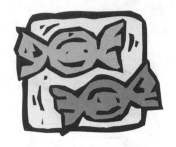

*I*s it okay to eat candy? I love it and *don't want to give it up.*

▼
TIP:

It is okay to eat anything as long as you don't eat too much and you know how much you're eating, so you can make adjustments to keep your blood glucose close to normal. More and more candy and sweets have labels with a nutritional analysis, including the amount of carbohydrate and fat, so it is easier to know how much you are eating. When you know that, you can compensate by eating less of something else, exercising, or taking more insulin (if this is an option).

Some people eat their favorite candy to treat low blood sugar. The challenge here can be controlling the number you eat, especially if you really like the candy and you're so low you aren't thinking clearly.

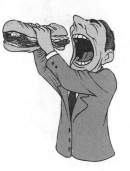

I'm confused about what I am supposed
to eat. What is a healthy diet for people
with diabetes?

▼
TIP:

The same diet that is healthy for everyone—one that includes
grains, beans, fruits, vegetables, low-fat dairy products, and
meats. You don't need special foods because of diabetes, but you
should do what you can to cut back on foods with lots of fat (like
lunch meats, salad dressings, cheeses, and fried foods), lots of added
sugar (like soft drinks), or both (like desserts and candies).

If you are taking insulin or other diabetes medication, the timing
of your meals could also be important for keeping your blood glucose
levels as close to normal as possible throughout the day. Keeping
track of how different foods affect your blood glucose can also help
you choose a healthy meal plan.

Seeing a registered dietitian (RD) can make this process easier
and more effective. An RD can work with you to see what type of
foods you like, what you don't like, and what would work best for
your diabetes management. Together, you can come up with a meal
plan that works for you.

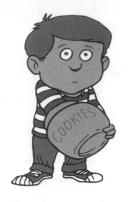

*S*ometimes *I can't stop eating. Is this
because of my diabetes?*

▼
TIP:

It could be. There are many reasons why people can't stop eating.
Sometimes it is more mental than physical. Since eating provides
an immediate satisfaction, some people eat to cope with emotional
needs that have little to do with physical hunger. And because eating
doesn't truly satisfy these needs, these feelings often return very
quickly and the person will keep eating. If diabetes makes your life
feel less satisfying, it could contribute to your problem.

Another group of people physically can't tell when they've eaten
enough. For some reason or another, their bodies don't signal that
they're full and they continue to eat long after they've eaten more than
they need.

Still other people eat to protect themselves from low blood
glucose. Some are so afraid of ever going low that they constantly
keep their levels really high. Dealing with these natural fears can
make a big difference. People who frequently go low need to adjust
their diabetes management plan, not overeat. Talk to your health care
provider about any issues that might be causing your overeating.

Chapter 3
BEING MORE ACTIVE

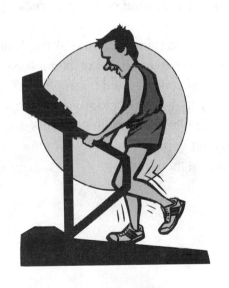

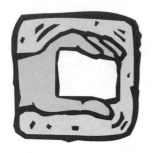

I don't like to carry things in my hands while I'm active, so it's a hassle to carry a fast-acting carb with me while I exercise. What can I do?

▼
TIP:

There are a few solutions to this problem:

- First, try carrying a fanny pack with a few carbs and perhaps a small glucose meter. Several companies make packs designed for athletes.
- You could also try carrying a couple of small tubes of cake icing in some wristbands. They are light, resistant to sweat and moisture, and contain a very concentrated form of glucose.
- Some athletes with diabetes actually place a roll of LifeSavers inside the webbing of their shoelaces. This doesn't add much weight and by being placed inside your shoelaces, you're not as likely to nibble on them randomly.

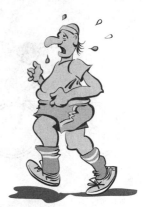

I worry that I will go low while exercising. How do I adjust my insulin so this doesn't happen?

▼
TIP:

Figuring out the best adjustment can take a bit of trial and error. First, ask your health care provider for advice. Second, do what serious and professional athletes do: Keep a training log. In your training log, you'll want to record the following things:

- Type of exercise
- Time of exercise
- Duration and intensity of your session
- What you eat before you start
- Most importantly, your blood glucose before you start and after you stop exercising

Since exercise can cause you to continue using glucose after you stop your session, it is important to measure your glucose about one hour after your session ends. By reviewing your training log, you will be able to see what did and did not work for you.

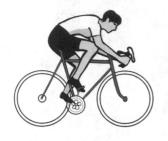

I don't want to run out of energy while I'm exercising. What should I eat to prevent this?

What foods you use depends on 3 things—the type of exercise you are doing, the duration and intensity, and your blood glucose level before exercising. If your blood glucose is below 150 mg/dl before you exercise, it is probably a good idea to eat about 15 grams of carbohydrate. This could be a serving of starch, fruit, or milk. You might also consider using foods that you really like, but usually don't eat because they have a negative impact on your blood sugars. One athlete we know enjoys eating a Snickers bar before his workouts. As he says, "I know there are better sources of energy, such as sports drinks, but I really like Snickers. So the way I see it, if I need to scratch my chocolate itch, I might as well do it when I know that the exercise will burn up most of the glucose!"

*H*ow can I exercise regularly when I
work all day?

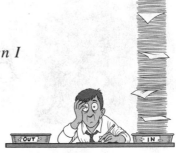

▼
TIP:

First of all, remember that *exercise* really means *activity*, so lots of things you don't consider to be exercise actually are. Just as important, you don't have to be active for large blocks of time to reap the benefits. Several short "bursts" of activity in a day can be just as good for you.

Try to make the most of opportunities to be active during the normal course of your day. Take the stairs instead of the elevator. Park at the far end of the parking lot and walk to the store. Set aside 10 minutes of your lunchtime for a brisk walk. You may be pleasantly surprised with your total daily activity level if you take advantage of opportunities like these.

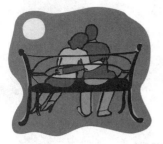

How many calories do I burn when my wife and I are intimate?

▼

TIP:

Sex is exercise, just like running or swimming. Like all exercise, the number of calories you burn making love depends on the duration and intensity of the activity, as well as your weight (the more you weigh, the more calories you burn doing the same activity). The average caloric consumption during lovemaking has been calculated at 250 calories an hour.

If your blood glucose tends to go low during sex or immediately after, you might want to check your level just before or after you make love. If you are low or headed in that direction, it's best to eat something. This can briefly interrupt your loving interlude, but it can also help prevent the more serious interruption of a low glucose episode.

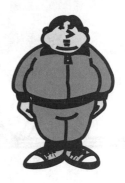

*W*hat can you suggest for a person who really dislikes exercise?

▼
TIP:

First, we will remove the word *exercise*. Researchers have found that you don't really need to exercise. Just any old kind of physical activity is good enough, if you do it regularly. As little as 30 minutes of moderate activity (like brisk walking) a day can do you good. Try to find an activity that you actually like doing. The possibilities are endless—walking the dog, swimming, dancing, or even playing with a child or grandchild.

Try to pair that activity with something else you like to do. For example, if you regularly talk to a friend on the phone or over the back fence, go for a walk with that person instead. Or, if it's feasible to walk to work or the store instead of taking the bus or driving, give that a try.

You can also set some activity goals or milestones, and reward yourself as you progress and reach them. You decide on the reward. Eventually, you may find you are feeling better and are actually enjoying the activity, and the activity itself becomes its own reward.

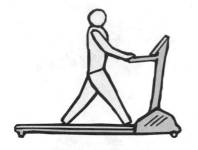

Is it safe to exercise if I have heart problems?

▼
TIP:

If you have heart problems, the American Diabetes Association recommends you have an exercise stress test before you start exercising. An exercise stress test shows how a workout affects your heart and blood pressure. The test also helps to detect "silent" heart disease (heart disease that has no symptoms), which is more common in people who have diabetes.

During an exercise stress test, you walk on a treadmill while your heart function and blood pressure are monitored. You start at a slow pace and gradually build up until you get tired or something unusual shows up on the monitor. The test usually lasts a few minutes and rarely lasts longer than 20 minutes. After the test is done, the doctor who did the test will tell you about the results, including any problems that need treatment and any conditions you need to take into account when you exercise.

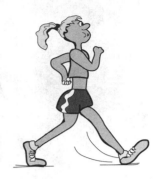

W*here can I find someone to walk with?*

▼
TIP:

Many people find it easier to exercise when they have company. Start by asking people you know who might be willing to join you. Check with family members, friends, and coworkers. Try to find someone dependable who is at about your level of fitness. If no one you know is interested or available, see if any of the malls in your area has a walking program, or look in your local paper for walking clubs. Almost all cities have several, for all ages and levels of fitness. Walking clubs are fun and the members are always happy to have you join them. You could also start walking at the track at a local school; you are almost certain to find other walkers there. Seek and you shall find.

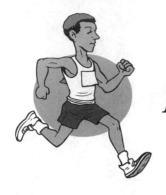

I want to compete in a 5-k run. What should I do to prepare?

TIP:

Competing can be fun and rewarding, as long as you stay safe. First, check with your health care provider to be sure that you're physically able to train for competition. Once you've been checked out, be sure your goals for the run are realistic. Your first goal should be to have fun, and your second should be to finish the run feeling good. Try to keep your time for the race lower on your list of priorities.

Next, you have to train so you will be ready to reach your goals. A healthy goal is to build up your weekly training mileage to between 10–15 miles a week. Start with runs of a mile or less and work up to 3 miles or a little longer (5 kilometers is about 3.1 miles). By the time of the race you should be able to run 5 km comfortably. Don't worry about the speed of your training runs. If you want to get some idea of what your race-day time will be, about 2–3 weeks before the race run 5 km as fast as you comfortably can and time yourself. You will probably run a bit faster on race day because your adrenaline will be flowing.

*C*an exercise cause my blood glucose
to drop hours later?

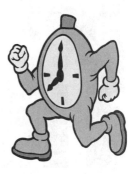

▼ TIP:

Yes. Depending on the intensity and duration of your activity, you can burn glucose for up to 24 hours after exercise. With long or hard exercise, you use sugars stored in your liver for fuel. After the exercise is over, your body wants to replenish those sugars as soon as possible. If there is no food available, the sugars are pulled from your bloodstream, which can cause hypoglycemia. To help prevent low blood glucose, check your blood sugar about every 45 minutes after a hard workout and gauge whether your blood sugar is going down, going up, or leveling off. If it is going down, eat a few carbs and keep checking until you level off.

*I*s it safe to exercise if my blood glucose is high?

▼
TIP:

This depends on how high and how much insulin you have on board. If your blood glucose is higher than 300 mg/dl, you should not exercise until you have taken some fast-acting insulin and your blood glucose level is below 250 mg/dl. The problem is this: If your glucose is high and you don't have enough insulin in your body to use the glucose, your cells will continue to signal they need glucose for fuel, and your liver will continue to put out that glucose. Without insulin to let the glucose into the cells, the glucose keeps building up in your blood, pushing your blood glucose levels higher and higher.

If you have enough insulin available, exercise may actually help lower your glucose. In fact, many athletes raise their blood sugar before exercise on purpose to create a bit of a buffer so they won't go low during their activity.

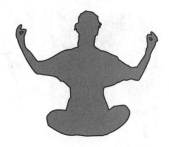

*H*ow *can I exercise if I don't get around very well?*

▼
TIP:

There are activities for everyone. Swimming or water aerobics are easy on your body, and there are chair exercises you can do sitting down. You can also try yoga or tai chi for no-impact exercise. Some of these activities require equipment (like a swimming pool), or some training (like yoga or tai chi), but others (like chair exercises) can be done anywhere at all with "equipment" you already have at home.

Try lifting cans of food while sitting in a chair watching television, or try waving around dishcloths while listening to music to increase your range of motion and your fitness. There are also books and videotapes on exercise available for people who have limited mobility. So look for ways to increase your activity despite your limitations. You will be glad you did.

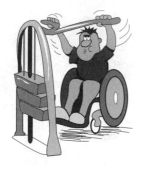

It's hard for me to get motivated about exercising. Will buying exercise equipment help me exercise more regularly?

▼ TIP:

It could, if you find something you really like. On the other hand, you don't want to spend lots of money on something that ends up being an expensive clothes rack. There are 3 keys to finding the right exercise equipment for you.

- First, decide on your activity goals. If you want to walk, the only equipment you'll need is a good pair of shoes and comfortable clothes. Strength training will require some free weights or a piece of equipment, perhaps one that lets you do a variety of exercises.
- Second, think about your space and money limitations. These will determine what, if any, equipment it makes sense to consider.
- Finally, try before you buy, especially if you're thinking about spending a lot of money. If you think a particular piece of equipment might be right for you, try it out at a friend's house, at the store, or at a local health club.

The right equipment can really help you stay active, so make sure the one you buy is the right one for you.

*S*tarting an exercise program isn't a problem. How do I stick with it?

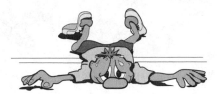

▼
TIP:

Y ou're in the same boat as a lot of people we know. Activity is like weight loss. Most people who want to lose weight have succeeded, often many times. But the trick is not losing weight—it's keeping it off.

Here are some keys to sticking with an activity program:

- Pick only things you like to do (or at least things you don't hate to do).
- Pick more than one activity (to avoid boredom, deal with weather problems, and cross-train).
- Be realistic. Don't expect to do what you could when you were in high school.
- Get company for your activity (to add to your motivation and pleasure).
- Make appointments with yourself to exercise (to help you stay on schedule).
- Reward yourself. Staying active is a major accomplishment, so regularly reward yourself for your effort.

Chapter 4
KEEPING BLOOD GLUCOSE LEVELS CLOSER TO NORMAL

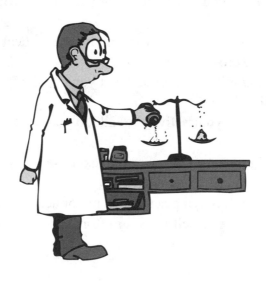

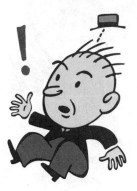

How can I do the same thing every day for a week and then suddenly get a blood glucose reading that is totally out of whack?

▼

TIP:

It would be wonderful if there were a precise formula for keeping blood glucose levels right where you want them; this much food, this much activity, and this much medication, and your blood glucose is always in range. But it doesn't work that way. No 2 days are exactly the same, so controlling diabetes requires constant monitoring and adjustment. Often, just when you think you have a plan that works reliably, something shifts; sometimes it's things you can't control or things you may not even recognize. Understanding yourself and the way you feel is the best tool for constant and complete management. If you know when your blood glucose is heading high or low—which takes regular monitoring—you can act on these ups and downs, and maximize your time spent in that lovely "normal" range.

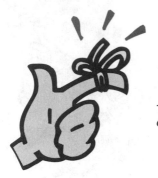

I have trouble getting blood out of my finger. Are there ways to make it easier?

▼

TIP:

B efore lancing your finger:

Wash it in warm water to get the blood flowing.
Shake your finger down like a thermometer.
Milk your finger.
Put a rubber band around your finger just tight enough to make the tip of your finger red. Remove the rubber band as soon as you draw blood.

Also consider these suggestions:

If no blood appears after you lance, wait about 5 seconds before squeezing. This gives the blood enough time to surface. If you squeeze too soon, you can sometimes have the opposite effect and decrease the flow.
Try lancets of different lengths to find the one that works best for you.
Try one of the alternate-site monitors to draw blood from your hands and arms.

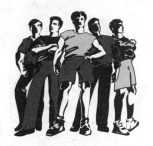

I *hate checking my blood glucose in public. What can I do?*

▼
TIP:

Your feelings are natural. Your diabetes is your business and it should not be anyone else's unless you want it to be. However, finding a private place to check your glucose can be difficult. Look for a quiet corner, or even a restroom stall if that is the only private place you can find. However, you may be surprised how few people even notice when you check your blood in public.

Some of the new blood glucose monitors are smaller, quicker, and quieter, and that can help make the process less stressful. Finally, if there is no place at all where you would be comfortable checking your glucose while you are out, check just before you leave the house, and check again as soon as you get home. That way you'll have at least some information for making decisions while you are out.

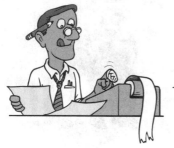

How can I afford to check my blood glucose as often as I should?

▼
TIP:

Monitoring your blood glucose can be expensive. The strips you use to check twice a day can cost as much as $700 a year. If you don't have good health insurance, you may have to pay all of that yourself. If you are having trouble paying for your strips, talk to your health care provider. Your provider could help you find a source for limited supplies of free strips, a less expensive strip to use, or different insurance plans that have better reimbursement for strips. You can also make the most of information you get from limited monitoring by checking at different times each day. For example, check before and after your breakfast one day, before and after lunch the next, etc. Remember, some information is always better than none at all. Talk to your health care provider to decide on the best monitoring schedule for you.

I don't like to carry my insulin and a syringe with me when I'm away from home. What should I do?

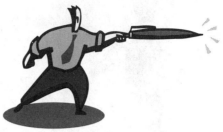

▼
TIP:

Fortunately, there are alternatives to a vial and syringe. One of our favorites is an insulin pen. An insulin pen is a small device that looks like a large fountain pen and enables you to easily take your insulin away from home—you just dial the dose you need. They are small, discreet, and protect your insulin vial from breaking. Insulin pens are the most popular way to deliver insulin in most other countries of the world, but they are just beginning to catch on in the United States. Your health care provider can tell you more about insulin pens and show you your options.

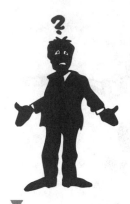

I have type 1 diabetes, use an insulin pump, and lead a pretty stable life. Do I really have to check my blood glucose 4–8 times a day?

TIP:

Not necessarily. However, be sure to talk with your health care provider before changing your glucose monitoring schedule. The safest days to reduce checks are very predictable ones, when your blood glucose before breakfast is close to normal. Take your normal boluses for any food you eat and pay close attention to any signs your blood glucose might be too high or too low. Check your level if you are not sure.

If your food or activity varies from usual, you should check more frequently. Finally, it's always wise to check your glucose before bed, just to confirm that the day has gone as expected, blood-sugar–wise.

My *doctor wants me to check my glucose*
more frequently, but it's always a
hassle. Half the time I can't find my meter,
and even when I know where it is, it's
usually not where I am. What can I do?

▼
TIP:

No one enjoys checking blood glucose. Different people dislike it for different reasons. If for you it's the fact your monitor is never where you are, getting extra monitors could help. Monitors are often provided free or at very low cost, because the companies that make monitors make their money on test strips, not the monitors themselves. So you might be able to get an extra monitor or two pretty cheaply. Keep the monitors where you are most likely to be using them. For example, keep one by your bed (good for testing when you get up or go to bed), keep another in your kitchen (good for testing before meals), and keep another where you work. If you work out of your car, be careful of extreme temperatures, both for your monitor and your strips. Do not keep them in the glove box or trunk, and carry them with you if it is very hot or very cold.

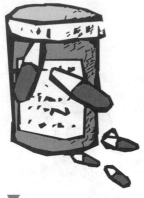

I'm taking several new diabetes medications and don't really understand what they are and how they work. How can I learn more?

▼
TIP:

There are lots of new diabetes medications available, and the number is growing rapidly. So it makes sense to stay informed about ones that might be right for you. New insulins are being introduced all the time, and we now have diabetes pills to help you control your blood glucose levels in different ways. There are pills that help you make more insulin, pills that control the release of glucose from your liver into your blood, pills that help your body use insulin better, and pills that slow the absorption of food. Since different medications help control glucose in different ways, many people take two or more diabetes pills to get the most benefit. Your health care provider is your best source of information about new diabetes medications, because your provider knows you and your diabetes.

You can find information on new diabetes medications from other places as well, including publications of the American Diabetes Association, such as *Diabetes Forecast*, and on the ADA web site (*www.diabetes.org*). Many pharmaceutical companies also maintain web sites with information about their new products.

My doctor wants me to start taking insulin, but when my mother started taking it years ago she developed complications. Will that happen to me?

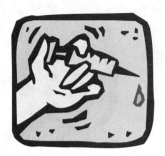

TIP:

No. We can't promise you won't get complications if you take insulin, but we can assure you that insulin itself does not cause complications. In fact, taking insulin will actually *reduce* your risk of getting complications. That's because complications are the result of having high blood glucose for a long time, and insulin can help *lower* blood glucose. So insulin usually cuts your risk of complications; it doesn't increase it.

You mention that your mother developed complications after she started taking insulin, but the insulin is almost certainly not to blame. Since complications are the result of years of high blood glucose, the truth is this: Your mother would almost certainly have developed complications if she had not started taking insulin, and the complications would have come sooner and been more severe. Please don't let your concerns compromise your health. If you take insulin when you need it, you can help prevent complications, not cause them.

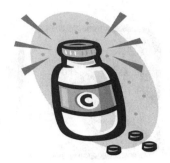

I'm looking for anything that might lower my blood sugar. Are there mineral supplements that could help?

▼
TIP:

Many minerals, including chromium, magnesium, selenium, and zinc, have been promoted by popular magazines and supplement companies as effective tools in controlling blood glucose. But there is currently no scientific evidence for these claims, so it is hard to recommend taking supplements. If you eat healthy foods, including lots of fresh fruits, vegetables, and grains, you should get all the minerals you need to stay healthy. From what we know now, taking supplements probably won't make you any healthier. Nor will it make your blood glucose any lower.

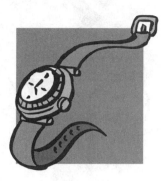

I'm so tired of checking my blood glucose. Will there ever be a way to check without sticking myself?

▼
TIP:

Several companies are working on so-called *noninvasive* blood glucose monitoring alternatives that work to get accurate blood glucose readings without the dreaded "poke."

The newest devices, however, are really only a step toward truly noninvasive monitoring. One looks like a wristwatch and you wear it on your wrist, just like a watch. You have to check your glucose the old-fashioned way once a day to set the watch, which then gives glucose readings three times each hour.

Another company has a monitor about the size of a pager that gets readings through a sensor inserted under your skin. The monitor records glucose levels every 15 minutes. Since the device is new, the company has only limited approval. Your doctor has to give you the monitors, and they can only be used for a few days. The device stores all your glucose readings during that time, but you can't see them until you visit your doctor at the end of your monitoring period. If further testing is positive, this may change.

Hopefully, like the process of sterilizing and sharpening syringes before an injection, "sticking" yourself will soon fade into history, existing only as a memory of the diabetes therapy of old.

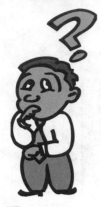

*W*ith dozens of blood glucose monitors on the market, how do I choose the one that's right for me?

▼
TIP:

Picking the right monitor is a little like choosing a car—you have to think of the features that matter most to you. And there are lots of features to choose from. Are you looking for the fastest monitor? There are some that complete the check in 5 seconds. Other monitors have larger screens that are easier to see if your vision is not good. Some use strips that are easier to handle if you have arthritis or nerve damage. Looking to get organized? There are monitors that have lots of data management capabilities, which can help you track your results more precisely and communicate these results to your health care provider. There are monitors that use very small drops of blood and others that let you test on your hand, arm, or leg, as well as your finger.

So you see, there are lots of options. To choose the monitor that's best for you, talk to your health care provider. Or better yet, talk to a diabetes educator; he or she will probably be up to date on all the latest models and have some available for you to see.

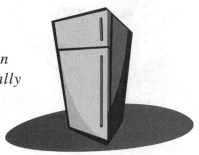

It is really hard to keep my insulin refrigerated all the time, especially when I travel. Do I always have to do this?

▼

TIP:

No. Your insulin should be fine for about 1 month as long as it does not freeze or get really hot—about 85°F. So as long as it is less than a month old, you only need to protect it from extreme temperatures. If you leave your insulin in a car on a hot summer day, keep it in a cooler—just make sure the insulin doesn't touch the ice, or it might freeze. You also need to be careful your insulin doesn't freeze in the winter. Keep it someplace safe. And do the same when you fly. Always keep your insulin with you; never put it in the luggage you check. Your luggage could get lost, and even if it arrives safely, your insulin could be frozen or exposed to extreme heat.

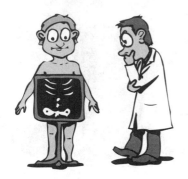

*D*o I really need to have an A1C check at the doctor's office if I check my blood glucose regularly at home?

▼

TIP:

The A1C check (also known as an HbA1c check) tells you your glucose control over a period of about 3 months. The glucose check you do at home tells you your level at that moment; the A1C tells you what your mean blood glucose has been over the last 90 days or so. The A1C check is a great tool because it gives a very clear, longer-term picture of your glucose control. That helps fill out the picture you get from your own glucose monitoring. For example, if your A1C level is 9%, your blood glucose averaged 210 mg/dl over the past 3 months. Unfortunately, this is about the average A1C of people with diabetes in the United States.

People who don't have diabetes have A1C levels somewhere under 6% (an average blood sugar of 90 mg/dl). As you can see, there is a big difference between normal blood glucose levels and the levels most people with diabetes have. The Diabetes Control and Complications Trial (DCCT) showed that lowering your A1C by just 0.5% can make a big difference in your diabetes management. Getting your blood glucose levels closer to normal is hard work, but every little bit you lower them helps. The A1C test lets you see where you stand. You can use that information to increase your chances for a longer, healthier life.

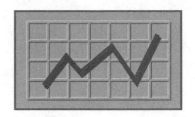

I'm really confused about what my blood glucose level should be.

▼
TIP:

The simple answer is, as close to normal as possible. The ADA recommends specific glucose goals for people with diabetes. They say you should aim for glucose levels that are 80–120 mg/dl before meals, for levels less than 160 mg/dl 2 hours after meals, and for levels that are 100–140 mg/dl before bed. As for A1C, they suggest you aim for a level of near or under 7%—an average glucose of about 150 mg/dl. The ADA has also set higher "take action" levels for each of these measures. For example, the "take action" level for A1C is 8% (an average glucose level of 180 mg/dl).

If your current glucose levels are higher than the ADA goals, or even if they're higher than the take action levels, don't lose heart. At least half of all people with diabetes in this country have A1C levels higher than the ADA take action level. The most important message is this: Every little bit helps. If you lower your glucose and keep it lower, you lower your risk of diabetic complications. That's as true for people who have A1C levels of 11% as it is for those whose levels are much lower.

Chapter 5
MANAGING HIGH AND LOW BLOOD GLUCOSE

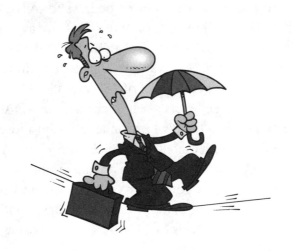

*H*ow can I treat a low blood glucose when I am at the theater or a concert without making lots of noise unwrapping candy?

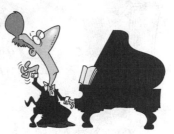

TIP:

*P*ut jellybeans (or some other "soft" candy) into a plastic sandwich bag. The plastic bag makes no noise when opened, and the candy won't make any noise when you chew it. Make sure you know how many candies you need to treat a typical low and make up a bunch of single-use "bean bags." That way you will have a ready source of tasty, portion-controlled carbohydrate whenever you need it. Keep one in your briefcase, car, bedside stand, and anywhere else it might come in handy.

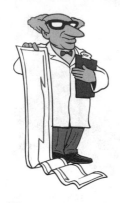

How can I resist taking too much insulin to treat a high blood glucose?

▼
TIP:

Instead of treating a high blood glucose in one big swoop, take it down in small steps. Trying to get your blood glucose down when it is high is a good thing. But overdoing it can push your level too low, and that isn't a good thing. So you have to think before treating— what has worked in the past and what hasn't? It would be great if you could go from a high glucose level to a normal one in one big jump, with a nice, soft landing. But it usually doesn't work that way; sometimes the landing is hard. Too often you end up low, and that hurts. To avoid that, get your blood glucose back where you want it in a couple of easier steps, instead of one giant, painful step. Take a little less insulin than is tempting, and then check your glucose level when the insulin should be working to see the results and make any adjustments. This approach should make it possible to get your blood glucose down while lowering the risk of going too low.

Why shouldn't I eat chocolate to treat a low?

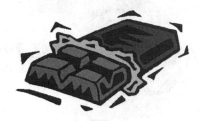

▼
TIP:

Many people are tempted to eat chocolate to treat a low, because they love chocolate and they feel they are making good of a bad situation. To some degree they are, but this approach has a downside. Chocolate contains a lot of fat, which is part of the reason it tastes so good. Unfortunately, your body absorbs foods that contain fat more slowly, so something sugary and fat-free will probably raise your glucose faster than chocolate. So, though it might be tempting to reach for the chocolates when you are low, other things will probably get you back to normal quicker. That doesn't mean you shouldn't enjoy chocolate. Just be aware of its limits as a treatment for low blood glucose.

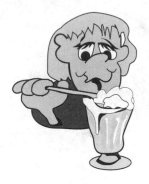

How can I avoid overeating when I am low?

It's easy to overeat when you are low, because a low blood glucose makes it very hard to think clearly. Everything you know about food and how much it takes to bring your glucose up without going too high goes out the window. Instead, you respond to something that is very clear: your body's cry of "feed me!" By the time you're thinking clearly again, you have usually eaten way too much.

A few things can help make it easier to resist temptation:

■ First, have unit-size low glucose treatment "kits" available. These can be anything that works for you, from a small box of raisins to a can of regular soda to a few jelly beans.

■ Second, when you are low, get one of your kits and take it somewhere away from other sources of food.

■ Third, eat what is in your kit and tell yourself something simple that helps you wait 15 minutes before taking any further action (unless, of course, you feel *worse*). An example: "I really want more but this is probably enough." Keep your phrase simple or you won't be able to keep it in mind when you are low.

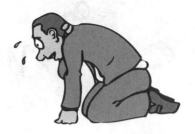

I *had a really bad low blood sugar*
and my doctor told me I needed
to get glucagon. What is glucagon?

▼
TIP:

Glucagon is an emergency treatment that is prescribed by your doctor for severe low blood glucose. It is injected when your reaction is so severe you can't treat yourself with food or drink, whether it's from an inability to swallow, confusion, or even unconsciousness. Since you won't be in any condition to give yourself glucagon when you need it, someone else should know when to give it and how to mix and inject the glucagon shot. It will usually raise your blood glucose in about 10–15 minutes.

Having glucagon (and someone who knows how to use it!) readily available can mean the difference between a scary few minutes and a much longer ordeal with 911 calls and trips to the emergency room. Keep in mind that glucagon raises your blood glucose by drawing on the glucose reserves in your liver, so you should eat something as soon as you can to replace those reserves. Unfortunately, some people feel sick to their stomach after taking glucagon, so eat lightly.

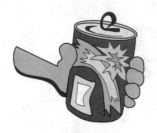

What is the best treatment for low blood glucose?

▼
TIP:

There are lots of choices. The ADA recommends you treat a low glucose level (less than 70 mg/dl) by eating or drinking something that contains 15 grams of sugar, preferably in a form that is absorbed quickly. Good choices include hard candy, jelly beans, fruit, fruit juice, regular soda, honey, table sugar, and glucose tablets or gel. Look up your favorite low blood glucose treatment foods to see how much of each equals 15 grams.

Check your glucose level 15 minutes after eating and treat again if you are still low. Try to avoid overtreating lows, and don't eat pure chocolate to treat lows because it contains lots of fat and relatively little sugar, so it takes longer to raise your blood glucose.

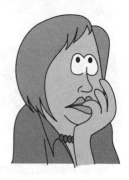

I *have to take a lot more insulin just before I get my period. Is that normal?*

▼
TIP:

Many women find they need more insulin in the days just before they start to menstruate, and that their insulin needs go back to normal when their periods begin. This isn't surprising, since estrogen levels increase just before a woman's period begins, and estrogen raises insulin needs. Everyone is different—your menstrual cycle might have a tremendous effect on your glucose levels or it might have none at all. Younger women tend to have this menstrual fluctuation most dramatically. If your blood sugars go up before your period, try to figure out when it starts to happen and try to pin down the amount of additional insulin you'll need until your period begins.

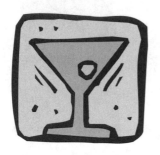

I got really low once when my friends and I were drinking, and they thought I was drunk. How can they tell the difference in the future?

▼
TIP:

First of all, drinking too much is never a good idea. Your friends should not be responsible for your low blood sugar or your diabetes. The signs of going low and being drunk are very similar, and it will be hard for them to tell which is at work, especially if they've been drinking too. If you take insulin, the problem can be even worse, because drinking, too much can lower glucose levels even more.

Do all you can to avoid going low when you are drinking. Eat a little something extra. Take a little less insulin. Check your blood glucose when you can. Once again, your friends should not be responsible for you, but some friends will want to know how to help. He or she must be sober and must be able to recognize changes in your behavior that indicate you might be low. Your friend should also know how to check your blood glucose level and know what to do if you are low or it's impossible to check your glucose. The easiest remedy in this situation is 4–6 ounces (about half of a glass) of regular (not diet) soft drink. This will be helpful if you're low and harmless if you've just had a little too much to drink.

*H*igh blood glucose levels after meals really upset me. Is there anything I can do to keep them down?

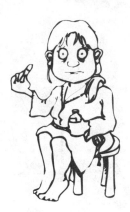

▼
TIP:

To avoid high glucose after a meal, you need information. Check your levels before eating and again 2 hours later. Do this for each meal a couple of times. If you take rapid-acting insulin with your meals, you can use your after-meal glucose levels to figure out how much more insulin you need to take before you eat. Be sure to talk with your health care provider before making changes in your plan— adding insulin can increase your risk of going too low. Some diabetes pills are especially effective for helping control after-meal glucose levels (for example, repaglinide [Prandin] and nateglinide [Starlix]). Talk to your health care provider about these pills if you are not already taking them. Taking a walk after eating can help, too. So can eating smaller, more frequent meals or eating meals with less carbo-hydrate, since carbohydrates contribute most to after-meal high glu-cose levels.

The fact you check your levels and know your after-meal blood glucose level is a good thing. Most people don't know because they rarely check. And unfortunately, most people have higher glucose lev-els after meals than they do before meals. Researchers say that after-meal glucose levels contribute to as much as one-third of A1C levels, the standard measure of long-term control.

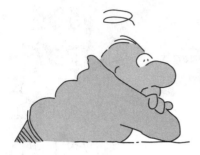

I strive for tight control, and I'm very scared of getting complications. How can I keep from getting really upset every time I get a high blood glucose?

▼

TIP:

Try not to worry. An occasional spike in your blood glucose is not likely to cause any harm. The problems come when your blood glucose stays high for long periods of time—days, weeks, and months. The best predictor of your chances for a long life, free of complications such as heart disease and stroke, is your average blood glucose level over a period of months (along with your blood pressure and lipid levels), not the number of blood sugar spikes. The A1C test gives the best estimate of your long-term control and risk of diabetic complications. Many studies have shown that whether you have type 1 diabetes or type 2, the lower your A1C, the lower your risk of developing complications. So your A1C level is the number to focus on, not a particular glucose reading. Focusing on individual blood sugar readings is misleading, and if you concentrate on the high ones it is likely to sap your motivation and energy. You need a realistic perspective to support the hard work required to manage your diabetes, and that perspective should be broader than your most recent glucose reading.

I was shocked at how high my last A1C was. How could it be high when my morning blood glucose checks are always close to normal?

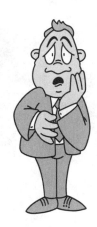

▼
TIP:

Your blood glucose levels can change quite a bit during the day, which means checking at a single time each day can give a very misleading picture of your overall control. The glucose checks you do at home are like photographs; they capture what is going on the moment they are done. On the other hand, an A1C reading is like a 3-month-long videotape; it captures everything that goes on during that period. As you can imagine, the videotape contains much more information about those 3 months than a daily photograph would.

For example, if someone took a single photograph of you each day at 3:00 A.M. for 3 months and then used the photographs to see what you did for those 3 months, it would look like you had been sleeping the whole time. In the same way, if your blood glucose tends to be lowest in the morning, those readings won't give an accurate picture of your overall control. Talk to your health care provider about checking at other times of the day to see when you are high, and what you can do to get your overall control in line with your good morning levels.

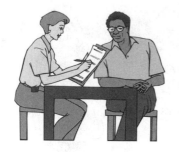

What should my A1C be to avoid complications?

▼
TIP:

There is no magic A1C number that guarantees you will not develop complications. However, the lower your A1C level, the less likely you are to get diabetic complications. It now seems that even slightly elevated A1C levels carry some increased risk for complications like heart disease and stroke. Unfortunately, very few people can get their A1C levels as low as they are in people who don't have diabetes; we don't have the tools to achieve this goal, and the amount of work and the increased risk of low blood glucose make it impossible for most people to manage. So all people with diabetes carry some increased risk of developing complications. Trying to be realistic, the American Diabetes Association says people with diabetes should aim for A1C levels of 7% or less. That's the equivalent of a 150 mg/dl average blood glucose. The ADA suggests that you take action and talk with your health care provider about changes in your treatment if your A1C is higher than 8% (the equivalent of a 180 mg/dl average blood glucose). The most important thing to keep in mind is this: Any improvement in your A1C reduces your risk of getting diabetic complications. A small improvement reduces your risk a little, and a big improvement reduces your risk a lot. But every improvement reduces your risk.

Chapter 6
UNDERSTANDING AND
AVOIDING COMPLICATIONS

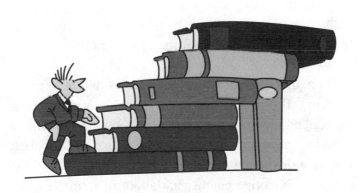

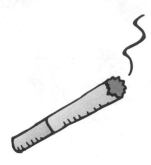

I don't think I can quit smoking. How important is it for me to stop?

TIP:

Very. Smoking is unhealthy for anyone, but smoking and diabetes is a truly deadly combination. Even if you didn't smoke, your risk of getting heart disease or having a stroke increases 2–4 times just because you have diabetes. Diabetes can cause blocked arteries, which leads to heart attacks and strokes. Smoking makes this even worse, and the risk of serious heart problems when you have diabetes *and* smoke is about 10 times greater than for someone who doesn't have diabetes or smokes.

You can't change the fact you have diabetes, but hard as it is, you can stop smoking. If you decide you are ready to stop smoking, there are many effective help programs available. Contact the American Lung Association in your area, or ask your physician or diabetes educator for help. He or she may refer you to a good stop-smoking program in your area. Nicotine patches and nicotine gum are also available from the drugstore, and they can help you deal with your nicotine addiction while you stop smoking.

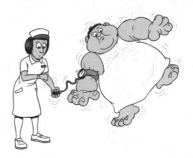

It's hard enough trying to control my blood sugars. Do I have to control my blood pressure and lipid levels as well?

▼
TIP:

Controlling your blood pressure and lipid (cholesterol) levels is as important as controlling your blood sugar, if not even more important. Heart attacks and stroke are the major causes of death among people with diabetes, and your risk of developing these complications is 2–4 times greater than for someone without diabetes. High blood pressure and abnormal lipids are major risk factors for these complications.

In addition to reducing stress, increasing activity, and eating heart healthy meals, there are excellent medications available to help you control blood pressure and lipids. The recommended levels for people with diabetes are lower than the levels for people the same age who don't have diabetes, due to the fact that people with diabetes are at a higher risk. Current goals for people with diabetes are:

■ Blood pressure <130/80
■ LDL cholesterol (the bad one) <100
■ HDL cholesterol (the good cholesterol) >45

Talk to your health care provider about your levels and anything you can do to improve them.

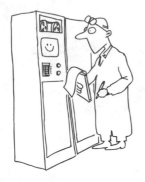

Is the trouble I'm having with my erections related to my diabetes?

▼
TIP:

Quite possibly, but maybe not. Millions of men who don't have diabetes still have trouble getting and keeping an erection. The causes may be physical or psychological or both. Still, problems with erections are more common in men with diabetes, and the causes are usually physical. Diabetes can affect the nerves and the blood vessels that control erections. Ask you doctor to help you identify what could be causing your erection problems. In addition to blood vessel and nerve damage, your doctor might talk to you about the possibility that depression or drinking too much alcohol could be contributing to your problems. They might even be a side effect of a medication you're taking.

There are many treatments available, such as improving blood glucose control, taking medications such as Viagra that make it easier to get and keep an erection, or using devices designed to do the same thing. Devices include simple elastic rings that prevent blood from flowing back out of the penis (and thereby prevent losing the erection) to penile implants that require surgery.

Ask your primary care provider for a referral to a physician who specializes in diagnosing and treating erection problems. Usually this will be a urologist.

*C*an diabetes affect a woman's sexuality?

▼
TIP:

Diabetes can affect a woman's sexual experience in a variety of ways. Some women have problems with vaginal dryness, and that can make intercourse uncomfortable. Having diabetes also increases your risk for infections, including vaginal infections. Nerve damage can dramatically reduce sensation and pleasure. Limited mobility, feeling unattractive because of weight, and feeling tired because of high glucose levels all contribute further to the challenges many women with diabetes face when it comes to their sexuality.

Fortunately, there are ways to deal with these challenges, though none is perfect and they all take work. Be sure to talk with your health care provider about your options. Vaginal lubricants can relieve dryness. Controlling your blood sugar and using a medication can help control yeast infections. Learning the touch you can feel and enjoy is very important if you have nerve damage. Building strength through exercise, and finding comfortable positions can help if you have limited mobility. Focusing on what makes you attractive—you know there are things that do—is the last and most important element of a plan for a more enjoyable sex life.

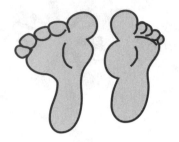

I've had a lot of trouble with my feet. They used to hurt and burn, but now I hardly feel them at all. Are things getting better?

TIP:

Probably not. It sounds as if you have neuropathy, or nerve damage, which is common in people who have had diabetes for many years. As nerve damage gets worse, people often notice the very symptoms you describe: lots of burning and pain at first, but then much less as time goes on. Many times people say they no longer feel their feet at all. While pain can be awful, when you lose feeling in your feet you also lose an important warning sign. Pain has a purpose. If your foot hurts when you step on a tack, for instance, you will quickly remove the tack and treat the wound. But when you don't feel pain you lose the protection it provides. You don't feel anything when you step on the tack, so unless you frequently check your feet, it can take a long time for you to realize you're in trouble and to take action. That delay can lead to infections, and infections can be especially hard to clear up when you have diabetes. So going from painful feet to feet you can't feel is not a good thing. Your feet hurt less, but that means you need to find other ways to protect them.

I have one diabetic complication and feel like lots more will follow. Does having one complication mean I will get others?

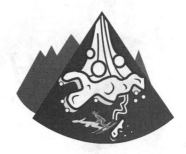

▼
TIP:

Not necessarily. It is true that higher blood glucose levels make all complications more likely, so if high glucose levels have led to one complication, they may very well lead to others. But you can use this correlation to your advantage. If your blood glucose levels go down, you lower your chances of getting another complication. Not only that, but getting your glucose levels down is one of the best ways to keep the complication you already have from getting worse.

Doing your best to stay healthy is hard because it takes so much time and effort. Keeping in mind why you try so hard can help maintain your motivation. Some people say that getting a complication made them see their lives with diabetes differently; the complication was both a blow and a wake-up call. It hurts and it makes them take a hard look at how they were managing their diabetes. Talk to your health care provider about things you can do to increase your chances of living the rest of your life with no more complications.

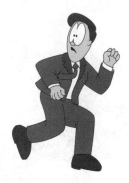

How can I stop worrying so much about high blood sugars? My fears make me keep my level too low much of the time.

TIP:

Keeping your blood glucose levels close to normal is a good thing. It helps you feel better day-to-day, and it cuts your risk for diabeteic complications. Unfortunately, it sounds as if you push so hard for the lowest possible glucose levels that it actually makes you feel worse. Being low a lot is a burden. It's embarrassing and it can be dangerous. People who are often low also tend to worry about it almost constantly. So they worry about highs and they worry about lows.

It's hard not to worry about your blood glucose levels, but sometimes it helps to look at the facts. First, what is your A1C level? If it is under 8%, your control is pretty good. If it is under 7%, it is very good. There is much room for improvement if your A1C level is higher than 8%. That would mean you are having lots of highs along with the lows. Talk to your health care provider about changes in your treatment plan that could help keep your glucose levels closer to normal throughout the day and cut down on your worrying.

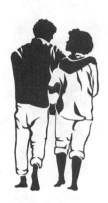

I think diabetes caused my wife's heart attack. Is there anything we can do to help avoid another one?

▼
TIP:

Having diabetes certainly made your wife's heart attack more likely. Heart disease is the leading cause of death in people with diabetes. There are things your wife—and you—can do to help protect her from another heart attack. She can try to live a healthier life by staying active, cutting the amount of fat she eats, controlling her weight, and taking medication (if prescribed) to help with other risk factors like her blood pressure and cholesterol levels. If your wife smokes, stopping is the most important thing she could do to keep her heart healthy.

Making these changes is hard, and that is where you come in. Give your wife the support she needs. Ask what you can do to help, whether it is preparing a healthy, tasty dinner or joining her for a walk after you have enjoyed your meal. You could also help your wife find useful diabetes resources, such as education classes, a good dietitian, or Internet web sites. Getting involved in a positive way like this can do you both good.

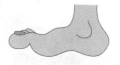
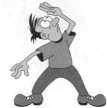

*H*ow can I check my feet every night like I am supposed to when my eyesight is so bad?

▼
TIP:

U nfortunately, you are not alone. As important as it is to check your feet every day, especially if you have any loss of feeling, many people have trouble checking themselves because of back, vision, or other problems. You may be able to rig up a system that lets you see your feet. Shining a flashlight on your feet or placing a lamp on the floor right by your feet while you check them could help. If you have trouble seeing the bottom of your feet, place a mirror on the floor and hold your foot over it.

If you still aren't able to check your feet yourself, ask family members or friends to help. It's hard to ask for help, but if there are people in your life who love you and have the time, it's worth asking. They might even appreciate the chance to do it. Talk to your health care provider about other ways to help your feet last a lifetime.

*W*ill a pill solve my sexual
problems?

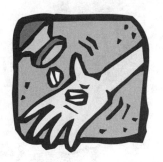

▼
TIP:

It could help. There is a pill called Viagra that men take to help them maintain erections. Studies show the pill is safe, and it seems to help many men who have diabetes. In one study, men taking Viagra said they had good erections about half the time they tried intercourse, while men taking a placebo medication said they had good erections only about 10% of the time.

Some people who use Viagra have side effects, especially headaches, flushing, and indigestion. People who take nitroglycerine for heart problems or any other nitrate medication should not take Viagra because their blood pressure could fall dangerously low. Researchers are still studying the effects of Viagra, including any benefits it might provide for women.

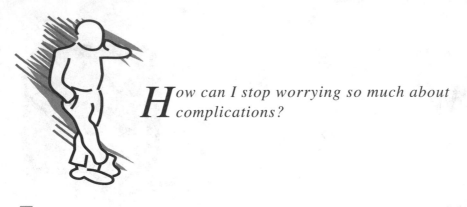

How can I stop worrying so much about complications?

▼

TIP:

First, do everything you can to prevent them. Keeping your blood glucose close to normal makes complications less likely, and that might help you worry less. Talk to your health care providers on a regular basis. They can help you take better care of yourself and check to see if you have any signs of complications, so any problems can be treated as quickly as possible. Knowing you have good care and good control can put a lot of fears to rest.

Share your feelings with family or friends who might be able to offer support. Consider joining a diabetes support group. There you will see that your feelings are not that unusual (and probably pick up some new tips for improving your glucose control). It can also help to connect with the sources of confidence and peace of mind that mean the most to you. Religious faith can be a tremendous source of strength and serenity, and so can the loving support of family and friends or the confidence you feel in yourself when you know you are taking good care of yourself.

Finally, consider this homily: "Worry never robs tomorrow of its sorrow; it only saps today of its strength."

*I*s it true that I have to give up alcohol?

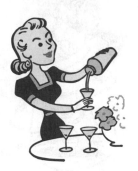

▼
TIP:

No. If your blood glucose control is good, having an occasional drink with meals should do no harm. The dietary guidelines published by the U.S. government say drinking moderately is okay as long as you don't drink and drive. Moderate drinking means one drink a day for women and two for men. One drink is 12 ounces of regular beer, 5 ounces of wine, or 1 1/2 ounces of 80-proof distilled spirits. These guidelines work for most people who have diabetes.

Having diabetes means you should also take special precautions when it comes to drinking. First, you need to fit the calories you are drinking into your meal plan to avoid going too high. That's important because alcohol contains almost as many calories per gram as fat does. Substitute alcohol calories for fat calories, with one drink equal to about 90 calories. Second, alcohol can cause very low blood glucose if you drink and don't eat anything. If you take insulin or pills that help your body make more insulin (sulfonylureas or meglitinides), it is safest to drink alcohol only with meals.

So it is okay to drink, but as with so many other things, it takes extra effort to do it safely when you have diabetes.

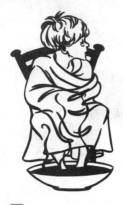

I'm worried about this sore on my foot that the doctor called a foot ulcer. What is a foot ulcer?

TIP:

An ulcer is an open sore. People with diabetes are more likely to get foot ulcers for three reasons. First, many people with diabetes have lost some feeling in their feet because of nerve damage, so they might not notice tiny cuts or cracks in the skin that could lead to serious problems. Second, many people with diabetes also have circulation problems, so it is hard to get oxygen, white blood cells, and antibiotics to the wound to help it heal. That's why many people with diabetes find that any wound, even the smallest one, can take a really long time to heal. In fact, without an adequate blood supply, foot ulcers may never heal. Finally, high blood glucose levels also hinder healing.

Foot ulcers can appear any place on your feet, though most often they are on the bottom or side of your big toe and on the ball of the foot. Prevention is essential. Pamper your feet. Keep them clean, dry, and protected from injury. Watch them like a hawk. If you see any sign of an open cut or sore, no matter how small, contact your health care provider immediately. You might also ask for a referral to a podiatrist, someone who specializes in treating foot problems.

*H*ow can I have diabetic
complications when I don't
feel bad?

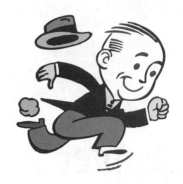

▼
TIP:

Unfortunately, you can feel fine without really being fine. For example, people with diabetes often have nerve damage, so they don't feel things that indicate serious problems. Like heart problems, for example. People who have diabetes are more likely to suffer so called silent heart attacks, serious heart damage they never even feel. Serious foot problems are also more common in people who have diabetes, in part for the same reason—nerve damage caused by the disease. Small foot injuries are often overlooked because the person doesn't feel bad. In fact, the person might not feel anything at all, even with a very serious foot ulcer.

So you can have complications and not feel bad. Just as important, you can have a very high risk of developing complications without feeling bad. Many people walk around for years with dangerously high glucose levels, and say they do not feel bad. So what you can't feel can hurt you. That is why it is so important to have regular checkups with your health care provider and verify that everything you can't feel is okay. That will help protect you from feeling bad for years to come.

Chapter 7
GETTING THE BEST
HEALTH CARE

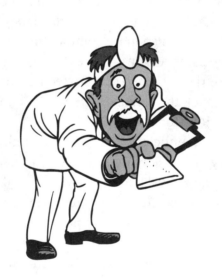

Should I be seeing any specialists for my diabetes?

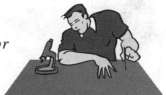

▼
TIP:

This is a terrific question with no clear-cut answers. Many primary care practitioners, or generalists, know a lot about diabetes and try to keep up to date. You are reading this book, so you are learning a lot about diabetes. If you believe your practitioner is not as up to date as you or is not giving you the care or answers you desire, you should look for another practitioner or request a referral to a specialist. Endocrinologists specialize in treating diseases of the endocrine system, including diabetes. However, not all endocrinologists specialize in diabetes, so try to find one who does.

No matter what, you should see an eye care specialist. If you are having problems with your feet you should see a podiatrist. You should also see specialists if you have problems with your heart, or have kidney or nerve damage. Diabetes educators can help you build your self-care skills, and mental health professionals can help you cope with the stresses of life with diabetes. Talk with your health care provider to be sure you have all the right players on your diabetes care team, and to decide how often you should see each of them.

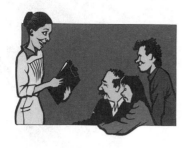

I just got diabetes and I am confused about what I need to do. Should I see a diabetes educator?

TIP:

Yes. A diabetes educator can help you get off to a good start living with diabetes. Among other things, a diabetes educator can help you learn

- How to check your blood glucose
- How and when to take insulin or diabetes pills (if this applies to you)
- How to recognize when your glucose is too high or low and what to do about it
- How to eat healthier and be more active
- How to quit smoking (if you are a smoker)

Diabetes educators are a great source of continuing support and helpful information and should be key members of your diabetes treatment team in the future, as well.

Many insurance plans, including Medicare, will pay for diabetes education. The ADA has a list of education programs they formally recognize on their web site (*www.diabetes.org*). Or call (800) DIABETES for information. You can also contact the American Association of Diabetes Educators (AADE) at (800) TEAM-UP-4 or *www.aadenet.org* to get the names of diabetes educators in your area. Your local hospital may also offer diabetes education programs or have a diabetes educator on staff.

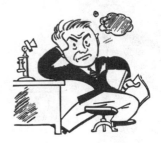

I can't find time during my doctor appointments to get my questions answered. What should I do?

▼
TIP:

- Write down the issues you want to discuss before your visit. Your health care provider has limited time, so stay simple and focus on the things that matter most. You might see if the person checking you in can place a copy of the list in your chart for the provider to see. Tell your provider right away that you have questions so there is time to get answers.

- Make sure your questions are complete and reflect your true concerns. A complete question might be, "Which protein source is lowest in fat?" or "How can I avoid being so worried about my heart?"

- Your physician may respond to faxes, though some prefer not to communicate this way. If your provider does respond to faxes (or phone calls), limit the exchange to 1 or 2 short, simple questions. E-mail may also be a possibility.

- Health care providers are experts in the medical management of diabetes; you are the expert in your life with diabetes. As they share their knowledge about diabetes with you, share with them your knowledge about your life and let them know what makes diabetes management more difficult. This is the best way to solve problems and reach your diabetes goals.

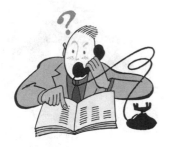

I just moved to a new city. How do I find a good diabetes doctor?

▼

TIP:

You could ask your previous doctor for a referral, contact a local hospital in your new city, or get in touch with the American Diabetes Association at (800) DIABETES. You could also find a diabetes educator in your new city and ask him or her. Call the American Association of Diabetes Educators' referral line, (800) TEAM-UP-4 (or go to the AADE web site, *www.aadenet.org*). Attending a diabetes support group (most local hospitals have them) and asking people about their doctors is also an option.

When you consider a new doctor, keep in mind the things that matter most to you. Important factors include

- Your insurance coverage
- How much the doctor seems to know about diabetes
- The doctor's personal style
- The availability of a diabetes treatment team (nurse, dietitian, and others)
- How easy it is to get to the office

A good diabetes doctor can be a tremendous resource, so do all you can to choose yours wisely.

I *don't like the way my* *diabetes is being treated.* *What can I do about it?*

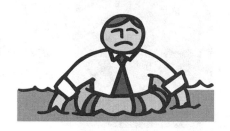

▼

TIP:

First, talk to your health care provider. Explain to him or her that you are not happy with your current treatment, explain why you are not happy, and ask what you can do to get your treatment more to your liking. Another option is to try "smart experiments," where you change elements of your diabetes treatment to get the most benefits and the least problems. One example would be switching your exercise to after dinner to see if it helps control evening blood sugars. The rules for smart experiments are:

■ Always discuss them first with your health care provider. He or she can help you refine your plan and point out any possible dangers.
■ Know the diabetes basics before you start. For example, how your diabetes medications affect your glucose levels, how to measure your blood glucose, and how to recognize symptoms of low and high glucose.
■ Start with one or two changes. Monitor frequently to check the results of your experiment.
■ Don't make big changes. Make smaller ones, especially at first.
■ Keep good records of what you are doing—changes in medication dose and timing, when you eat, exercise, and so on. This makes it easier to figure out what works best for you.

If you don't like how your diabetes is being treated, smart experiments could help.

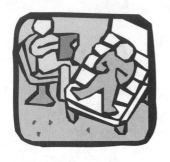

Should I see a mental health professional for my diabetes?

▼
TIP:

It could be a good idea. Many people who have diabetes feel "stressed-out" by the daily demands of their disease. Feeling overwhelmed is terrible, and it can trigger a negative spiral—if you feel overwhelmed, you probably can't find the energy to actively care for your diabetes, so your glucose control suffers. That means you feel worse physically and worry a lot about the long-term damage caused by those high glucose levels. And that creates even more stress.

So, doing anything you can to cut stress is very good. Doing things you enjoy and getting support from family and friends can help, and so can talking to a good counselor. If you have more serious emotional problems, like depression, the need for professional help is even greater. Working with a mental health professional who knows something about diabetes could help you feel better and get you back on track with your diabetes care. Unfortunately, there aren't many mental health professionals who specialize in working with people who have diabetes. To see if there are any in your area, ask you health care provider, contact your local hospital, call the ADA at (800) DIABETES, or call the AADE at (800) TEAM-UP-4.

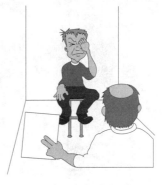

I'm having vision problems. Are there any specialists I should see?

Absolutely. Eye problems are a common complication of diabetes and an ophthalmologist (a doctor who specializes in eye care) can help preserve your sight. An ophthalmologist can tell if your eyes have been affected by diabetes. If so, an eye doctor can treat your eyes with laser therapy to protect your vision. Because it protects so many people from blindness, this treatment is one of the great advances in diabetes care over the past 30 years. Laser therapy works best if it is performed at the first sign of eye problems, which is why regular visits to the eye doctor are so important.

The ADA recommends you have a complete eye exam with an eye doctor every year if you were diagnosed with diabetes after you were 30 years old, or if you are younger and have had diabetes at least 5 years. Try to find an eye doctor who has experience treating people with diabetes. Ask your health care provider for a referral.

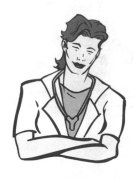

My mother had serious foot problems with her diabetes and I am afraid the same thing could happen to me. Should I see a foot doctor?

▼

TIP:

Yes. Foot care is very important when you have diabetes, and seeing a podiatrist (foot doctor) will help you keep your feet healthy. Because you have diabetes, you are more likely to have nerve damage (which means you can hurt your feet without feeling it) and circulation problems (which means any injuries to your feet take a really long time to heal). To help, a podiatrist can

- Show you how to care for your feet at home
- Help you with routine foot care, which can prevent more serious problems
- Treat corns, calluses, and small sores
- Help you keep your toenails safely trimmed
- Design supports to protect your foot from pressures that create sores
- Show you how to buy shoes that fit properly
- Perform foot surgery, to help save feet from even more serious harm

Ask your health care provider for a referral to a podiatrist if you have any questions or concerns about your feet. Local hospitals or the local ADA office can also help you find a podiatrist.

I'm worried my health insurance isn't good enough. What should be covered by my insurance plan?

▼
TIP:

T he ADA says your health care coverage should include the following:

■ Regular health care visits (yearly eye exams, as well as 4 visits a year with your regular doctor if you have type 1 diabetes, and 2 times a year if you have type 2 diabetes)

■ Lab tests (including tests of A1C, blood pressure, and blood fat levels, as well as tests to monitor any complications)

■ All the diabetes medications and supplies you need for good care (including blood monitors and strips)

■ Diabetes education provided by trained educators. After all, you provide most of your own diabetes care, and you need to know how to do it.

Unfortunately, many people with diabetes do not have this kind of coverage. Insurance companies are hesitant to cover people with conditions like diabetes because they can be costly to treat. Things are beginning to shift, and benefits are improving under both private and government health insurance plans. However, you might find that your coverage is still not good. If you are not getting what the ADA recommends, you are not getting what you deserve. Talk to your health care provider or contact the ADA for help getting the coverage you need.

Chapter 8
GETTING THE SUPPORT
AND INFORMATION
YOU NEED

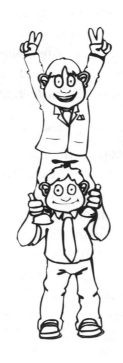

*H*ow can I get my family to be
more supportive when it comes
to my diabetes?

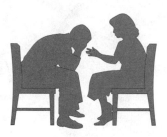

▼
TIP:

Many people who have diabetes are looking for more and better support from their families. Some feel their families don't take their diabetes seriously enough, don't understand the challenges of diabetes management, or don't accommodate their diabetes needs. Some feel their families even tempt them to take worse care of themselves. Other people feel their families go to the opposite extreme, forming a "diabetes police" that tries to control everything they do.

You need your family's positive support to live well with diabetes, but each person's need for this support is different. To help get the support *you* need, answer these three questions:

- What does my family do that makes my life with diabetes easier?
- What does my family do that makes my life with diabetes harder?
- What could my family (realistically) do differently to help me manage my diabetes?

Once you have answered these questions, talk with your family. Let them know how much you appreciate the help they are already providing, try to understand their feelings, and work to get more support one step at a time.

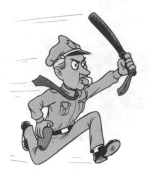

*M*y husband has become the "diabetes police" and he's on me about everything I do and don't do. How can I get him to stop trying to control my diabetes?

▼
TIP:

Keep in mind that your husband probably does this because he loves you and is worried that something bad will happen if he doesn't stay on your case. Unfortunately, this "diabetes police" approach does not work for either of you. You feel harassed, your husband feels frustrated and helpless—something has to change.

First, try to identify anything your husband does that actually helps you manage your diabetes. He seems to be looking for ways to help. Getting him to do more of the things you appreciate might shift the way you are relating to each other about diabetes management.

Once you know what you want from your husband, talk to him about it. Let him know that you appreciate his love and concern for you, but that his "policing" isn't helping. Be as specific as you can about what you want and need. Ask him to talk about how he *feels* ("I get really upset when I see you go for that second helping of dessert") instead of what you *do* ("How could you eat that when you know what it will do to your glucose?"). Talking about feelings and what your husband is already doing to help are good ways to get him to turn in his diabetes police badge for good.

*B*oth my sister and I have diabetes, but she seems to take much better care of herself. How can I deal with this?

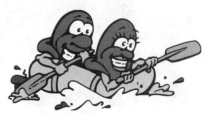

▼
TIP:

Many of us have siblings we envy for one reason or another—success, looks, or even the fact that they manage their diabetes better. While this can be a source of frustration, it can also be a source of motivation. Try to identify the things you admire about the way your sister manages her diabetes. Does your sister's approach help you see how you might manage your own diabetes better? If so, think about a step-by-step approach to working in some of those things into your own diabetes care.

It can also help to be clear about what you are already doing right when it comes to managing your diabetes. There are probably things you overlook when you are comparing yourself to your sister. There might even be some things you do better than she does.

Once you are feeling more confident about your own diabetes management, talk with your sister. You might be surprised to hear that she struggles with her diabetes more than you realize. Hopefully, you can both do better, and turn your shared situation from a source of sibling stress into a source of sibling strength.

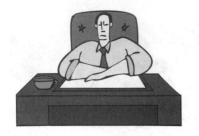

Should I tell a prospective employer I have diabetes?

▼
TIP:

This is up to you. Job discrimination against people with diabetes has dropped over the years. According to current laws, you can only be denied a job if you can't perform the essential duties of the job even if the employer makes reasonable accommodations to help you (like providing breaks for you to check your glucose, have snacks, and go to the bathroom more frequently). Unfortunately, the new laws only cover people who work for companies that employ at least 15 people, and proving hiring discrimination is tough. Still, employers can get into big trouble if they reject a person who has diabetes and then hire a less qualified person.

Many employers will not ask about your health. In fact, it is illegal to do so unless they ask all prospective employees the same question. If your employer does ask, you don't have to tell them. However, you could lose some of your legal protections against job discrimination if you lie about having diabetes before you are hired.

Many people say it is best to tell because work is less stressful when they aren't trying to hide something as important as diabetes. It is also easier to take better care of your diabetes at work when you can do it openly.

Is it okay to keep the fact I have diabetes to myself?

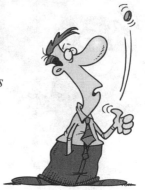

▼
TIP:

Once again, this is up to you. First, keep in mind that diabetes is pretty common now, so many people know a little about diabetes. Second, diabetes is not a disease to be ashamed of. It is not caused by improper behavior.

Most people are curious about something that they may have heard about, but don't really understand. They will naturally have questions. Humor can be a useful tool to help break the tension you may feel talking about your diabetes. For instance:

"I would have never known you had diabetes!"

"Well they stopped making us wear the scarlet Ds a long time ago!"

It may be uncomfortable, but it's a good idea to let people you spend lots of time with (like your coworkers) know you could go low (if this is a possibility), how you act when you are low, and how to help you treat the low if you can't do it yourself. If you pick the right people to tell, you will probably get some understanding right away, and possibly some needed help in case of an emergency later.

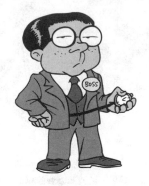

*M*y boss gives me a hard time when I take a break to get a snack because my blood glucose is low. What can I do?

▼
TIP:

Your boss's behavior is illegal. As long as you are able to get your work done, you should be allowed reasonable accommodations, including breaks for snacks, glucose checks, and more trips to the restroom. You should also be allowed to keep food and diabetes supplies nearby and be allowed to work a standard shift instead of a swing shift. If you're not getting these things, your boss is breaking the law.

Consider making your own accommodations (but none that compromise your health!) to make it easier for your employer to follow the law and meet your needs. If your boss refuses to cooperate, talk to the human resources department at your company. Provide the following to anyone you talk to:

■ Information about diabetes
■ What you do to manage your diabetes
■ Specific accommodations you require
■ The company's legal obligation to provide those accommodations under the law

If all else fails, you might contact organizations dedicated to fighting job discrimination, such as the ADA, your union (if you belong to one), your state human rights commission, the Equal Employment Opportunity Commission, the U.S. Department of Labor, or your local employment office.

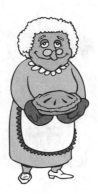

*W*hat should I say to a friend who tempts
me with things I shouldn't eat, saying a
little bit won't hurt me?

▼
TIP:

*F*irst, be sure your friend understands why you don't want to eat
what he or she is offering. Be as specific as you can. Maybe you
are afraid of a high glucose, or worried you would not be able to stop
after eating a little bit. Or it could be that you simply don't want
anything to eat. Whatever your reason, give it. That should stop your
friend from tempting you. If she keeps it up, see if you can find some
written material that might get through to her. Your health care
provider may have some suggestions. Or take your friend to a
diabetes support group meeting where she is sure to hear that your
feelings about being tempted are shared by other people who have
diabetes.

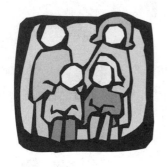

I *have type 2 diabetes and I worry*
about other family members getting it.
Is there any way it can be prevented?

▼
TIP:

The short answer is yes. A recent study was conducted using people who were overweight and had a condition called impaired glucose tolerance (IGT), sometimes called pre-diabetes. People with IGT have high blood sugar levels but not high enough to be called diabetes. About half of all people with IGT eventually develop type 2 diabetes.

There were 3 groups. One group received coaching in a healthy lifestyle designed to help them lose weight. Their goal was to be active (for most, this meant walking) 30 minutes a day, 5 days a week, and to lose 7% of their weight and keep it off. The 2 other groups took pills. One group took a medication called metformin (Glucophage) and the other group took placebo pills that looked just like the metformin but had no active medication.

The results of the study were impressive. People in the group who made lifestyle changes were 58% less likely to develop diabetes during the study than the people in the placebo medication group. Metformin also helped prevent diabetes during this study, but it was only half as effective as lifestyle changes. So, yes, it is possible to prevent diabetes, though we don't know for how long.

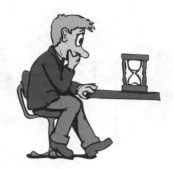

I've been waiting for a diabetes cure for years. When will it come?

▼
TIP:

That depends on what you mean by a cure. Pretty soon we should see some new tools that make it much easier to keep blood glucose levels closer to normal throughout the day. This wouldn't be a true cure, but it would help people with diabetes lead better, healthier lives. Along with better pills, better insulins, and better devices for delivering insulin, we could soon have glucose monitors that could be implanted in your body. Connecting an implanted glucose monitor to an insulin pump would create an artificial pancreas, which could do almost as good a job as a real pancreas.

A true cure for diabetes is still some years away. To cure diabetes we need to solve the two problems that cause diabetes: insulin resistance (problems using insulin effectively), and destruction of the beta-cells that make insulin. People with type 2 diabetes have both problems, while people who have type 1 diabetes have problems only with beta-cell destruction. We don't yet have a cure for diabetes, but we have made a lot of progress toward this goal in the past few years. You may see the day when diabetes is a disease of the past.

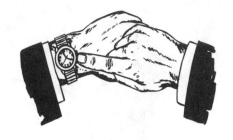

*M*y blood sugars seem to shift by the minute but I can't check my blood that often. I've heard it is possible to monitor blood glucose levels continuously. Is this true?

TIP:

Several companies have developed continuous glucose measuring systems. One such device is the GlucoWatch Biographer, which is worn like a watch and measures glucose under the skin. It displays readings every 20 minutes for 12 hours, and stores up to 4,000 readings. The GlucoWatch can be programmed to signal if glucose levels rise above or fall below preset levels, or if glucose levels fall rapidly. You still have to check your glucose the old-fashioned way every 12 hours to calibrate the device, and the readings represent what your glucose level was 15 minutes before, so they're not exactly current. For more information, go to *www.glucowatch.com.*

Another company has developed the Continuous Glucose Monitoring System (CGMS). The CGMS is currently available by prescription and is mostly used short term to help people adjust insulin doses. A sensor is placed just under the skin and attached to a monitor, which is worn on your belt or carried in your pocket. The sensor records glucose levels every 5 minutes and is usually worn for up to 3 days. When the test is complete, the health care provider downloads data from the monitor into a computer. These data show when the person is high and low and what insulin adjustments would help. For more information, go to *www.minimed.com.*

I use my computer to get a lot of diabetes information because it's so easy. Is the information about diabetes on the Internet reliable?

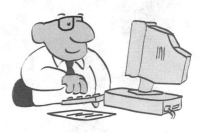

▼

TIP:

Not always. Though there is an amazing amount of valuable information on the Internet, a good portion of it is bunk. Along with lots of valid and helpful information, you will also find personal experiences that don't apply to you and outrageous claims designed to sell you a product. Separating the good from the bad can be difficult. The American Diabetes Association (*www.diabetes.org*) and the American Association of Diabetes Educators (*www.aadenet.org*) are good places to start when you want information, because they sponsor reliable sites. Many other organizations also sponsor web sites featuring the latest diabetes research and other helpful information. There are also chat rooms where you can "talk" to other people who have diabetes and share experiences. You can learn a lot in a chat room, but keep in mind that you are hearing peoples' personal experiences, and these experiences might not apply to you. Before you act on something you see on the Internet concerning your diabetes, talk with your health care team to be sure it is right for you.

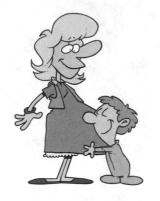

If I had gestational diabetes when I was pregnant will I get type 2 diabetes?

TIP:

Not necessarily, but your risk does go up. The fact you had diabetes when you were pregnant means your pancreas has trouble keeping up with your insulin needs. About half of all women who have gestational diabetes will eventually develop type 2 diabetes. But there are things you can do to cut that risk. Studies show that if you change your lifestyle by eating more carefully, increasing your activity level, and losing weight, your risk of developing type 2 diabetes goes way down.

Changing your lifestyle is hard, but these changes are the same ones you should make if you get diabetes. Making those changes now could protect you from ever developing diabetes. Talk with your health care provider to learn more about your risk of getting diabetes and how to avoid it.

Chapter 9
DEALING WITH EMERGENCIES, TRAVEL, AND ILLNESS

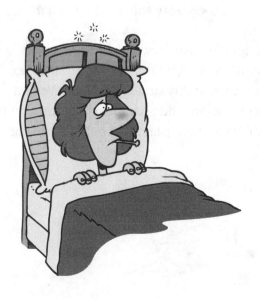

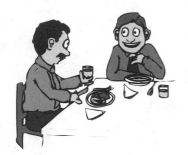

What should I do if I forget to bring my insulin when I go out to eat at a restaurant?

▼
TIP:

Things like this happen sometimes. If you can't go back to get your insulin, you have a few options to help minimize the potential negative impact on your glucose.

- Select foods that have less impact on your glucose level. Carbs have the biggest impact, so try to steer clear of those.
- Eat less of what you order. You can almost always take home the remaining food for a tasty snack when you are better prepared to deal with it!
- Exercise after the meal. Try taking a brisk walk.
- Take a shot of rapid-acting insulin as soon as you can after the meal. If you choose this strategy, make sure that you check your blood glucose before and an hour or so after you take the insulin. Also, don't overcompensate; it is better to be conservative.

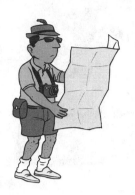

*W*hen I travel, I'm always afraid I'm going to forget something. What diabetes supplies should I take when I'm away from home?

▼

TIP:

*P*ack twice as much of everything you would normally need if you were at home. This includes

- Blood glucose monitor and strips
- Medication
- Syringes or pump supplies if you use insulin
- Ketone testing strips
- A source of fast-acting carbohydrate (in case you experience a low blood sugar)
- If you are traveling during a mealtime, enough food to cover that meal

Extra food is a good idea in case you get stranded at an airport or your car breaks down. If you have to go through airport or border security, a letter from your doctor explaining why you carry syringes can be helpful. Check with the American Diabetes Association website (*www.diabetes.org*) for current recommendations for travel.

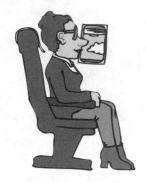

I'm never sure how to adjust my insulin when I travel. What adjustments should I make when I cross time zones?

▼

TIP:

This depends on your insulin regimen, where you are going, and how long you will be gone. We'll assume you use either an insulin pump or a combination of long-acting and rapid-insulin injections. If it's a short trip across one or two time zones, it might be best to take your basal insulin (basal rate for pump or long-acting insulin by injection) at the same hour of the day in the time zone that you usually take your insulin back home. For instance, if you live in Kansas and you're visiting New York, where it's an hour ahead, take a 9:00 A.M. basal at 10:00 A.M. Then, simply take your boluses or mealtime shots of rapid-acting insulin when you eat.

Another option is to continue taking your basal insulin at the same time you would at home, without taking into account the time difference. This means less adjustment, but you might end up with problems controlling your glucose if there is a big time difference. If you try this approach, check your glucose frequently. You may have to make adjustments with your rapid-acting insulin to help keep your glucose levels close to normal.

I'm feeling stressed about traveling by plane with my insulin and syringes, especially since September 11. What should I do?

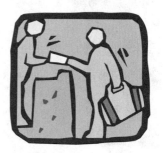

▼
TIP:

You do **not** need a prescription for your insulin or syringes. You simply need proof that what you are carrying is insulin. For proof, the Federal Aviation Administration (FAA) says you should keep the box that your insulin came in (or the plastic bag your boxes came in, if your insulin came from a mail-order pharmacy). These packages should have the information the FAA requires—"a professional, pharmaceutical pre-printed label which clearly identifies the medication." So don't throw away the original box or bag for your insulin if you plan to travel by plane. You can also carry lancets on the plane, as long as they are capped and you are also carrying "a glucose meter that has the manufacturer's name embossed on the meter."

Since September 11, 2001, the FAA has issued new security measures that apply to people with diabetes. Each airline might enforce these measures slightly differently, so it is best to check with your airline before traveling. You can also go to the ADA website (*www.diabetes.org*) for the latest guidelines. More than likely, you won't have any problems. But like always, it is best to be prepared.

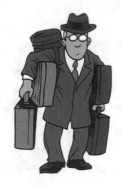

I'm afraid my insulin pump will set off alarms in airports. Is this possible?

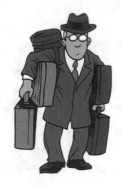

▼
TIP:

Reports vary. Some detectors may be more sensitive than others. Some people say their pump always sets off the alarm, others say that it occasionally sets it off, and still others say it never does. Insulin pumps are made mostly of plastic, so even if you do set off an alarm, your pump might not be the cause. If you are carrying or wearing anything else that could have triggered the alarm, you could remove or point out those things first. If there are no other potential causes or the security guards ask to search you, tell them that you have diabetes and you are wearing a medical device that delivers insulin. Offer to show them the pump and how it works. Carry a letter from your doctor saying (as simply as possible) that you need the pump and how the pump works.

As always, when it comes to coping with diabetes, a little planning and a little common sense will take you a long way.

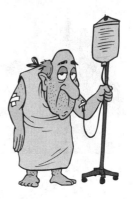

Why is it so much harder to control my blood glucose when I am sick?

▼

TIP:

Being sick stresses your body, and stress can raise your blood glucose. Any kind of stress—physical or mental—can have that effect. So when you are sick, you have to take extra precautions to be sure your blood glucose doesn't go too high.

It's hard when you are not feeling well, but when you are sick you need to monitor more closely. The ADA recommends that you check your blood glucose and urine ketone levels every 4 hours. If your blood glucose level is high, it's a sign you need more insulin. If your urine ketones are 3+ or higher, it's a sign you need more insulin and probably some fast-acting carbohydrate like regular soda, as well.

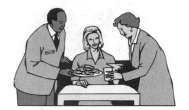

*W*hat are the best foods to eat
when I am sick?

▼
TIP:

S ince you need to stick to your regular diabetes medication when
you are sick, it's important to eat something, even when you can't
eat regular food. Most people find that things like regular soda, fruit
juice, sherbet, frozen juice bars, pudding, applesauce, and ice cream
are the easiest to eat, but anything with calories that you can keep
down will do.

Dehydration is a real risk if your blood glucose stays high for a
long period of time. So fluids like soda and juice are especially good
when you are sick because they help protect you from dehydration.
Broth and vegetable juices are also good because they help replace the
minerals you lose through vomiting and diarrhea.

*A*t what point should I call my doctor
when I am sick?

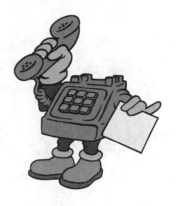

▼
TIP:

Your doctor is the best person to answer this question. Be sure to talk with him or her to see if the guidelines we discuss below apply to you. Generally, here are some things that should probably prompt you to call your doctor when you are sick:

■ Not being able to hold down fluids. If you go more than 12 hours without being able to hold down fluids, you are probably getting dehydrated and you could get really sick without proper care.
■ High urine ketone levels. Urine ketone levels that stay at 3+ or higher are another source of potentially serious problems.

Hopefully, you will rarely get so sick you need to call your doctor. But it is good to know the signs that signal you need help, so you will know when to make that call.

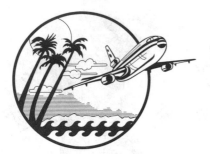

Why is it so hard to control my diabetes when I travel?

▼
TIP:

Travel often throws your diabetes management plan for a loop. Everything changes—you eat all your meals in restaurants, your activity level is probably changed and inconsistent, and unexpected stresses that push up your glucose levels lurk everywhere.

Here are some suggestions for making good control a little easier when you travel.

- At restaurants, ask about the ingredients of the menu items so that you can avoid post-meal highs or lows.
- Frequent blood glucose monitoring can help you catch potential problems early, thus preventing highs and avoiding lows.
- Travel with workout clothing. Most hotels have exercise facilities and you can ask the hotel staff about safe places to walk outside the hotel.
- Always wear comfortable shoes when you travel so that you can walk briskly at every opportunity.

TIPS FOR A HEALTHY PREGNANCY WITH DIABETES

▲

A project of the
American Diabetes Association

▼

Written By

Patti B. Geil, MS, RD/LD, FADA, CDE
Laura B. Hieronymus, MSEd, APRN, BC-ADM, CDE

TIPS FOR A HEALTHY PREGNANCY WITH DIABETES

▼

TABLE OF CONTENTS

Chapter 1
PRIOR TO PREGNANCY

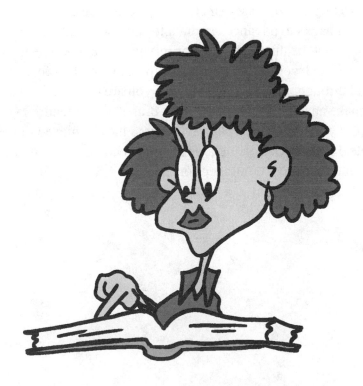

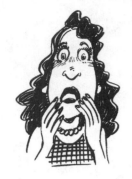

I have type 1 diabetes. Will I be able to have a baby?

▼
TIP:

Yes, with the right planning and preparation. Not too long ago, it was common for a woman with diabetes to be told she should never consider having a child. High blood glucose levels during pregnancy caused problems for the mother (worsening of diabetic complications) as well as the baby (increased risk of fetal death and birth defects). Thanks to advances in diabetes and neonatal care, a normal pregnancy and healthy baby are entirely possible *if* you keep your blood glucose levels as near normal as possible both before conception and throughout your pregnancy. If you are considering having a baby, make an appointment with your diabetes care team to discuss your pregnancy plans. Until you have achieved the best possible diabetes control and are ready to become pregnant, be sure to use a reliable form of contraception.

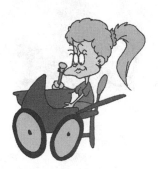

I have diabetes and want to become pregnant soon. My physician would like me to participate in a prepregnancy planning program. What does this involve?

▼

TIP:

In a prepregnancy planning program your medical team will discuss with you the importance of normal blood glucose levels both before and during pregnancy, the potential risks of pregnancy for you and your baby, genetic counseling, and contraceptive advice. You should also work with a diabetes nurse educator and registered dietitian to outline a plan for achieving normal blood glucose levels. This plan will include an intensive insulin regimen, careful nutritional management, physical activity, and frequent monitoring of blood glucose levels. Research has shown that better blood glucose control before and during pregnancy lowers the risks to both mother and baby. A prepregnancy planning program is the best way to ensure that both of you are as healthy as possible.

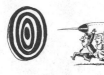 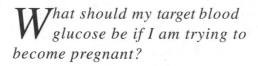

*W*hat should my target blood glucose be if I am trying to become pregnant?

▼

TIP:

As close to normal as possible, especially before you conceive and in the first trimester of your pregnancy. The following goals for self-monitored blood glucose before conception have been recommended by the American Diabetes Association:

	Whole Blood Goals	Plasma Goals
Before meals:	70–100 mg/dl	80–110 mg/dl
2 hours after meals:	<140 mg/dl	<155 mg/dl

Adapted from "Preconception Care of Women with Diabetes," *ADA Clinical Practice Recommendations*, 2003.

Overall, your goal should be to attain the lowest A1C level you possibly can at least three months before you get pregnant, without risking excessive hypoglycemia. The A1C test measures blood glucose control over a longer period of time (about 4 months) than a finger stick self-check of blood glucose. Research shows that if you can keep your A1C less than 1% above the normal range before your pregnancy, your chance of developing complications is dramatically reduced. The normal range is considered to be less than 6%, although this figure may vary. Near-normal blood glucose levels are necessary to reduce risks and promote a healthy pregnancy outcome.

I have heard that the risk of your child having birth defects is high if you have diabetes. Is this true?

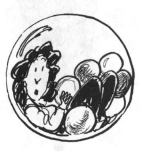

▼

TIP:

Not necessarily. This depends on your blood glucose level. If blood glucose levels are high during conception and the crucial first 8 weeks of pregnancy, the rate of birth defects and miscarriage in the first trimester can approach 65%. Common birth defects involve the heart, skeletal, and nervous systems. Since the majority of pregnancies are unplanned, it is likely that birth defects and miscarriage will occur more commonly in women with diabetes *if* they have high blood glucose when they conceive.

The good news is that research shows if you keep normal blood glucose levels before and during the early weeks of pregnancy, your risk of birth defects is similar to that of someone without diabetes. Control before conception is key!

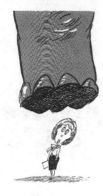

*W*ill my blood glucose control affect
my ability to carry a baby to full
term?

TIP:

More than likely, yes. Elevated blood glucose levels put you at a
higher risk for miscarriage, particularly in the first 3 months of
your pregnancy. High blood glucose levels during this critical first
trimester can cause the rate of miscarriage to be 30–60%, depending
on how high the blood glucose is at the time of conception. High
blood glucose can also cause early labor and/or birth. Babies born too
early, before their lungs are fully developed, can have a serious
breathing problem called respiratory distress syndrome.

Most women with diabetes have uneventful pregnancies and carry
their babies to full term without any problems. But complications can
occur more frequently in your baby if you have had diabetes for a
long time or if you develop a condition such as toxemia, which causes
high blood pressure and swelling. It's important for you to have close
follow-ups during your pregnancy, preferably with a high-risk pregnancy program. A successful pregnancy with diabetes requires an
investment of effort, time, and money.

I've had trouble getting pregnant and my doctor mentioned polycystic ovary syndrome (PCOS). Is this a form of diabetes?

▼

TIP:

Not necessarily, but the two are linked. Polycystic ovary syndrome, or PCOS, is the most common cause of infertility among women in the United States, affecting 5–10% of all women in the childbearing years. PCOS keeps the body from ovulating, which means eggs aren't released from the ovaries for fertilization and pregnancy cannot occur. The condition is linked with insulin resistance, a condition in which the body resists the action of the hormone insulin, as well as obesity and excessive male hormones.

Because it is linked to insulin resistance, PCOS is also associated with type 2 diabetes. Fifty percent of women with type 2 diabetes develop PCOS and 30% of obese women with PCOS develop glucose intolerance or type 2 diabetes by age 40. Women with type 2 diabetes and/or PCOS are also more susceptible to cardiovascular disease.

If you are diagnosed with PCOS, an oral contraceptive or a medication such as metformin may be prescribed to reduce insulin resistance. Healthy eating and physical activity for weight control should also be part of a program intended to restore your fertility. Should you become pregnant, you may be at risk for gestational diabetes due to your underlying insulin resistance and the added insulin resistance that normally occurs with pregnancy, especially after the 16th week of your pregnancy.

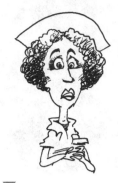

*S*ix months ago I was told I have pre-diabetes. Is it okay for me to have a baby?

▼

TIP:

Yes, but once again, only if you take the appropriate precautions. Pre-diabetes, formerly referred to as *impaired glucose tolerance*, means that your blood glucose levels are above the normal range, but not high enough for you to be diagnosed with type 2 diabetes. Most people with pre-diabetes are well on their way to diabetes unless lifestyle changes, such as increased physical activity and improved nutrition, are made.

If you have pre-diabetes and you want to become pregnant, pre-pregnancy planning is essential. Work with your health care team to determine your overall health and to stay up to date on your blood glucose levels. Working with a registered dietitian (RD) is helpful as well. An RD can establish nutrition needs, a healthy body weight, and provide physical activity tips that will benefit your overall health and work to normalize your blood glucose levels prior to conception.

Because insulin resistance occurs normally in pregnancy due to hormonal changes, you will need medical guidance from someone with expertise in diabetes and pregnancy to help you manage your blood glucose levels throughout your pregnancy.

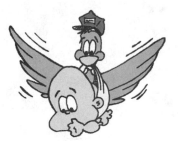

I am 28 years old and have had type 1 diabetes since I was 13. Is it okay for me to have a baby?

▼

TIP:

Yes, but be sure to meet with your physician to discuss the issue beforehand. Your physician should discuss the following with you:

- Current contraception methods, to ensure you attain normal blood glucose levels before you get pregnant
- Risks of pregnancy, to both you and your child
- The importance of maintaining normal blood glucose levels for several months prior to pregnancy. Studies have shown that intensive management of diabetes and normal blood glucose levels before pregnancy can lower the risk of complications to nondiabetes levels.
- Genetic counseling, which can determine your baby's risk of developing diabetes. Your age at the time of pregnancy can influence this risk. If you have type 1 and are less than 25 when you conceive, the chance of your baby developing type 1 diabetes is about 4%; if you're older than 25 years, the chance decreases to about 1%.
- Any complications you may have. Having complications does not automatically mean you can't have a child, but if you do have complications, understanding how they will affect your pregnancy and how your pregnancy will affect your complications is essential.
- Your level of commitment. Having diabetes means pregnancy will be a lot more work. If you're not committed to an increased level of medical and obstetric supervision, the ability and willingness to perform frequent blood glucose testing, and undergoing prompt follow-ups to treatment plans, you may not be ready for pregnancy. If, however, you feel like you can meet these extra demands, a happy and healthy pregnancy may be in your future.

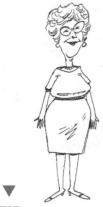

My mother has diabetes. Does this increase my risk of developing gestational diabetes?

▼
TIP:

Yes. Women who have a strong family history of diabetes are at a higher risk for developing gestational diabetes mellitus, or GDM (see page 1090). GDM first occurs during pregnancy and usually disappears after the birth of the baby. Almost 7% of all pregnancies are affected by GDM and your chances of developing it increase if you

- Have a family history of diabetes
- Have previously had a very large baby or stillbirth
- Are overweight
- Had an earlier pregnancy with GDM
- Are older than 25 years of age

Because of your high-risk status, your physician should immediately evaluate you for GDM with glucose testing if you do become pregnant. If there's no sign of GDM at your first screening, you should be checked again 24–28 weeks into your pregnancy, which is when GDM is most often detected.

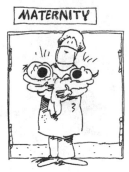

I *had gestational diabetes with my last pregnancy. Will I have it again?*

▼

TIP:

Although any pregnant woman can develop gestational diabetes, because of your previous history of GDM, you are more likely to develop it than others. Gestational diabetes occurs when the pregnancy hormones produced by your placenta cause your body to become resistant to insulin. You may become unable to produce enough insulin to meet your body's needs, so your blood glucose levels slowly rise and reach levels above normal by about 24–28 weeks into your pregnancy. At this point, a healthy meal plan, physical activity, and maybe even insulin injections will be needed to keep blood glucose levels in control and prevent complications in your baby.

If you do become pregnant, your physician should evaluate you for GDM with blood glucose testing as soon as possible. It may be necessary to repeat the blood glucose screening as your pregnancy progresses, particularly between 24–28 weeks.

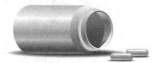

I've been told I need to take a prenatal vitamin before trying to become pregnant. Why?

▼
TIP:

You want the best possible nutritional status before, during, and after pregnancy for your health and for the health of your child. Folic acid is especially important before pregnancy. It reduces the risk of certain birth defects, such as cleft palate and spina bifida. All women of childbearing age, whether they have diabetes or not, are advised to get 400 mcg of folic acid per day from fortified foods, supplements, or a combination of both for a period of time before becoming pregnant.

Iron is another important nutrient. If a woman has iron-deficiency anemia when she becomes pregnant, it may be difficult to build up her iron stores during pregnancy.

Eating whole grains, vegetables, and fruits as part of healthy daily eating is the best guarantee that you will have all the nutrients you need. Women most likely to benefit from taking supplements are those who don't eat healthfully, are underweight or constantly trying to lose weight, or abuse alcohol or drugs. Seek professional nutrition guidance so you get the vitamins and minerals you need and don't get too much of the ones you don't need.

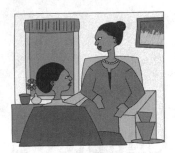

I have had type 1 diabetes for 14 years. My diabetes educator suggested that I begin using an insulin pump before I try to become pregnant. Why?

▼

TIP:

Maintaining as near-to-normal blood glucose levels as possible for at least 3 months before conception—and throughout pregnancy—lowers the risk of complications for both you and your baby. Women with type 1 diabetes who are planning to get pregnant often watch their meal plan more closely, check blood glucose levels more often, and take up to 4 injections daily or use an insulin pump. An insulin pump allows you to get near-normal glucose levels by delivering insulin as needed to match up with the food you eat, the action of pregnancy hormones, and blood glucose levels that fluctuate more as pregnancy progresses. You could wait to begin insulin pump therapy until after you become pregnant, but using it for glucose control before pregnancy gives you time to learn how to use it well. With an insulin pump, you need to be committed to doing blood checks often, counting carbs, and learning to adjust your insulin dose. To succeed, you need to be motivated and to have strong support at home and the doctor's office.

Chapter 2
EXPECTING THE BEST:
DIABETES & PREGNANCY

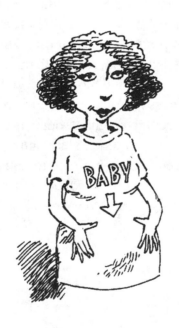

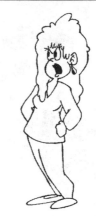

I've heard that pregnancy hormones
affect blood sugar levels. Is this true?

▼

TIP:

Yes. The placenta is a flat, circular organ that links the unborn
baby to the mother's uterus during pregnancy. It produces *contrainsulin* hormones, such as human placental lactogen, prolactin,
estrogen, and progesterone. The production of these hormones, along
with increased levels of cortisol, can affect your body's sensitivity to
insulin, whether it is insulin produced by your own body, insulin
injected by syringe or pen, *or* insulin infused by an insulin pump.
Although these hormones are essential to a healthy pregnancy, this
hormonal "aggravation," along with the weight you'll gain as your
pregnancy progresses, can contribute to a rise in blood glucose levels,
particularly after the 18th week of your pregnancy.

The best way to ensure your glucose levels are under control is to
know where your glucose levels are at all times. Frequent self-glucose
monitoring (up to 8 times a day when you are pregnant) can help
identify changes in blood glucose levels. This will help you and your
diabetes health team make the necessary changes for the best blood
glucose control throughout your pregnancy.

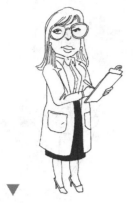

I am pregnant and my doctor says I am at risk for gestational diabetes. What does that mean?

▼
TIP:

Gestational diabetes mellitus, or GDM, means your blood glucose levels are higher than normal for a pregnant woman. Unless you already have diabetes (in which case there's no need to screen for diabetes—you already know), your obstetrician should consider whether or not you need a GDM screening based on your risk for developing GDM.

Low Risk (probably will not be screened for GDM):
- Member of an ethnic group with low prevalence of GDM
- No known diabetes in first-degree relatives
- Younger than 25 years old
- Weight normal before pregnancy
- No history of abnormal glucose metabolism
- No history of poor pregnancy outcome

Average Risk (usually screened for GDM at 24–28 weeks):
- Any woman who does not meet all of the "Low Risk" conditions but is not considered "High Risk"

High Risk (should be screened for GDM early in pregnancy and again at 24–28 weeks):
- Marked obesity, strong family history of type 2 diabetes, personal history of GDM, glucose intolerance, or glucose present in the urine
- Various ethnic groups with a high prevalence of GDM (includes Native American, African American, and Hispanic women)

*M*y doctor says I need to be screened for gestational diabetes. What does that involve?

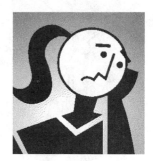

TIP:

G enerally, the screening for GDM goes as follows:

Initial Screening:
- Fasting is not required.
- You will take 50 grams of a glucose solution.
- A laboratory will analyze your glucose reading.
- If your glucose reading is higher than 130 mg/dl, an oral glucose tolerance test (GTT) is recommended.

Diagnosis and GTT:
- Fasting is required.
- A laboratory will analyze your fasting glucose reading.
- You will then take 100 grams of a glucose solution (sometimes 75 grams).
- A laboratory will analyze your glucose levels at 1, 2, and 3 hours after you take the glucose solution (or just 1 and 2 hours after taking 75 grams of solution).

Sometimes this procedure will be modified. In high-risk populations, a health care professional might skip the initial screening and go straight to the GTT, usually because it's less expensive. Some medical professionals suggest a GTT only if your initial screening is higher than 140 mg/dl, instead of the 130 mg/dl level listed above. It's important to remember that all glucose readings should come from laboratory analysis. Readings from finger stick methods are not good enough to make a diagnosis.

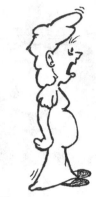

I've just found out I have gestational diabetes and I'm worried about birth defects. What are the chances that my baby will have a birth defect?

▼

TIP:

This depends. Birth defects have been linked to poor blood glucose control in a number of studies. Because the development of vital organs (such as the spine, heart, and brain) occurs mostly by the 8th week of pregnancy, it is essential that women with preexisting diabetes have near-normal blood glucose control before conception to decrease the risk of birth defects. Gestational diabetes (GDM) makes things a little tricky, however, since it isn't diagnosed until pregnancy has already begun. Although GDM is typically diagnosed during the late 2nd or early 3rd trimester of the pregnancy, it is possible that blood glucose levels may have been high earlier in the pregnancy. If blood sugar levels were normal as vital organs were developing, then the risk of birth defects would be similar to any pregnant woman without diabetes—about 3–6%. However, if glucose levels were less than optimal during this period, then the risk for birth defects may be increased. It's always a good idea to discuss any concerns you have about birth defects with your health care team.

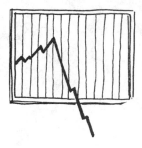

I have been experiencing hypoglycemia without realizing it while I am pregnant. Is this common?

TIP:

Many women experience "hypoglycemia unawareness" during pregnancy, although you do not have to be pregnant for this to happen. This condition generally only affects women who are using insulin to control their diabetes, since they are the ones at risk for hypoglycemia (low blood sugar). Hypoglycemia unawareness can be especially common during pregnancy because hypoglycemia can be more common. When you're pregnant, the recommended goals for glucose control are lower than goals for the nonpregnant person with diabetes. Your brain may get comfortable with lower levels of blood glucose and be less sensitive to the warning signs you get when you're "too low" (usually 60 mg/dl or less). In addition, there's also the possibility that the fetus can deplete carbohydrate and calorie stores in your blood, which can also cause hypoglycemia.

Work with your diabetes health care team to lower your risk of hypoglycemia. Checking your blood glucose up to 8 times a day is often recommended. This can help you identify blood glucose patterns, as well as "at-risk" times for hypoglycemia. Having a "Glucagon Emergency Kit" (see page 1119) on hand is also an important part of your diabetes plan. Your health care team can provide a prescription for the kit and show you how it's used.

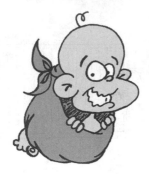

*W*ill severe hypoglycemia affect my baby?

TIP:

There is very little data that supports a direct connection between hypoglycemia (low blood sugar) and fetal danger. However, this does not mean that hypoglycemia is not dangerous. Symptoms of severe hypoglycemia, which include confused or hostile states of mind, lack of coordination, fatigue, and even passing out, can increase the risk of an accident, which may be harmful to both you and the fetus.

Hypoglycemia is a risk for all women with diabetes who take insulin. Hypoglycemia unawareness, a condition where you do not recognize low blood glucose, may also be exaggerated during pregnancy, especially in women with type 1 diabetes (see page 1093). Women with diabetes who are pregnant—especially those on insulin therapy—are asked to monitor their blood glucose levels up to 8 times daily. You are advised to treat blood glucose levels of 60 mg/dl or below whether you have symptoms or not. You should check blood glucose levels before you drive, as well.

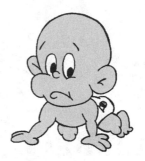

My doctor says, based on the results of my amniocentesis, I need to take steroid injections. She also mentioned something about respiratory distress syndrome. What does all of that mean?

TIP:

An *amniocentesis* is a procedure in which your health care professional (usually your obstetrician or perinatologist) will take a sample of amniotic fluid from your uterus. The sample is then analyzed to determine if your fetus is at risk for respiratory distress syndrome, a condition that affects your newborn baby's ability to breathe. There are studies that indicate that the risk of respiratory distress syndrome is greater in infants whose mothers have diabetes. Because of this risk, women with diabetes will usually have at least one amniocentesis before delivery to determine if the fetus' lungs are mature. If the results show immature fetal lungs, then a steroid, such as dexamethasone, is usually given by injection on 2 consecutive days to help the fetal lungs mature. The procedure should be monitored very closely since dexamethasone can cause hyperglycemia (high blood sugar). You may need to change your insulin dosages during the course of the therapy to counteract the steroids. If time permits, your physician may repeat the amniocentesis at a later date before starting any steroid therapy.

Chapter 3
PREGNANCY AND NUTRITION: MORE THAN JUST EATING FOR TWO

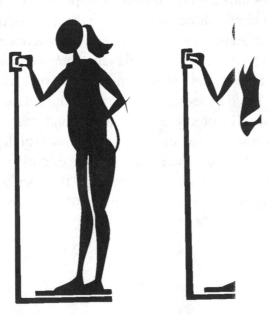

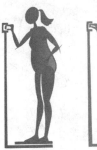
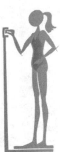

*H*ow much weight should I gain *during my pregnancy?*

▼
TIP:

As a woman with diabetes, there are no special issues regarding your weight gain, as long as you are eating a nutritionally healthy diet and your blood glucose levels are within the recommended ranges. Weight gain during pregnancy is normal, even necessary for successful outcomes, yet many women (even those without diabetes) worry about pregnancy-related weight gain. Basically, the amount of weight you should gain is based on your body mass index (BMI) and your weight before pregnancy. Your BMI is a combination of weight and height. To determine your BMI, multiply your prepregnancy weight by 705, divide this number by your height in inches, and then divide this number by your height again. Or just check a BMI chart.

The basic guidelines for pregnancy-related weight gain are as follows:

BMI	Recommended Weight Gain
Less than 19.8	28–40 pounds
19.8–26	25–35 pounds
26.1–29	15–25 pounds
More than 29	15 pounds
Exceptions	
Twin pregnancy	34–45 pounds
Triplet pregnancy	About 50 pounds

As always, check with your diabetes care team for the amount of weight gain that's right for you.

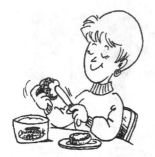

I have type 2 diabetes and was quite overweight when I became pregnant. Should I try to lose a few pounds for a healthier pregnancy?

▼
TIP:

No. It's true that women who are overweight during pregnancy may experience more medical problems, such as hypertension (high blood pressure) and preeclampsia (hypertension and swelling caused by pregnancy). However, pregnancy is not the time to lose weight. Cutting down on calories can cause your body to burn fat stores, resulting in ketones, which could be harmful to your baby. Although you shouldn't be dieting, you should limit your weight gain to about 15 pounds while you are pregnant. Hold your weight gain steady and vow to yourself that you'll drop the pounds after the baby is born.

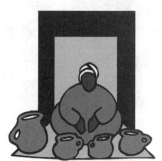

My obstetrician says I'm gaining weight too quickly. Is there an ideal rate of weight gain during pregnancy?

▼
TIP:

There is no "ideal" formula for weight gain. However, weight gain should be gradual and follow a predictable pattern. During the 1st trimester, you should gain 2–5 pounds *total*. Almost all of this weight is gained as your uterus and breasts enlarge, your blood volume expands, and the placenta and amniotic fluid is formed. During the 2nd and 3rd trimesters, a healthy rate of weight gain is 1/2 to 1 pound a week. The last trimester is when the baby is growing the most. If your weight gain slows during the last trimester there's a higher risk you'll deliver the baby before it is due.

Throughout your pregnancy, your goal should be to keep your weight gain steady and your blood glucose under control. If you notice any sudden weight gain or loss during your pregnancy, check with your health team to rule out any serious problems. A registered dietitian with expertise in pregnancy and diabetes can work with you to design a healthy eating plan for you during pregnancy.

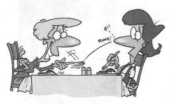

I've often heard that pregnant women are eating for two. How much extra food should I be eating?

▼

TIP:

Eating for two doesn't mean you should be eating twice as many calories each day! Generally, the recommended calorie intake for an active pregnant woman is 2400–2800 calories—about 300 more calories a day than usual. However, because your baby's health is so closely linked to your own, you should pack as much nutrition as you can into each meal. It's important to eat a healthy variety of foods from each food group. The table below is based on the Diabetes Food Pyramid. It shows the different food groups and example servings from each. Talk with your dietitian about how many servings from each food group you should eat to meet your daily calorie goals. Foods with an * are sources of carbohydrate; your intake of these should be based on your blood glucose levels.

Food Group	Examples of a Serving
*Grains, Beans, and Starchy Vegetables	1 slice of bread 1/3 cup cooked beans 1/2 cup cooked cereal
*Vegetables	1 cup raw vegetables 1/2 cup cooked vegetables 1/2 cup vegetable juice
*Fruits	1 small apple 1/2 medium banana 1/2 cup apple juice
*Milk	1 cup milk 1 cup yogurt
Meat and Others	2–3 ounces of cooked lean meat, poultry, or fish 1/2 cup tofu
*Fats and Sweets	Variable serving sizes; use with caution
Alcohol	Do not drink alcohol while you are pregnant!

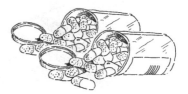

*A re there any vitamin supple-
ments I should be taking while
I'm pregnant?*

▼

TIP:

Maybe. If you make healthy food choices from a variety of food groups, you will generally receive all the vitamins and minerals you need. However, certain vitamins and minerals may require special attention.

- **Folic Acid**—You should consume at least 400 micrograms of folic acid every day, whether it is from foods, supplements, or both. Folic acid can be found in legumes, green leafy vegetables, liver, citrus fruits and juices, and whole-wheat bread.
- **Iron**—A routine, low-dose iron supplement of 30 milligrams a day is recommended for all pregnant women. You can also find iron in lean red meat, fish, poultry, dried fruits, and iron-fortified cereals.
- **Zinc and Copper**—Iron can interfere with the absorption of other minerals, so if you are taking an iron supplement you should also be taking 15 milligrams of zinc and 2 milligrams of copper daily. You can find these minerals in most prenatal vitamin and mineral supplements.
- **Calcium**—If you are 14–18 years old, you should be getting at least 1,300 milligrams of calcium daily; if you're 19–50 years old, you should be getting 1,000 milligrams. Dairy products are the best source of calcium.

There are some specific pregnancy cases where it is highly recommended you take a supplement. If you smoke or abuse drugs or alcohol, have iron deficiency anemia, rarely or never eat meat, or are pregnant with more than one fetus, then you should probably be taking a supplement. Talk with your diabetes care team to see which minerals or vitamins you require during pregnancy.

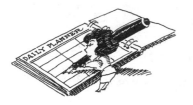

Can I use carbohydrate counting to plan my meals while I'm pregnant?

▼
TIP:

Yes, carbohydrate counting is an excellent way to plan your meals while you are pregnant. Carbohydrate has the biggest effect on your after-meal blood glucose levels, so an adequate and consistent level of carbohydrate is an important factor in keeping your blood glucose levels under control and your pregnancy healthy. Carbohydrates are found in grains, vegetables, fruit, milk, and sweets.

Work with a registered dietitian (RD) to plan a diet that has the correct amount of carbohydrate for your pregnancy. Generally, 40–45% of your calories should come from carbohydrate, although this can vary from person to person. An RD can figure out a more specific number for you and your needs. An RD can also help you learn more about portion size, which is critical to carbohydrate counting. If you are taking insulin, whether through injections or through a pump, you'll need to know how much carbohydrate you are eating to adjust your insulin doses. If you do intend to plan your meals with carbohydrate counting, remember that self-monitoring of blood glucose levels is very important.

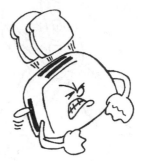

*M*y registered dietitian told me to limit the amount of carbohydrate I'm eating in the morning. Why?

▼

TIP:

B ecause pregnant women don't handle carbohydrate as well in the morning as they do at other times of the day. This is due to the increase of pregnancy hormone levels in the morning, which work against insulin. Basically, pregnant women tend to be more glucose intolerant in the morning. Many meal plans for pregnant women will have 30 grams of carbohydrate for breakfast—equal to 1 slice of toast and 1 cup of milk (8 ounces). If this isn't satisfying your hunger, try adding protein to your morning meal. Protein doesn't affect your after-meal glucose levels that much, and it is filling.

Check your blood glucose levels often. If your after-breakfast glucose levels are within target range, you may be able to add a small amount of carbohydrate back to your breakfast. If your blood glucose levels are high, you might need to reduce your morning carbohydrate intake or begin doing some moderate exercise after breakfast.

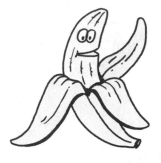

Can I have snacks between meals?

TIP:

Of course. Snacks provide a constant source of nutrition for your growing baby and help you avoid extreme changes in blood glucose levels. In addition, smaller and more frequent meals and snacks can help prevent the heartburn and nausea that usually go hand in hand with pregnancy.

Unfortunately, many pregnant women with diabetes skip meals or snacks, thinking this will help keep their blood glucose under control. Do not do this! Going long periods of time without food can cause your body to burn fat, which leads to the presence of ketones in your bloodstream and "starvation ketosis." This can have a very negative impact on your baby's brain development. Your baby also requires a steady source of glucose 24 hours a day, not just while you're awake. This makes a bedtime snack very important.

Check your blood glucose often throughout the day and work with your registered dietitian to develop a meal plan that is right for you. Most pregnant women find that a meal plan of 3 meals a day with 3 between-meal snacks is best. Snacks that contain protein, such as peanut butter or low-fat cheese, can help satisfy hunger without having a big impact on blood glucose levels.

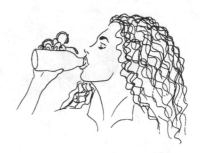

*I*s it safe for me to use artificial
sweeteners while I'm pregnant?

▼
TIP:

For the most part. The effects of artificial sweeteners on pregnancy have been well studied. Currently, the Food and Drug Administration (FDA) has approved 5 nonnutritive, artificial sweeteners as being safe for use during pregnancy. But keep the following in mind.

- **Saccharin** crosses the placenta and can remain in fetal tissues, although it does not appear to be harmful. You should still probably avoid this sweetener.
- **Acesulfame-K** also crosses the placenta, but once again, there doesn't appear to be any harmful side effects. There are no specific recommendations for using this sweetener during pregnancy.
- **Aspartame** must be present in very large amounts to cross the placenta, but it appears to be safe if you keep your intake within the FDA guidelines. Women with phenylketonuria should use aspartame with caution.
- **Sucralose** appears to be a safe sweetener during pregnancy. The FDA has concluded that sucralose poses no reproductive risk.
- **Neotame** is the most recent FDA-approved sweetener. Research shows that it is safe for use in pregnant and breastfeeding women.

Nutritive sweeteners, such as fructose and sorbitol, contain carbohydrate that must be counted in your meal plan. Remember to read your food labels closely and talk with your medical team about your use of sweeteners.

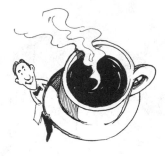

Do I need to limit caffeine intake while I'm pregnant?

▼

TIP:

It might not be a bad idea. Caffeine can cross the placenta and affect your baby's heart rate and breathing, although no studies in humans have found that caffeine is linked with birth defects. However, most health care professionals recommend that pregnant women keep their caffeine intake to about 300 milligrams a day. The following chart lists the amount of caffeine found in common foods and beverages.

Beverage	Serving Size	Amount of Caffeine
Percolated coffee	5 ounces	85 mg
Instant coffee	5 ounces	60 mg
Espresso	1 ounce	40 mg
Leaf/bag tea	5 ounces	30 mg
Soda/cola beverage	12 ounces	36 mg

Discuss your use of caffeine with your health care team and learn what they recommend for you and your situation.

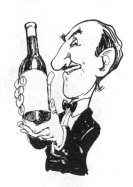

Will it hurt the baby if I have an occasional alcoholic drink while I'm pregnant?

▼
TIP:

Yes! If you are pregnant or may become pregnant, you should not drink alcohol. Period. Alcohol crosses the placenta, so your baby will be exposed to any alcohol you drink. Heavy drinking during pregnancy seriously increases the risk of mental retardation, learning disabilities, and major birth defects, a condition known as *fetal alcohol syndrome*. Even moderate drinking (no more than 1 serving of alcohol a day) has been linked to lower fertility rates and fetal growth problems. Beer, wine, and other alcoholic beverages carry a warning label about the dangers of drinking while pregnant. So save the champagne to celebrate after your baby is born!

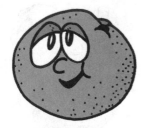

*F*ruit seems to help the constipation
I've had since becoming pregnant,
but it has a lot of carbohydrate. Is there
something else I should be using?

▼
TIP:

Not necessarily. Constipation is a normal part of pregnancy. Pregnancy hormones tend to relax digestive muscles and slow down the digestion process. Iron supplements can also lead to constipation. If fruits tend to relieve your constipation troubles, then by all means, keep eating fruit. Just be sure to count the carbohydrate as part of your overall meal plan. Fruit probably helps because it has fiber and fiber-rich foods, such as legumes, whole grains, bran, and vegetables can help aid in digestion. All of these foods contain carbohydrate. If you're looking for a noncarbohydrate approach, try drinking 8–12 cups of water a day and getting moderate daily exercise. These activities can help keep you regular. If the problem persists, check with your health care team for other options.

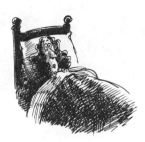

I have suffered from morning sickness throughout my pregnancy. Would it be safe for me to try an herbal remedy?

TIP:

No. Until the safety of herbal remedies with pregnancy is proven, it's best to avoid using them. There have been very few scientific studies done looking at the safety of alternative therapies. While herbal remedies sound safe because they are "natural," some may cause severe side effects, such as increased bleeding.

The bigger concern here is the effect morning sickness can have on your diabetes. Morning sickness is a very normal part of pregnancy, though its causes are still not understood. We do know that it tends to be worse when your stomach is empty, so you may find relief by just eating smaller meals more frequently, avoiding offensive odors, drinking more water, and getting more fresh air. Depending on how well you tolerate carbohydrate, your health care team may suggest you eat a carbohydrate food, such as rice cakes or saltines, before getting out of bed in the morning. These snacks will also help prevent ketonuria, which can make morning sickness worse.

Nausea can also be a sign of hypoglycemia, and hypoglycemia can make nausea worse, so be prepared to check your blood glucose often. If you're taking insulin, you may need to adjust your dosage on a meal-to-meal basis while you figure out which foods you can stomach. If your morning sickness and vomiting become severe, your medical team may suggest you be hospitalized to avoid dehydration and electrolyte imbalances.

There is a silver lining to all of this, however. Morning sickness usually disappears after the 3rd month of pregnancy *and* women who have morning sickness are less likely to have a miscarriage or premature birth.

My obstetrician told me to avoid certain types of fish while I'm pregnant. Why?

▼
TIP:

Because some types of fish contain methyl mercury, which can be harmful to developing nervous systems. Your obstetrician's worries are backed by the Food and Drug Administration (FDA), which has released information on the dangers of eating certain types of fish while you are pregnant, planning to become pregnant, or nursing. Methyl mercury occurs naturally in the environment, but is also a by-product of industrial pollution. Generally, methyl mercury is found in large, long-lived fish, such as the shark, swordfish, king mackerel, and tilefish. These fish should be avoided while you are pregnant. It is probably safe to eat up to 12 ounces of cooked fish per week, so long as they are smaller types of fish. You may want to contact your local health department to find out if there are any special warnings about toxins in fish caught or sold in your area.

I heard a news report about something called "listeriosis" and how it is especially dangerous for pregnant women. What is it and should I be worried?

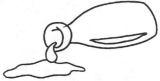

TIP:

Listeriosis is a food-borne illness caused by the bacteria *listeria monocytogenes* and is especially dangerous for pregnant women and their unborn babies. It can cause premature delivery, miscarriage, fetal death, and severe illness or death in a newborn who has been infected. Pregnant women and their unborn babies are 20 times more likely than other healthy adults to get listeriosis. With that in mind, it's best to be cautious. To reduce your risk of getting listeriosis, avoid foods that are more likely to be carrying the bacterium, such as soft cheeses (feta, Brie, Camembert), unpasteurized milk, hot dogs, lunch meats, and deli meats. Signs of the illness include flu-like symptoms and problems with the nervous system, such as headache, stiff neck, and confusion. Antibiotics are the recommended treatment. If you think you have listeriosis, talk with your medical team immediately. A blood test can confirm whether or not you have the illness.

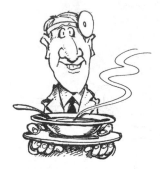

*W**hat is a registered dietitian and where can I find one?**

▼
TIP:

A registered dietitian (RD) is the nutrition expert on your diabetes care team, the one who will help you develop a meal plan specifically tailored to your needs as a pregnant woman with diabetes. An RD with experience in pregnancy and diabetes will be especially helpful. Your primary doctor may recommend an RD, or you may find one at a local hospital, outpatient clinic, or health department. The following resources may also be helpful:

- To find a registered dietitian in your area, call the American Dietetic Association at (800) 877-1600, or visit their web site at *www.eatright.org*.
- To find a diabetes education program that has been approved by the American Diabetes Association, call (800) 342-2383, or visit their web site at *www.diabetes.org*.
- To find a diabetes educator, call the American Association of Diabetes Educators at (800) 832-6874, or visit their web site at *www.aadenet.org*.

Chapter 4
MANAGING MEDICATION DURING PREGNANCY

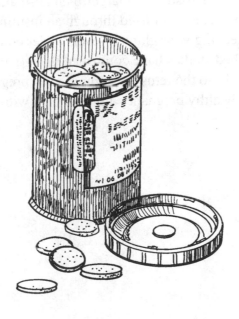

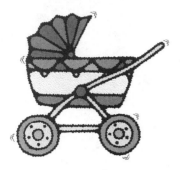

Will insulin therapy have a negative effect on my baby?

TIP:

No. Insulin therapy has been used safely to reach and/or maintain the best possible glucose control in pregnancy for years. We know that glucose crosses the placenta to the fetus. The effects of hyperglycemia (high blood glucose) during pregnancy are well documented and include a higher incidence of birth defects, increased rate of miscarriage, and macrosomia (a larger than normal fetus). Insulin therapy, whether injected or infused through an insulin pump, has an essential role in keeping your glucose levels under control for you and your baby. Published studies have confirmed that good blood glucose levels lower the risks to the fetus throughout your pregnancy. Insulin is a vital part of a healthy pregnancy for a woman with high blood glucose.

I *have gestational diabetes and my doctor says I need to take insulin. My mother takes pills for her diabetes. Why can't I?*

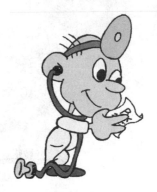

TIP:

Because you are pregnant and your mother is not (we're assuming). Oral medications can often be used to treat type 2 diabetes, depending on an individual's needs. However, oral glucose lowering agents have generally not been recommended *during pregnancy*. If your blood glucose control is not meeting the recommended goals for diabetes and pregnancy, the medication of choice is insulin therapy. Insulin therapy should be recommended if blood glucose levels exceed the following:

	Whole Blood Goals	Plasma Goals
Fasting	≤95 mg/dl	≤105 mg/dl
1 hour post-meal	≤140 mg/dl	≤155 mg/dl
2 hours post-meal	≤120 mg/dl	≤130 mg/dl

Adapted from "Gestational Diabetes Mellitus," *ADA Clinical Practice Recommendations,* 2003.

Most health care professionals recommend insulin therapy if blood glucose levels fall outside the above ranges within a 1- to 2-week period. The type of insulin therapy used during pregnancy will vary depending on your individual needs, your safety, and the experience of your health care professional.

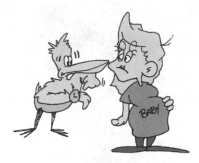

My A1C is 6.8% on 2 shots of insulin a day. My diabetes team is recommending 3 to 4 injections a day now that I am pregnant. Why?

▼

TIP:

First of all, congratulations on your efforts to control your blood glucose! A 6.8% A1C level is very good. It is important to note, though, that the goals for diabetes control are different when you are pregnant. When you're pregnant you want the lowest A1C possible, without putting yourself at an excessive risk for hypoglycemia. Normal A1C is usually considered below 6%, though individual lab analysis may vary. Your diabetes team is probably recommending 3–4 injections daily to help you fine-tune your insulin regimen. This might be to help you control your after-meal blood glucose a little better, or it might be to lower your risk of hypoglycemia, or it might be both. Self-monitoring of blood glucose (up to 8 times daily) is recommended to continuously evaluate your diabetes care plan and assist with any necessary changes in a prompt manner.

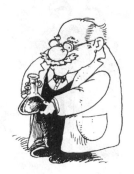

*M*y *endocrinologist is recommending
an insulin pump to help me control
my diabetes while I am pregnant. How
will it help?*

▼
TIP:

By providing very tight blood glucose control. An insulin pump is
a mechanical device attached to tubing and an infusion set that
infuses insulin directly under your skin. The pump sends insulin
through the tubing/catheter at a preprogrammed, continuous (basal)
rate, as well as in larger insulin amounts (bolus) programmed by the
user to cover any carbohydrate intake from snacks or meals. Many
health care professionals recommend the use of insulin pumps during
pregnancy because they feel that pump therapy closely mimics the
insulin release of a normal pancreas. Ideally, you would start pump
therapy *before* pregnancy to achieve good glucose control before you
conceive.

Insulin pump therapy has been used safely in both type 1 and type
2 diabetes. The ability to adjust and deliver insulin in increments
smaller than 1.0 unit makes it easier to fine-tune insulin delivery during very insulin-sensitive periods (such as the 1st trimester, especially
in type 1 diabetes), as well as in insulin-resistant states, which occurs
in type 2, gestational diabetes (GDM), and during the 2nd and 3rd
trimesters in type 1 diabetes. You will want to evaluate the expense of
insulin pump therapy and determine your health care coverage for the
device and supplies. The expense may not be as feasible if you have
gestational diabetes, since GDM usually disappears once the baby is
delivered, making insulin pump therapy a short-term investment.

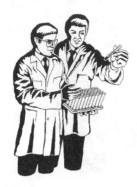

I don't have type 1 diabetes, but my doctor says I will need insulin during my pregnancy. Why?

TIP:

Because insulin is the best and safest way to control your blood glucose while you're pregnant. Many women have successfully used nutrition, exercise, and diabetes pills to manage type 2 diabetes. However, oral diabetes medications are usually not used during pregnancy because of the possible risk of complications. More research is needed to determine whether or not diabetes pills are safe for women who are pregnant. Insulin, on the other hand, has been safely used to manage diabetes in pregnancy for years.

Ideally, you should start an intensive insulin regimen (3–4 injections daily) or perhaps insulin pump therapy *before* you are pregnant to get your blood glucose under control. Keep in mind that insulin resistance increases in type 2 diabetes during pregnancy, as well as in type 1 and gestational diabetes in the 2nd and 3rd trimesters. This is a result of weight gain and contrainsulin hormones produced by the placenta. Remember to increase your self-blood glucose checks up to 8 times a day to keep yourself and your diabetes care team aware of where you are in your control.

O nce I became pregnant I started intensive insulin therapy. My doctor told me I needed to have a medication called glucagon *available just in case I needed it. What is glucagon?*

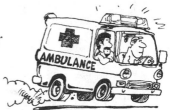

TIP:

G lucagon is a hormone injection used as an emergency treatment for hypoglycemia (low blood sugar). During pregnancy, you run a higher risk of hypoglycemia due to lower blood sugar goals, lower sensitivity to the symptoms of hypoglycemia (hypoglycemia unawareness), and the use of your glucose stores by the fetus. Glucagon is used when you have severe hypoglycemia in which you are unable to swallow, perhaps confused, or have passed out due to hypoglycemia. It works by causing the liver to make glucose and usually takes effect within 15 minutes. Once you are alert and able to eat, monitor your blood glucose levels carefully and eat a carbohydrate snack, such as crackers. Keep in mind that a full syringe of glucagon will be too much for anyone weighing less than 120 pounds. In this case, it's best to give 1/2 of the shot and then wait 15 minutes before giving the rest.

A glucagon kit is recommended for anyone with type 1 diabetes, regardless of whether or not you are pregnant. If you have type 2 or gestational diabetes, your diabetes care team should assess whether or not you need glucagon. A prescription is required to obtain glucagon at the pharmacy and your physician may want to write the prescription for a "Glucagon Emergency Kit" that contains a syringe and is ready to be mixed and injected. Since you will be in no shape to give yourself glucagon when you need it, your family members or significant others will need to be fully educated on how to give you a glucagon injection and know the location of the kit, which is usually refrigerated.

Chapter 5
BABY STEPS: PHYSICAL ACTIVITY DURING PREGNANCY

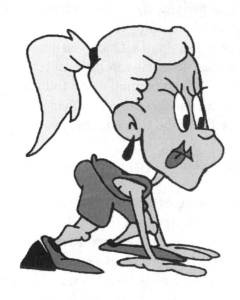

*S*hould I exercise while I'm
pregnant?

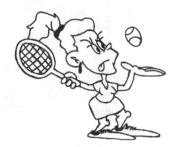

▼

TIP:

Y es. The American College of Obstetricians and Gynecologists
recommends 30 minutes or more of moderate exercise on most,
if not all, days of the week for pregnant women who don't have medical or obstetric complications (see page 1122 for a list of complications that would keep you from exercising). If your physician has
evaluated you and finds that your diabetes is well controlled without
complications, physical activity can provide a variety of benefits in
terms of both your pregnancy and your diabetes.

Moderate exercise helps you prepare for the physical demands of
labor and childbirth. Exercise can help improve your muscle tone, circulation, and heart function, as well as provide you with a feeling of
mental and physical well-being. Women who are physically fit find
that their recovery after childbirth is faster and easier. Exercise also
helps increase the efficiency of your body's own insulin, meaning that
if you do require insulin during pregnancy, exercise may allow you to
use a smaller dose.

Discuss a program of physical activity during pregnancy with
your physician and diabetes team. They can notify you of any special
limitations or considerations, as well as provide you with specific
guidelines for taking care of your diabetes as you exercise.

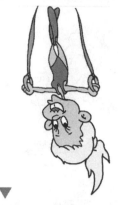

A *re there any pregnancy-related complications that would prevent me from exercising?*

▼ TIP:

Y es. Exercising with some complications could put you and your child at undue risk. Such complications include

- Significant heart or lung disease
- Being at risk for premature labor
- Experiencing premature labor during your current pregnancy
- Multiple gestation (twins or more) at risk for premature labor
- Persistent 2nd- or 3rd-trimester bleeding
- Placenta previa (a condition where the placenta would precede the Baby's exit from the womb after 26 weeks into the pregnancy)
- Ruptured membranes
- Incompetent cervix
- Preeclampsia/pregnancy-induced hypertension (high blood pressure)

Having any of these conditions is an indication that you should not participate in aerobic exercise while you're pregnant. If you have been diagnosed with any of the above, or feel that you may be at risk, talk with your diabetes health care team about the precautions you should take.

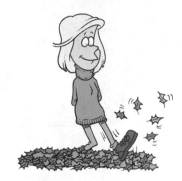

I wasn't physically active before my pregnancy. What is the best exercise for a diabetic pregnancy?

▼

TIP:

B ecause you were relatively inactive before your pregnancy, it is wise to have your obstetrician evaluate you and make recommendations for specific types of physical activity during your pregnancy. Physical activity provides many pregnancy health benefits and assists in blood glucose control. Walking is considered one of the best forms of physical activity for pregnant women. Brisk walking will provide you with a good total-body workout and should be relatively easy on your joints and muscles. Swimming, water aerobics, and prenatal stretching classes offer other opportunities for you to gradually begin a program of physical activity. Arm exercises might be another option. If you have your physician's OK, your goal should be to accumulate 30 minutes or more of moderate exercise on most, if not all, days of the week. Be sure to check your blood glucose before, during, and after your exercise session and make adjustments in your meal plan if needed.

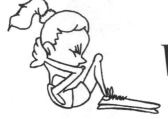

*W*hich exercises should I avoid now that I'm pregnant?

▼

TIP:

Anything that puts your body under unnecessary stress. Pregnancy means many changes in your body, which means changes in your ability to exercise. Pregnancy hormones cause the ligaments that support your joints to become relaxed, so you should avoid jerky, bouncy, or high-impact motions. Because you are carrying extra pounds (most of them in the front of your body), your center of gravity has shifted. This may place stress on the joints and muscles in your pelvis and lower back. In addition, those extra pregnancy pounds will mean that your body has to work harder during exercise than before. Don't overdo it!

Although you and your physician should go over your plans for physical activity, in general, it is best to avoid activities with a high risk of falling (gymnastics, horseback riding, downhill skiing, tennis, racquetball, etc.), those with a high risk of injury to your abdomen (ice hockey, soccer, and basketball), and, if you're not used to exercise, exercises that put stress on your lower body (bicycling, strength training with your legs, etc.). In addition, you should avoid scuba diving because the fetus is at increased risk for decompression sickness during this activity.

Certain forms of exercise may involve uncomfortable positions and movements that may be harmful for pregnant women. For example, after the 1st trimester, the expanding uterus may affect circulation to the fetus, so it's best to avoid exercises that require you to lie flat on your back.

Although physical activity is good for both your pregnancy and your diabetes, be careful and choose the best form of exercise for your health and that of your baby.

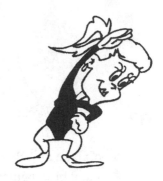

W *hen is the best time for me to exercise?*

▼
TIP:

T his depends on your diabetes. In most cases, exercise lowers blood glucose by helping your body's cells become more sensitive to insulin. It may be best to take part in physical activity directly after a meal when your blood glucose level will be at its highest. Women with gestational diabetes may find that taking a walk after breakfast is especially helpful in controlling their morning rise in blood glucose. If you are taking insulin, you should avoid vigorous physical activity at the time your insulin is reaching its peak. Remember that exercise can have a blood glucose–lowering effect for up to 24 hours after you've stopped exercising, so continue to check your blood glucose frequently.

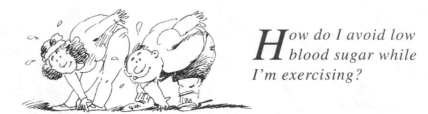

*H*ow do I avoid low
blood sugar while
I'm exercising?

▼
TIP:

D on't take any chances. Being pregnant can make you more prone
to low blood glucose (hypoglycemia), and you may experience
hypoglycemia if you delay a meal, skip a snack or meal, or exercise
more than usual. To prevent hypoglycemia, check your blood glucose
frequently—before, during, and after physical activity if necessary.

- **Before you exercise**—Check your blood glucose. If it is over
  240 mg/dl and you take insulin, follow up by checking your urine
  for ketones. If ketones are present, this means you do not have
  enough insulin in your system. You may need more insulin, so contact your health care team and do not exercise until your ketone levels have returned to trace or negative amounts.

    If your blood glucose is less than 100 mg/dl before you
  begin a 30-minute session of physical activity, eat a small snack
  with 15 grams of carbohydrate such as 1 small muffin, 1 small
  piece of fruit, or 1/2 an English muffin.
- **While you are exercising**—Be alert for the signs of hypoglycemia,
  such as headache, shakiness, confusion, sweatiness, irritability,
  fatigue, hunger, and personality change. Check your blood glucose.
  If it is below 70 mg/dl, treat it with 10–15 grams of carbohydrate.
  Good sources are glucose tablets or gel, 4 ounces of fruit juice or
  regular soft drink, 6–8 ounces of fat-free or low-fat milk, or 5–7
  Lifesavers. Recheck your blood glucose within 15 minutes and
  treat again if necessary. Do not resume exercising until your blood
  glucose is back to at least 100 mg/dl.
- **After you exercise**—Physical activity continues to have a blood
  glucose–lowering effect up to 24 hours after you've exercised.
  Continue to monitor your blood glucose on a regular schedule and
  be alert for the signs and symptoms of hypoglycemia.

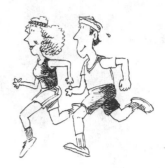

I have type 1 diabetes and routinely jog 6 miles a day. I just found out that I am pregnant. Can I continue my daily jog?

▼

TIP:

Physical activity is highly recommended for pregnant women with diabetes, particularly if you have been in good shape before becoming pregnant. Check with your physician for a complete evaluation as soon as possible. If your diabetes is under control, without complications, it is likely you'll be able to continue your routine, as long as it is comfortable and safe for you and the baby. At some point, you may need to switch to a more low-impact form of exercise, such as brisk walking. If you have a history or risk of preterm labor or fetal growth restriction, your obstetrician may advise you to reduce your activity in the 2nd and 3rd trimesters.

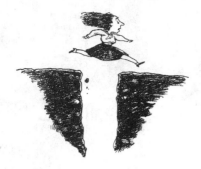

I would like to continue exercising while I'm pregnant, as long as it's safe. What are some warning signs that I should stop exercising?

▼
TIP:

B e alert for the following warning signs that you should stop exercising while you're pregnant:

- Signs and symptoms of hypoglycemia (low blood sugar)
- Vaginal bleeding
- Shortness of breath before you exercise
- Dizziness
- Headache
- Chest pain
- Muscle weakness
- Calf pain or swelling
- Preterm labor
- Decreased movement of the fetus
- Amniotic fluid leakage
- Uterine cramping without bleeding

If you do experience any of these symptoms, stop exercising and contact your health care team.

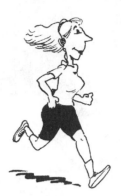

I was just told I have gestational diabetes. The diabetes educator told me that exercise would help control my blood glucose levels. How?

▼
TIP:

Physical activity lowers blood glucose by helping the body cells become more sensitive to insulin, which helps control your blood glucose. Gestational diabetes (GDM) is a form of diabetes that appears during pregnancy and usually disappears after the baby is born. Its exact cause is unknown, but it may be related to pregnancy hormones that block insulin's action in the mother's body, causing insulin resistance. If insulin is not working efficiently, glucose builds up in the blood. This can potentially cause complications in the baby, such as large birth weight, low blood sugar, breathing difficulties at birth, and jaundice. Treatment for gestational diabetes is geared toward keeping blood glucose levels as close to normal as possible and involves a healthy eating plan, physical activity, and insulin, if necessary.

Taking a brisk walk for 20–30 minutes after meals can be a big help in controlling blood glucose, particularly since glucose levels are highest after meals. Pregnancy hormones are often at higher levels in the morning, making women with gestational diabetes more prone to higher blood glucose values in the morning. In this situation, a brisk walk after breakfast can be very helpful in keeping blood glucose levels in control.

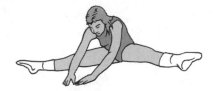

What should be included in a good exercise routine for a pregnant woman with diabetes?

▼

TIP:

Lots of things. Pregnant women with diabetes reap many benefits from exercise, such as improved muscle tone, circulation, and heart function, as well as a feeling of mental and physical well-being. Exercise also helps your body use its own insulin more efficiently, meaning that if you do require insulin during pregnancy, exercise may allow you to use a smaller dose. If you have been evaluated by your physician and have been given the OK to include more physical activity in your daily routine, be sure to consider the following points:

- Check your blood glucose levels before, during, and after an exercise session.
- Always have a fast-acting form of carbohydrate and/or a snack available to treat low blood sugar.
- If it's been some time since you've exercised, start slowly and work up to the recommended goal of 30 minutes a day of moderate exercise, such as brisk walking or light arm exercises.
- Drink plenty of water before, during, and after an exercise session.
- Always begin each exercise session with a warm-up period that includes such activities as careful stretching.
- Don't go overboard. As a general rule, your pulse should not go over 140 beats per minute during your exercise session.
- After you exercise, allow enough time to cool down and reduce your activity level gradually.

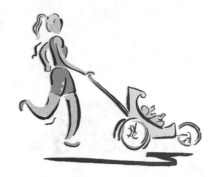

*H*ow can I become more physically fit after the baby is born?

TIP:

B y resuming the activity schedule you had before you were pregnant. Just remember to take it slowly. Many of the changes your body experiences during pregnancy persist from 4–6 weeks after you have your baby. Plus, your body will require time to recover from the hard work involved in labor and delivery.

Because physical activity is so beneficial to your general health and diabetes control, it is very important to resume an exercise routine after you check with your physician. Although recovery may be a bit longer after a cesarean delivery, your prepregnancy exercise routines should be resumed gradually as soon as it is physically and medically safe. A quick return to physical activity after childbirth will help you get your body back into shape and has been linked to a reduced risk of postpartum depression.

If you have had gestational diabetes during your pregnancy, it is important for you to realize that you are at high risk for developing type 2 diabetes later in life. For this reason, you should continue to follow a healthy meal plan and lose any excess weight you may have gained. Physical activity is especially beneficial for you because exercise helps your body use glucose more effectively, and this reduces your risk for developing type 2 diabetes.

Chapter 6
A CLOSE CHECK ON
DIABETES CONTROL

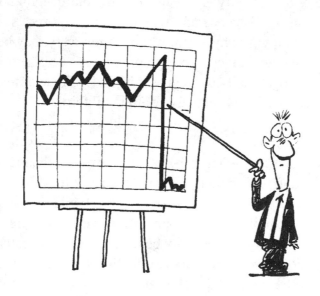

I had diabetes before I was pregnant. Now that I am pregnant, how often should I monitor my blood glucose?

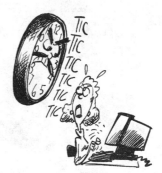

▼

TIP:

Most health care professionals recommend that a woman with preexisting diabetes (both type 1 and type 2) who becomes pregnant monitor her blood glucose levels up to 8 times daily. In terms of your day-to-day routine, you should probably monitor

- Before each meal
- 1 or 2 hours after each meal
- At bedtime
- Occasionally at 2–3 A.M.

Monitoring your blood glucose frequently gives you detailed information about your blood glucose control, helps you identify changes in your control (such as hypoglycemia or hyperglycemia), gives you information about the effects of meals and other events (such as exercise) on your blood glucose, and provides you with feedback for changes in your insulin therapy.

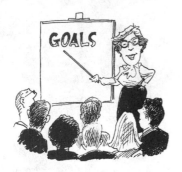

*W*hat are the blood glucose goals for women who are pregnant?

▼

TIP:

When women who do not have diabetes are pregnant, their blood glucose levels tend to be lower than non-pregnant levels. It follows that when a woman who has diabetes gets pregnant, she'll aim for lower glucose levels as well. The following table gives the recommendations for diabetes and pregnancy blood glucose goals from the American Diabetes Association. Whole blood values reflect a blood sample that is taken and measured by a meter using a whole blood sample. A plasma value would be a serum-blood sample for glucose taken by a laboratory (or a finger stick value using a meter that converts the whole blood reading to a plasma-correlated value). Plasma values usually read approximately 10–15% higher than whole blood values.

Blood Glucose Goals for Diabetes and Pregnancy

Timing	Whole Blood Value	Plasma Value
Fasting	60–90 mg/dl	69–104 mg/dl
Before meals	60–105 mg/dl	69–121 mg/dl
1 hour after meals	100–120 mg/dl	115–138 mg/dl
2 A.M.–6 A.M.	60–120 mg/dl	69–138 mg/dl

Adapted from *Medical Management of Pregnancy Complicated by Diabetes*, 3rd ed., ADA, 2000.

Discuss appropriate blood glucose goals with your health care team.

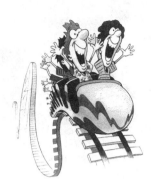

What should my A1C (hemoglobin A1C) be while I am pregnant?

▼

TIP:

An A1C (hemoglobin A1C) is a blood test that can predict average blood glucose levels for about 8–12 weeks. People without diabetes generally have an A1C of less than 6%, though this usually drops to less than 5% during pregnancy. Women with diabetes should strive for near normal A1Cs prior to, as well as during, pregnancy. Studies show that if you can keep your A1C to 1% above normal or lower, the risk of birth defects is about the same as for someone without diabetes. Keep in mind that the rates of each complication continue to decrease the lower A1C test levels go. It is essential for you and your diabetes care team to establish the lowest possible A1C goal for you, without putting you at excessive risk for hypoglycemia. Fine-tuning all areas of your diabetes treatment plan will be helpful in achieving this goal.

I have gestational diabetes and I'm monitoring my blood sugars 2 hours after each meal. Why is that important?

▼

TIP:

Since you didn't have diabetes before you were pregnant, it is helpful to see how eating affects your blood glucose control. It is essential for you to partner with a registered dietitian (RD) to develop a meal plan that is right for you. Even if you closely follow the meal plan, normal pregnancy hormones, as well as the weight you're bound to gain while pregnant, will cause your blood glucose levels to fluctuate. *Do not* stop eating or skip meals to control your blood glucose. Insulin therapy may be necessary to control your glucose levels. See page 1115 for guidelines on beginning insulin therapy with GDM.

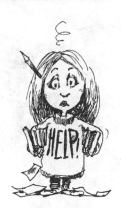

My doctor wants me to report blood glucose results on a weekly basis. Is this really necessary?

TIP:

Yes! Most health care teams like to study blood glucose results on a 1–2 week basis during pregnancy. Depending on how often you have appointments, the physician who is managing your diabetes may have you call, fax, or e-mail in your blood glucose numbers if you are not seeing him/her during a particular week. If you have 2 blood glucose numbers in a 1-week period that are higher than the recommended goals, quick adjustments to your treatment plan need to be made. For women with gestational diabetes (GDM), blood glucose numbers that do not meet goals may indicate you need to start taking insulin. For women with type 1, type 2, and GDM who take insulin, adjustments are typically needed at least every 2 weeks, although this may vary from person to person. Because of the effects of contrain-sulin hormones, as well as other factors that "aggravate" blood glucose levels, close monitoring and frequent adjustments to your treatment plan will probably be necessary throughout your pregnancy.

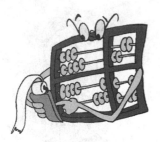

I have gestational diabetes and have been monitoring my blood sugar levels for about 4 weeks. All of my readings have been within recommended goals. Do I need to keep checking?

▼

TIP:

Yes. Your good glucose control is good for both you and the baby. As your pregnancy moves along, your need for insulin will increase. This is due, in part, to a continuing increase in the hormones produced by your placenta and various other maternal hormones. As these hormones and the weight in your abdomen increase, so does the need for insulin. Women with preexisting diabetes will need double or sometimes even triple the insulin they did before they were pregnant. You will need to monitor your blood sugar levels to be sure that your body can cope with these increasing demands for insulin. If your blood glucose starts to rise, it allows you and your diabetes team to immediately modify your treatment plan as necessary to keep you and your baby healthy!

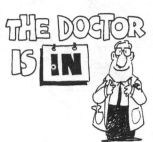

I am pregnant and have gestational diabetes. After lunch my blood glucose was 145 mg/dl. My friend with diabetes says that blood glucose level is OK, but my doctor says it isn't. Who's right?

▼

TIP:

In a way, both your friend and your doctor are right—depending on the situation. When it comes to goals for pregnant women with diabetes, your doctor has the right answer. Your reading of 135 mg/dl is higher than the recommended pregnancy goal. See page 1134 for the American Diabetes Association's blood glucose goals for pregnancy.

Your friend, on the other hand, may be thinking about the *recommended* goals for glucose control, without regard to pregnancy. The normal goals for people with diabetes who are not pregnant are slightly higher than pregnancy goals. Discuss any concerns you have with your health care team. When your glucose levels are outside the recommended range for pregnancy and diabetes, your treatment plan should probably be adjusted.

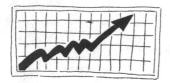

My A1C was 9.0% when I got pregnant. Will my baby be OK?

▼

TIP:

This depends on what you're doing about it now. A number of studies have shown that a high A1C level in early pregnancy can lead to a 2–5 times higher risk of birth defects and miscarriages. Generally, the higher the A1C, the greater the risk for these complications. It's recommended that you get your blood glucose under control *before* you are pregnant. In fact, normalizing blood glucose levels before and during pregnancy reduces your risk of pregnancy-related complications to that of the nondiabetic population. Now that you are pregnant, it is absolutely necessary that your blood glucose be controlled. Ideally, you should work with a team of health care professionals to help you manage your diabetes during pregnancy. This team should include

- Your primary care physician or endocrinologist
- An obstetrician
- A nurse educator (preferably a certified diabetes educator, or CDE)
- A social worker
- A registered dietitian
- A pediatrician or neonatologist

There are a variety of tests designed to check for birth defects, including ultrasonography and amniocentesis. If you plan to become pregnant again in the future, work with your health care team and have your blood glucose under control *before* pregnancy!

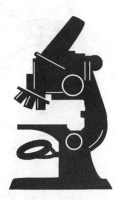

I have gestational diabetes, I'm 36 weeks
pregnant, and I'm using insulin. My
doctor just did a fructosamine test to
monitor my blood glucose control. What
does this mean?

TIP:

A *fructosamine* test shows the amount of glucose attached to your
protein molecules, which is a good indicator of your continuous
glucose levels over a 2-week period. Some health care professionals
use the results of this test to monitor short-term changes in glucose
control, mostly to see how well adjustments to your plan are going.
When it comes to pregnancy and diabetes, you want to achieve good
control as quick as you can. A fructosamine test is a good way to get
reliable, continuous blood glucose readings over a relatively short
period of time.

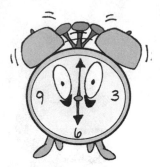

My diabetes team recommends urine ketone testing every morning. Is this necessary?

TIP:

Yes. Ketones appear when your body can't break down the glucose in your bloodstream *or* if there is not enough glucose available to meet your energy needs. When this happens, your body begins to use stored fat for energy, which results in ketones (acid substances) in your bloodstream. Ketone testing each morning can help you detect a condition called "starvation ketones," which means there is not enough glucose in your bloodstream for you and the fetus. If the condition persists over a few days, your diabetes health care team may recommend an increase in calories, perhaps with your bedtime snack. A condition called "ketoacidosis" can occur if ketones get built up in your bloodstream. Prompt troubleshooting of high blood glucose levels is essential while you are pregnant, since ketoacidosis can occur very quickly and at lower blood glucose levels than normal. Regular ketone testing done each morning, as well as when you have high blood glucose, can help prevent a serious medical situation.

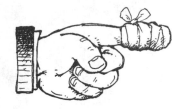

I have type 2 diabetes and have been using my forearm for blood glucose checks. I just found out I am pregnant and my doctor recommended finger stick glucose checks instead. Why?

▼

TIP:

Because the finger stick method is more accurate. Your blood glucose readings change during the course of the day, due to things such as food, medication, illness, stress, and exercise. Glucose circulates through your body in the bloodstream, first through your arteries, then to the capillaries (such as in your fingers), and finally your veins. The blood in your arteries has the highest glucose levels, followed by capillary blood, and then the blood in your veins. Blood also flows faster in your fingers than it does in alternative sites, such as your thigh, calf, forearm, upper arm, or hand. So what does this mean? It means that alternative site glucose values can lag behind finger stick glucose values; changes are seen sooner in a finger stick sample. When your blood glucose rises after a meal, or you suffer a sudden onset of hypoglycemia, you'll notice more quickly by using finger stick samples. This is especially important when you're pregnant, since the recommended goals for glucose control are "tighter" than normal. This includes glucose values both before and after eating (see page 1134 for diabetes/pregnancy glucose goals). In addition, hypoglycemia is often more frequent and more severe during pregnancy. Because of this, your doctor may prefer you use the finger stick method to get the fastest, most reliable reading possible.

INDEX

101 Tips for Improving
Your Blood Sugar

▼

Pills. *See* oral medication
Pneumonia vaccinations, 85
Prandin, 121
Precose, 122
Pregnancy, 120
Protein foods, 67

R
Reactions, hypoglycemic, 41, 46–47, 50–51
Rebound effect, 53
Records, diabetes management, 10
Regular insulin, 20, 34–35, 38, 44, 60–63, 65–67, 69, 79–80, 82, 98–100
Resource Guide, 70
Restaurant meals, 55, 92
Rezulin, 122
Risk factors, 120, 123

S
Saccharin, 90
School, 119
Screening for diabetes, 120
Sexual activity, 30, 102
Sickness, 64, 77–83
    fevers, 80
    hyperglycemia and, 78, 83
    medical help for, 81
    vaccinations, 85
Skin, sterilizing, 15
Sleeping
    hyperglycemia and, 38
    hypoglycemia and, 49, 51
Smoking, 117
Snacks. *See also* Meal(s)
    bedtime, 45, 49, 51, 91, 102
    between meal, 95, 100
    day care and, 119
    preexercise, 99, 101
    school and, 119
Soft drinks, 93, 98
Sorbitol, 90
Stomach, slow emptying of, 25

Storage, of insulin, 68
Stress, 83
Stroke, 13, 22, 30, 50, 116
Sugar, 16, 38, 41, 46, 91, 93–94, 98
Sugar-free foods, poor taste of, 90
Sulfonylureas, 121, 122

T
Table sugar, 94
Taste, of sugar-free foods, 90
Teeth, care of, 111
Test strips, 15, 18
Thinking ability, hypoglycemia and, 43
Thirst, 29
Tight control, 23, 47, 50, 107, 110, 112, 123
Time zones, 20
Touchup dosing, 66
Trips
    across time zones, 20
    blood glucose measuring and, 18
    insulin storage and, 68
    preparing for, 16
Twins, 11
Type 1 diabetes, 6, 8, 11, 24, 75, 110, 124
Type 2 diabetes, 6, 9, 24, 75–76, 110, 123–124

U
Ultralente insulin, 34, 36, 63, 65–66, 91
Urination, frequent, 29
Urine ketones, 9, 78, 81
United Kingdom Prospective Diabetes Study (UKPDS), 116
U.S. resident, 8

V
Vaccinations, 85
VA clinics, 123
Viral infections, 11, 64, 77–83
Vision problems, 29–30, 114

101 Tips for Staying Healthy with Diabetes

pre-existing condition exclusion, 148

Health management. *See also* Doctor visits
coworkers and, 132
test guidelines, 228

Heart disease
cholesterol and, 217
fat intake and, 220
homocysteine and, 183
hot tubs and, 218
risk of, 211, 221
saunas and, 218
Syndrome X, 221
testing for, 214
waist/hip ratio and, 195

Hemoglobin, glycosylated, 197, 236

Hepatitis, 165

Herbal remedies, 182

Heredity, as cause of diabetes, 133, 146

High blood glucose. *See also* Blood glucose levels
damage from, 174

Historical background, diabetes, 140, 144

Homocysteine, 183

Hospitalization
blood glucose control and, 237
surgery, 234

Hot tubs, 218

I

Impaired glucose tolerance (IGT), 238

Incontinence, 219

Infections
eye, 202
foot, 152, 216
from IUDs, 232
postoperative, 234
skin, 153

Infectiousness, of diabetes, 133

Insoluble fiber, 179

Insulin

allergic reaction to, 172
birth control pills and, 232
blood glucose testing and, 173
discovery of, 140
driving commercial vehicles and, 155
low dosages for children, 235
weight gain and, 176

Insulin-dependent diabetes. *See* Type 1 diabetes

Insulin pumps, 134, 167

Internet, diabetes information on, 157

IUD (intrauterine device), 232

K

Kaopectate, 154

Ketoacidosis, 156, 192, 237

Ketones, 156, 192, 237

Kidneys
assessments of, 137
blood pressure medication and, 223
failure of, 143
problems during pregnancy, 199, 203
protein and, 206
transplants of, 169

L

Langerhans, Paul, 140

Laser therapy, 198
exercise following, 207

Leg cramps, 204

Lomotil, 154

Loperamide, 154

Losartan, 223

Low blood glucose, 166. *See also* Blood glucose levels

M

Macular edema, 198

Magnesium supplements, 184

Meal planning. *See also* Diet
adherence to, 193
frequency of meals, 194

Medical costs, 148

insulin pumps, 167
pancreas transplants, 169
Medical visits. *See* Doctor visits
Medications. *See also* individual
  medications
  for colds, 161
  contraceptives, 168
  for depression, 162
  for high blood pressure, 223
  new. *See* New products
  sexual problems and, 213
  stopping, 175
  tiredness and, 229
  weight gain and, 176
Melatonin, 185
Metamucil, 179
Metformin, 151
Meyer, Jean de, 140
Mineral supplements. *See*
Supplements, dietary
Minkowski, Oskar, 140
Monounsaturated fats, 220

N

Nerve problems
  bladder function, 219
  constipation, 225
  gustatory sweating, 208
  painful neuropathy, 204
  postural dizziness, 212
New products, 145
  blood glucose levels and, 175
  for blood pressure problems, 223
  for complication prevention, 197
  for Type II diabetes, 151
Nicotine patches, 211
Non insulin-dependent diabetes. *See*
  Type II diabetes
Nutrition. *See* Diet

O

Obesity, 221. *See also* Weight control

P

Painful neuropathy, 204

Pancreas, 134, 140, 146
  transplants, 169
Podiatrists (DPMs), 215–216
Polyunsaturated fats, 220
Postural dizziness, 212
Prayer sign, 205
Precose, 151
Prednisone, 170
Pregnancy
  blood glucose control and, 236
  diabetes during, 139
  high blood pressure and, 199
  kidney disease and, 203
  risks, 199
Prevention
  of complications, 174, 200
  of diabetes, 146, 238
Products, new. *See* New products
Prostate exams, 219
Protein, 206
Pseudophilin, 179
Psychological problems. *See*
  Depression
Psyllium, 154, 225
Puberty, 160

R

Retinopathy, 198, 207
Rollo, John, 144

S

Saturated fats, 220
Saunas, 218
Sexual problems, 213, 230
Shoes, fitting of, 210, 233
Sick-day planning, colds, 161
Skin care. *See also* Foot care
  infections, 153
  rashes, 172
Sleep
  disturbances of, 227, 229
  melatonin and, 185
Smoking, 211
Sodium, lowering intake of, 188, 226
Soluble fiber, 179

Spilling protein, 206
Standards of Medical Care For Patients with Diabetes Mellitus, 228
Stiffness, in hands, 205
Stomach problems, 201
Stress tests, 214
Strokes, homocysteine and, 183
Summer camps, 160
Supervisors, diabetes disclosure and, 132
Supplements, dietary, 178
  folic acid (folate), 183
  ginseng, 181–182
  herbal remedies, 182
  magnesium, 184
  melatonin, 185
  vanadium, 182
Support groups, 141
Surgery, 234, 237. *See also* Transplants
Sweating, gustatory, 208
Syndrome X, 221
Syringes, low dose, 235

T
Teenagers, diabetes care and, 160
Testosterone, 213, 231
Tetracycline, 154
Thyroid problems, 135
  constipation and, 225
Tiredness, 166, 227, 229
TOPS (Take Off Pounds Sensibly), 191
Transplants
  of insulin-producing cells, 134
  of pancreas, 169
Triglyceride levels, 220, 221
Type I diabetes
  causes of, 133, 146, 149
  ketoacidosis, 192
  occurrence, 147
  prevention of, 146
Type II diabetes
  causes of, 133, 146
  dietary fiber and, 179

ginseng and, 181–182
new therapies for, 150
occurrence, 147
prevention of, 146, 238
stopping medication, 175

U
Urine leakage, 219
Urine testing, 156

V
Vaginal dryness, 231
Vanadium, 182
Viral conjunctivitis, 202
Vision. *See* Eye problems
Vitamin supplements. *See* Supplements, dietary

W
Waist/hip ratio, 195
Weight control, 176
  age and, 224
  diet/weight reduction programs, 191
  and IGT, reversing, 238
  obesity, 221
  Syndrome X, 220
  waist/hip ratio, 195
Weight Watchers, 191
White classification, 199
Wine, 164
World Wide Web, diabetes information on, 157

Y
Yawning, 166
Yeast infections, 153
Yohimbine, 213

101 Foot Care Tips

▼

Car, 282
Carpeting, 295
Certified diabetes educator (CDE), 265
Charcot's joint, 263, 332, 362
Chlorine bleach, 279
Cholesterol, 352–353
Circulation, *see* Blood circulation.
Cold feet, 348, 350
Color, 348
Complications, 256, 259, 260, 261, 264
Corn removers, 316
Corns, 257, 262, 267, 269, 271, 305, 315, 317
Cotton balls, 279
Counseling, 365
Crutches, 328
Custom-made shoes, 296, 301–302, 308, 365

D
Debride (dead tissue), 328
Deformity, 267, 294, 296, 301, 303, 306–308, 315, 322, 332, 335, 362, 365
Diabetes Control and Complications Trial (DCCT), 264
Diabetes educator, 265
Diabetic bullae, 311
Diuretics, 283
Doppler machine, 354
Drysol, 342
Dye, 354

E
Emery board, 286, 318
Erectile dysfunction, 335
Evening primrose oil,337
Exercise, 261, 271, 272, 322–324, 343, 349–350, 352, 360

F
Fainting, 334
Fever, 279, 330
Fireplace, 350
Fitting shoes, 265, 296, 299, 308
Flexibility, 270
Food, 261

Foot bath, 274, 275
Foot color, 348, 351, 364
Foot odor, 281, 303
Foot swelling, 282–284
Foot surgery, 265, 266
Footwear, 263, 266, 295–299, 307
Fruits, 272
Fungus, 258, 272, 290, 314, 342

G
Gait, 263, 271, 306, 345
Gangrene, 364
Gastroparesis, 335
Germs, 258, 275, 280, 310
Glasses, 269
Green clay poultice, 316, 318
Gout, 361

H
Hair growth, 348
Hammertoes, 262, 266, 294, 315, 335
Health care providers, 265, 268, 271, 276, 277, 278, 281, 290, 291, 301, 311, 318, 320, 327–330, 337, 354–355, 358, 360
Heart, 282–283, 335, 355
Heart attacks, 353, 356–357
Heating pads, 350
High blood pressure, 282, 304, 356
High blood sugar, 258, 313, 327, 330, 333, 337
High pressure areas, 303, 318, 326, 361
Hispanic Americans, 259
Hot peppers, 337–338
Hot water bottles, 350
House shoes, 295, 350
Household chores, 323
Hypertension, *see* High blood pressure.
Hypoglycemia awareness, 335

I
Inactivity, 271, 282, 352, 357, 360
Infection, 256, 258, 275, 279, 281, 289, 292, 310, 313, 316, 330, 340, 351, 362–364
Ingrown toenails, 257, 262, 267, 291–292

Running, 322
Running shoes, 262–263, 294, 322, 324

S
Sandals, 280, 322
Scans, 354
Senior centers, 269, 286
Sensory nerves, 332, 335, 344
Sexual functioning, 334
Skin, 258, 262, 267, 276, 278, 226, 332, 338, 342–343, 351
Skin oils, 275, 276
Shoehorn, 270
Shoes, 262, 263, 268, 271, 280, 281, 294, 296–299, 310–311, 317–318, 324, 327, 340, 342, 354
Shower, 274
Smoking, 352, 355, 357
Soaking, 275, 327
Soap, 274, 276
Sock puller, 270
Socks, 262, 268, 277, 280, 281, 284, 300, 310–311, 322, 327, 340, 342, 350–351
Sores, 267
Space heater, 350
Sponges, 270
Stair climbers, 322
Stomach, 335
Stretching, 270, 322–323, 337
Strokes, 353, 356–357
Sulfonylureas, 337
Support hose, 284, 249
Surgery, 262, 286, 312, 315, 317–320, 329, 348, 358, 362–364
Sweating, 276, 332, 335, 342–343, 350
Swelling, 282–283, 304, 312, 360–362
Swimming, 280, 322–323

T
Temperature, checking, 274, 351
Tests, 336, 351, 354
Tetanus, 313
Thyroid disease, 336
Toenails, 262, 269, 286–292, 314
Towels, 274, 280

Triglycerides, 353, 357
Tuning fork, 267, 334, 336
Type 1 diabetes, 260, 264
Type 2 diabetes, 260, 264

U
Ulcer, 256, 257, 259, 263, 265, 281, 290, 294, 296, 301, 303–354, 322, 326–330, 350, 354, 360–361, 363, 365
Unexplained high blood sugar, 313, 330
United Kingdom Prospective Diabetes Study (UKPDS), 264
Upper body exercises, 323
Uric acid, 361

V
Varicose veins, 349
Vascular surgeons, 265, 329
Vascular surgery, 348
Vegetable oils, 277
Vegetables, 272
Veins, 249
Vision problems, 269, 286
Vitamin deficiencies, 336
Vomiting, 334

W
Walking, 322–323, 344–345, 348–350, 357
Warning signs, 267
Wart, 319
Water, 322
Water pills, 283
Weight, 263, 353, 357
Weight lifting, 323
Wheel chair, 328
Wool, 277
Wounds, 267, 275, 281, 310, 326, 328, 330, 338

X
X ray, 312, 354, 363

Y
Yoga, 270, 323

101 Medication Tips

▼

Dehydration, 406
Dexatrim, cautions concerning, 464
DiaBeta, 373, 413
Diabetes
  complications of, 436–445
  different causes of, 372
  preventing, 482
Diabetic neuropathy, treating, 437–438
Diabinese, 373
  and alcohol use, 448
Diarrhea,
  while taking acarbose, 400
  while taking metformin, 406, 408
Diet, 379, 464–465
Digoxin, patients taking, 394
Discomfort of injections, 381, 413
Diuretics, patients taking, 395, 452
Dizzy feeling, 488
Doses, 385, 414, 420–422, 433, 479
Drugs. *See* Medications
Dry cough, treating, 444

E
Erectile dysfunction, treating, 442
Estrogen, 449–450
Exercise, adjusting medications with, 390, 426

F
Fatigue. *See also* Liver function
Fear of injections, 381, 413
Feet
  tingling and burning in, 437–438
  treating corns, calluses, or blisters, 461
Fenofibrate, patients taking, 450
Fever, while taking metformin, 406
Furosemide, patients taking, 394

G
Gastroparesis, treating, 440, 472
Generic names of medications, 373
Glimepiride, 373
Glipizide, 373–374, 376

taking, 388, 397, 412
Glucocorticoids, and diabetes, 447
Glucophage, 373, 377, 421
  and kidney function, 406
  side effects of, 408
  taking, 387, 389, 397
  taking maximum dose of, 413
Glucose. See Blood glucose
Glucose meters, 383, 476
Glucose tablets, 404
Glucotrol, 373
  taking, 397, 412
Glyburide, 373–374, 376, 383
  allergies associated with, 395
  taking, 396
  taking maximum dose of, 381, 413
  weight gain while taking, 401
Glynase, 373
Glyset, 373, 377
  missing a dose of, 385
  taking, 387, 389

H
Half-life of medications, 396
Headaches, morning. See Hypoglycemia
Heart disease, and diabetes, 443, 445
High blood pressure, and diabetes, 443, 445
Holiday eating, adjusting medications during, 386
Home testing, 383
Humalog, 415–418, 425
Humulin, 425
Hydrochlorothiazide, patients taking, 452
Hypoglycemia, 398
  monitoring symptoms of, 397, 403, 434, 451
  reducing risk of, 414, 421–422
  treating, 404
  while taking repaglinide, 409
I
ID bracelet, 481
Impotence, treating, 442

Miglitol, 373–374, 376–377
  missing a dose of, 385
  taking, 387, 389
Multivitamins, patients taking, 453

N
Names of medications, 373. *See also*
  individual medications
Nasal congestion, treating, 459
National Institutes of Health,
Diabetes Prevention Program of, 482
Nausea, 440
Nervousness. *See* Hypoglycemia
Niacin, and diabetes, 447, 453
Nonprescription medications,
    454–468, 476
  sugar content of, 460
  warnings labels on, 455, 462
Nonsteroidal anti-inflammatory
  agents (NSAIDS), and diabetes, 462
NPH insulin, 414–415, 418, 425, 430,
  434

O
Obesity, 421, 445
Oral medications, 375, 421
  switching to, 423
Orinase, 373
Over-the-counter medications,
    454–468, 476

P
Peripheral vascular disease, cautions
  for patients with, 449
Pharmacist, consulting with, 441,
  456–457, 462, 470–471, 473,
  475–480
Phenylpropanolamine, cautions
  concerning, 464
Polycystic ovary disease, patients
  with, 402
Postmenopausal patients, 450
Potency of medications, 376
Prandin, 373, 377
  missing a dose of, 385

missing a meal with, 398
side effects of, 409
taking, 387, 389
toxic potential of, 480
Precose, 373, 377
  missing a dose of, 385
  taking, 387, 389
Pregnancy, and diabetes, 392
Premixed insulin, 418
Propulsid, cautions for patients
  taking itraconazole, 472
Protease inhibitors, and diabetes, 447

R
Rapid-acting insulin, 415–418
Red pepper cream, 438
Regular insulin, 415–418, 424–425
Repaglinide, 373–374, 376–377
  missing a dose of, 385
  missing a meal with, 398
  side effects of, 409
  taking, 387, 389
  toxic potential of, 480
Rezulin, 373, 421–422
  cautions for patients taking, 471
  side effects of, 402, 405
  taking, 387

S
Sexual side effects, treating, 442
Shakiness. *See* Hypoglycemia
Side effects of medications, 377, 382,
  399–409, 476–477
Site of action of medications, 374
Sites for injections, 429, 435
Skin, yellowing of. *See* Liver
  function
Smoking, and diabetes, 466
Sore throat. *See* Liver function
Sporanox, cautions for patients taking
  cisapride, 472
Statins, cautions for patients taking,
  473
Stomach pain, 440
  while taking acarbose, 400

while taking metformin, 408
Strength of medications, 396
Sulfa antibiotics, patients allergic to, 395
Sweating. *See* Hypoglycemia
Syndrome X, 445

T
Tarry stools, 458
Testing blood glucose, 383
Therapeutic interchange, 479
Thiazide diuretics, patients taking, 395
Tingling in feet, 437–438
Toenail infection, treating, 472
Tolazamide, 373
Tolbutamide, 373
Tolinase, 373
Treatments, differing, 372, 376–377
Tricor, patients taking, 450
Triple therapy, 382
Type I diabetes, medication for, 372
Type 2 diabetes
  in the elderly, 391
  insulin use for, 410–427
  medication for, 372–373, 375–377, 397
  and overweight, 377
  treating, 379

U
Ultralente insulin, 425

V
Vaginal yeast infections, treating, 463
Velosulin, 425
Viagra, cautions for using, 442
Vitamins, recommendations concerning, 453, 465–467
Vomiting, 458
  while taking metformin, 406

W
Warfarin, cautions for patients taking, 457, 466, 473

Warnings labels, on non-prescription medications, 455
Water pills, patients taking, 395, 452
Weak feeling, 458
Weight gain, 421, 433
  while taking glyburide, 401
  while taking repaglinide, 409
Weight loss products, cautions concerning, 464
Wrist bracelet, 481

Y
Yeast infections, treating, 463
Yellowing of skin. *See* Liver function
Young children, keeping medications from, 480

101 Nutrition Tips

▼

101 Weight Loss Tips

▼

101 Tips for Aging Well
with Diabetes

A

Acarbose, 743
Albumin, 791
Alcohol, 777, 788, 794, 832
Alpha-1-receptor blockers, 753
Alpha-glucosidase inhibitors, 743–744
Amputation, 757, 784–785
Andropause, 793
Angiotensin-converting enzyme
    (ACE) inhibitors, 753, 755, 792
Appetite, 820
Arnica oil, 775
Artherosclerosis, 752
Arthritis, 757, 775, 798
Aspirin, 750, 752

B

Beta-blockers, 750, 753
Biguanides, 743–745
Blood fats. *See* Lipids
Blood glucose, 760
    factors that influence, 733, 750
    meters, 804, 806, 807
    target levels, 732, 822
    testing, 805–807
Blood pressure, 809
Borderline diabetes, 728

C

Calcium antagonists, 753
Calcium channel blockers, 750
Calories, burning of, 770
Carbohydrate, 761
    counting, 760
Celebrations, 829
Certified diabetes educator (CDE), 737,
    740
Cholesterol. *See* Lipids
Chromium, 755

Companionship, 826
Complications, 730, 781
Confusion, 800
Cooking, 830
Corticosteroids, 750
Cortisone, 750

D

Deformity, 784
Depression, 799, 820, 828
Diabetes,
    incidence of, 729
    future of, 741
    what is, 726
Diabetes management plan, 724, 746,
    802
    with illness, 818
Dialysis, 791
Diuretics, 750

E

Eating healthy, 759
Education, 725
Educator, 737, 749, 787, 804
Eldercare Locator, 740
Ephedrine, 750
Estrogen, 777, 796, 797
Exercise, 772, 775
    benefits of, 768, 771
    for seniors, 769, 771
    insulin and, 773
    types of, 770
    with type 2 diabetes, 774
Expense, 740
Eye exam, 782–783, 812
Eyesight, 782–783

F

Fad diets, 831

Organization, 738, 739, 756
Osteoporosis, 777

P

Personality change, 799–800, 828
Phenothiazines, 750
Phenytoin, 750
Physical examination, 802, 812
Physicians, working with, 814–815
Pills, 743–746, 753
  cutting of, 751
Pioglitazone, 743
Pneumonia vaccine, 754
Potassium, 755
Prandin, 743–744, 750
Prednisone, 750
Pseudoephedrine, 750

R

Registered dietician (RD), 759, 765, 831
Repaglinide, 743
Resources, 740
Retinopathy, 772, 775, 782, 783, 790
Retiring, 824
Rosiglitazone, 743

S

Sex drive,
  in men, 793–794
  in women, 797–798
Sluggish stomach function. *See*
  Gastroparesis
Smoking, 736, 759, 772, 777, 788, 792,
  794–795
Stroke, 780, 808
Sugar, 761
Sulfonylureas, 743–745, 750, 773
Syringe magnifiers, 749

T

Testosterone, 777, 793–795
Thiazide diuretics, 753
Thiazolidinediones, 743–745
Thromboxane, 752
Traveling, 739
Triglyceride, 744, 810
Type 1 diabetes, 727
Type 2 diabetes, 727, 774

V

Viagra, 795
Vitamins, 755

W

Water, 763
Weight, 776, 823
Will planning, 827

Y

Yoga, 774, 775

101 Tips for Simplifying Diabetes

▼

101 Tips for Coping with Diabetes

▼

Tips for a Healthy Pregnancy with Diabetes

About the American Diabetes Association

The American Diabetes Association is the nation's leading voluntary health organization supporting diabetes research, information, and advocacy. Its mission is to prevent and cure diabetes and to improve the lives of all people affected by diabetes. The American Diabetes Association is the leading publisher of comprehensive diabetes information. Its huge library of practical and authoritative books for people with diabetes covers every aspect of self-care—cooking and nutrition, fitness, weight control, medications, complications, emotional issues, and general self-care.

To order American Diabetes Association books: Call 1-800-232-6733. http://store.diabetes.org [Note: there is no need to use **www** when typing this particular Web address]

To join the American Diabetes Association: Call 1-800-806-7801. www.diabetes.org/membership

For more information about diabetes or ADA programs and services: Call 1-800-342-2383. E-mail: Customerservice@diabetes.org www.diabetes.org

To locate an ADA/NCQA Recognized Provider of quality diabetes care in your area: www.ncqa.org/dprp/

To find an ADA Recognized Education Program in your area: Call 1-888-232-0822. www.diabetes.org/recognition/education.asp

To join the fight to increase funding for diabetes research, end discrimination, and improve insurance coverage: Call 1-800-342-2383. www.diabetes.org/advocacy

To find out how you can get involved with the programs in your community: Call 1-800-342-2383. See below for program Web addresses.

- *American Diabetes Month:* Educational activities aimed at those diagnosed with diabetes—month of November. www.diabetes.org/ADM
- *American Diabetes Alert:* Annual public awareness campaign to find the undiagnosed—held the fourth Tuesday in March. www.diabetes.org/alert
- *The Diabetes Assistance & Resources Program (DAR):* diabetes awareness program targeted to the Latino community. www.diabetes.org/DAR
- *African American Program:* diabetes awareness program targeted to the African American community. www.diabetes.org/africanamerican
- *Awakening the Spirit: Pathways to Diabetes Prevention & Control:* diabetes awareness program targeted to the Native American community. www.diabetes.org/awakening

To find out about an important research project regarding type 2 diabetes: www.diabetes.org/ada/research.asp

To obtain information on making a planned gift or charitable bequest: Call 1-888-700-7029. www.diabetes.org/ada/plan.asp

To make a donation or memorial contribution: Call 1-800-342-2383. www.diabetes.org/ada/cont.asp